Jerry Baker's

GROW YOUNGER
Live Longer!

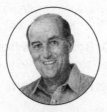

jerrybaker.com

Jerry Baker's

GROW YOUNGER
Live Longer!

Anti-aging secrets and solutions for a longer, happier, and healthier life!

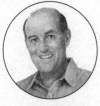

jerrybaker.com

Published by American Master Products, Inc.

Executive Editor: Kim Adam Gasior
Managing Editor: Cheryl Winters-Tetreau
Writer: Vicki Webster
Design and Layout: Alison McKenna
Copy Editor: Nanette Bendyna
Production Editor: Sydney Francois
Illustrator: Deborah Cowder
Indexer: Nan Badgett

Publisher's Cataloging-in-Publication
(Provided by Quality Books, Inc.)

Baker, Jerry, author.
  Grow younger, live longer! : anti-aging secrets and
solutions for a longer, happier, and healthier life! /
Jerry Baker.
  pages cm
  Includes index.
  ISBN 978-0-922433-23-0

  1. Older people--Health and hygiene. 2. Aging--
Prevention. 3. Longevity.   I. Title.

RA564.8.B35 2017   613.0438
                         QBI17-802

Printed in the United States of America
2 4 6 8 9 7 5 3 hardcover

⫸ CONTENTS

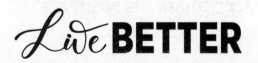

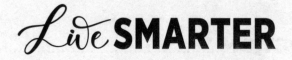

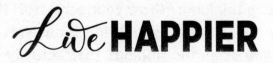

Live HAPPIER

>>> INTRODUCTION

I know what you're thinking: "Grow younger?! Me?! Ha!" Well, think again, friend! In these pages, you'll find thousands of tips, tricks, tonics, and proven scientific findings that actually will make you feel, look, and act years—even decades—younger than your birth certificate says you are.

> LIVE BETTER, SMARTER, AND HAPPIER!

It's never too late to start turning back the clock—and you can actually have a lot of fun doing it. This book is crammed full of super solutions for improving your health, boosting your happiness, and lengthening your life. For instance, you'll discover how you can look and feel years younger by doing everyday household chores, get a whole new burst of enthusiasm and purpose by reconnecting with old pals, and make your stress level plummet simply by pitching some unwanted junk. You will also learn how to:

- Develop healthy habits that will keep your weight down and your energy up—and could extend your life by as much as 8 to 10 years (Chapter 1).

- Relieve aches and pains using safe, natural remedies, so you can stay healthier, more active, and younger—physically, mentally, and emotionally (Chapter 2).

- Erect an inner fortress to fend off or alleviate the effects of chronic conditions ranging from asthma to type 2 diabetes, heart disease, and stroke (Chapter 3).

- Help your brain keep your body young by maintaining a happy, upbeat attitude; bidding bye-bye to stress and anxiety; and keeping your cogitating mind clear and razor-sharp (Chapter 4).

- Eat your way to a younger you by packing your diet with delicious anti-aging foods (Chapter 5).

> " You're never too old to become younger.
> —Mae West (1893–1980) "

VIII

- Look your youthful best—from the top of your head to the tips of your toes—your whole life long (Chapter 6).

- Keep your joints jumpin', your mood up, and your libido lively—simply by moving your body every chance you get, just as the longest-living people on the planet do (Chapter 7).

- Build and nurture one of the most youth-enhancing marvels of all: a network of loving and supportive friends, neighbors, and family members—human and otherwise (Chapter 8).

- Devise a savvy strategy for retaining your physical, financial, and emotional independence—right up until the final curtain falls (Chapter 9).

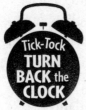

And that's just the beginning! In every chapter, you'll find fantastic features, like **Tick-Tock Turn Back the Clock**, which delivers timely tips and dynamite discoveries that'll help you rewind your biological timepiece. For example, just 20 minutes after you smoke for the last time, your blood pressure and heart rate should return to normal, or nearly so (page 36). And regular ballroom dancing—the kind that requires you to move in sync with a partner—can reduce your risk for dementia by 76 percent (page 144).

Mind Over Myth demolishes rampant misconceptions that can lead you down paths that at best simply waste your time and money. Sneak preview: You often hear that in order to see any beneficial results from physical activity, you have to exercise long and hard. The truth of the matter is that all it takes to stay healthy and grow younger is 30 minutes a day of moderate physical activity, like you get from taking a brisk walk or washing your car. Plus, you don't have to get your whole half hour at one time. Two 15-minute or even three 10-minute sessions will do the trick just fine (page 238).

: MIND OVER MYTH :

Centenarian Secrets present highly helpful nuggets of knowledge that have kept legions of folks charging along in fine fettle well into their golden years—and can do the same for you. For example, engaging in sex at least several times a week can make you look four to seven years younger—and live longer, too (page 291). And here's good news for you ladies: Studies show that drinking as little as one cup of tea per day may preserve your bone density well into your senior years (page 183).

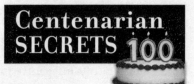

Fountain of Youth offers up easy-to-make formulas that perform youth-enhancing feats of all kinds—from soothing tired feet and achy muscles to enhancing your good looks and helping you kick bad habits. Two cases in point: The Nourishing Facial Scrub on page 199 will make your skin look softer, livelier, and younger than you ever thought possible. And Cravin'-Kickin' Oil Mix (page 39) will not only help you stop cigarette cravings cold, but will also help detoxify your system and heal the pre-

Fountain of Youth

mature aging and other damage smoking has done to your body.

Last, but far from least, **Rejuvenating Recipes** are packed with both anti-aging power and delectable flavor. Just to whet your appetite, Sour Cherry Salsa on page 50 is a delicious (and versatile) way to relieve the debilitating pain and stiffness of arthritis. And Sweet-and-Sour Onions (page 208) pack a potent load of compounds that keep your skin looking younger and prettier longer.

Rejuvenating Recipe

So what are we waiting for? Hop on the Grow Younger Express and take a fun-filled journey to a healthier, more beautiful, more youthful you!

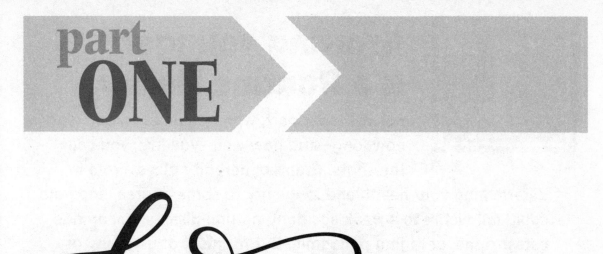

part
ONE

Live BETTER

Let's face it: No one goes through life without picking up a few aches and pains, and for most of us, the older we get, the more often they arrive and the longer they linger. And chronic conditions, ranging from annoying allergies to life-threatening diseases, can befall anyone at any age. The good news is that there are ways to minimize the effects of virtually all of those woes—or even avoid them entirely. In this part, you'll find time-tested tips and high-tech tricks to help you in both of those endeavors, so you can lead a long, happy, and productive life. The process begins—where else?—with making healthy habits part of your daily routine.

CHAPTER 1

Growing Younger Is a Routine Matter

For the most part, when it comes to deciding how long—and how well—you live, you call the shots. Granted, heredity plays a role in determining your health and longevity to some degree, and you could fall victim to a freak accident, natural disaster, manmade catastrophe, or raging pandemic. But for most of us, many of the choices we make, day in and day out, can be the difference between a long, healthy, active life—and a shorter, sicker one that you wouldn't wish on your worst enemy.

>>> LOSE WEIGHT—FEEL GREAT!

And younger, too. Think about it: Have you ever seen a centenarian—or anyone even approaching the 100-year mark—who was overweight? Probably not. That's because one of the keys to living to a ripe (and happy) old age is to stay slim and trim. If you're one of the two out of three Americans who are overweight, that may be a depressing thought. But it shouldn't be. Rather, it should simply be a resounding call to action because no matter how many extra pounds you're carrying, it's possible to lose them. And if you go about it the right way, the process can be a whole lot of fun.

> Shed 10 Pounds and Reap 10 Benefits

There's no doubt about it: If you're extremely overweight (as statistics show the average American woman is), getting your weight down to a healthy number can seem downright impossible. Well, here's a piece of news that should give you a major incentive to launch your slenderizing effort: You don't need to drop your whole load to see an improvement in your health and well-being. Losing just 10 pounds through a healthy diet and moderate exercise will deliver these 10 remarkable results:

- Lower LDL (bad) cholesterol by more than 10 percent

- Cut your risk of a heart attack by more than 50 percent

- Lower your chances of getting type 2 diabetes by 60 percent

- Lessen your risk for dementia, Alzheimer's disease, and stroke

- Improve sleep and cut your chances of developing sleep apnea

- Decrease your blood pressure, protecting your heart and kidneys

- Reduce the levels of carcinogenic hormones your body releases—especially the ones that cause breast and uterine cancer

- Ease joint pain and cut your odds of developing osteoarthritis by 50 percent (If you already have OA, tossing 10 pounds will reduce the stress on each knee by a full 40 pounds!)

- Improve your sex drive and help relieve erectile dysfunction

- Reduce the dosages for all the medications you may be taking, thereby easing any troublesome side effects—and saving money to boot!

> " Age is an issue of mind over matter. If you don't mind, it doesn't matter.
>
> —Mark Twain (1835–1910) "

❯ Slim Down and Beef Up Your Bank Account

Yep, it's true! The exact dollars and cents vary greatly from one person to the next, but here's a general rundown of the economic benefits of losing weight—and keeping it off:

Lower health-care costs. Because of the serious—and expensive— conditions that go hand in hand with obesity, most private insurers charge higher premiums for obese applicants. For the same reason, if you have health-care coverage through your work, there's a chance your share of the cost will be higher if you weigh much more than you should. Add that to your out-of-pocket costs for weight-related conditions, and the money you spend on prescription and OTC meds, and shaving pounds is likely to save you a hefty sum each month.

Lower clothing costs. The bigger a garment is, the more fabric is required to make it. That's why plus-size clothes cost more. Even if you sew your XXL duds at home, you're shelling out more for the material than you would if you wore a smaller size.

Lower food costs. Logic says that when you eat less food, you buy less food. Plus, if you regularly consume a lot of fast food and junk-food snacks, as most overweight folks do, you could save a bundle by eliminating or cutting back on the stuff. You'll save even more at the checkout counter if you adopt an eating style that focuses less on meat and more on less expensive protein sources such as legumes, eggs, and dairy products (see "To Get—and Stay—Slim, Don't Diet" on page 8).

Higher earnings. A recent study at the University of Florida found that women who weighed 25 pounds more than average earned close to $14,000 less per year than their healthy-weight counterparts. At first glance that may smack of unfair discrimination, but according to the renowned management consulting firm McKinsey & Company, there are solid business reasons to support the numbers: Obese

Blast Belly Fat and Live Longer

And better, too! That's because the most ominous kind of fat is the type that collects at your abdomen. Most of it is what scientists call visceral, or deep, fat. We need some of it to cushion our organs, but if you gain too much weight, your body runs out of safe places to store visceral fat. So it stashes the excess inside your organs (like your liver) and in layers around your heart. A "spare tire" is a huge red flag for the ugliest by-products of obesity, namely high blood pressure and breast and colon cancers.
Note: *If you're a woman and your waist size is 35+ inches, or if you are a man with a waist of 40 inches or more, you're on a fast track to big trouble. So start slimming down now!*

Tick-Tock **TURN BACK** the **CLOCK**

people have higher rates of absenteeism, are far more likely to need short-term disability leaves, and tend to be less productive on the job than people who tip the scales at healthy weights.

❯ 5 Sweet Side Effects of Slimming Down

With so many people overweight, it's no wonder that obesity has become a hot topic in scientific research circles. And the guys and gals in white lab coats are coming up with some astonishing ways that losing weight can improve your life. Just consider this small sampling:

1. Keep your brainpower sharper. A 10-year study published in the journal *Neurology* examined the cognitive powers of people who were normal weight, overweight, and clinically obese. Over that time frame, the test scores of the obese subjects declined 22.5 percent faster than those of the normal-weight folks.

2. Remember faces better. Researchers at Umeå University in Sweden discovered that after six months of dieting, overweight women were better able to remember faces of people they'd just met. The scientists reckon that weight loss improves the brain's ability to store new memories and access the stored information.

3. Stay happier. According to research at Leiden University Medical Center in the Netherlands, people who are either overweight or obese are significantly more likely than their slimmer counterparts to suffer from clinical depression.

4. Have healthier skin. According to an article in the *Journal of the American Academy of Dermatology*, obesity causes a whole raft of un-

The Fat Fine Print

So how do you know when you've crossed the line from unpleasant plumpness to full-blown obesity? Medical pros base that determination on your body mass index (BMI), a number arrived at by dividing your weight in pounds by your height in inches, squared. Then multiply that number by 703. If you'd rather not do the math, you can find out exactly where you rank by checking the Body Mass Index Table on the website of the National Heart, Lung, and Blood Institute.
http://www.nhlbi.nih.gov/guidelines/obesity/bmi_tbl.htm

MYTH: A detox (cleansing) diet is a dandy way to slim down quickly for a big event, like a wedding or a body-baring beach vacation.

REALITY: You'll lose weight rapidly, but most of it'll be water, as it is with other crash diets. When you resume your normal eating patterns, the numbers on the scale will shoot right back up again. Even worse, fasting and aggressive cleansing methods used in these routines often deliver unpleasant side effects, such as constipation, aches, pains, fatigue, brain fog, flu-like symptoms, and even colon damage. Some plans incorporate herbs and other supplements that can produce serious interactions with any drugs you may be taking. Detox diets are especially dangerous for people who have such underlying health conditions as diabetes or high blood pressure.

sightly and uncomfortable skin problems, including infections, pimples and other blemishes, breakdown in collagen structure (which keeps skin supple), and impaired wound healing. Plus, all that weight increases your risk for psoriasis and excessive hair growth.

5. See better, longer. A review in the *Survey of Ophthalmology* links obesity directly to three vision problems that are associated with aging eyes: cataracts, glaucoma, and macular degeneration.

❯ Don't Fall for Diet Delusions

No matter how overweight you may be, don't be taken in by this trio of rampant misconceptions:

Wheat is wicked and gluten is ghastly. A lot of folks—including the authors of some highly successful diet books—would have you believe that the instant you eat a slice of bread or a forkful of spaghetti, your belly will blow up like a balloon. Nonsense! Eating too much wheat will make you gain weight—just the same as an excess of any other food will. On the other hand, eaten in moderation, whole wheat is a valuable part of a healthy diet. As for the gluten that wheat contains, unless you have celiac disease, it's perfectly harmless.

Going organic will make you lose weight. The notion has sprung up in certain circles that chemicals in food make you fat, and if you simply switch to an all-organic diet, your poundage will plummet.

Hogwash! While it is true that eating organically grown food will help you avoid a lot of harmful toxins, shoveling down (for instance) a pint of chocolate ice cream will have the same effect on your waistline regardless of whether the originating cows ate pesticide-free grass or genetically modified grain.

Diet food can make you drop pounds. Baloney! All those "miraculous" weight-loss cookies, bars, and other pseudo-foods that you see in stores and on the Internet are the solid equivalent of diet soda (see "Say No to 'Diet' Drinks and Sweeteners" on page 186). They're highly processed products made from artificial sweeteners, artificial flavorings, and worthless fillers that trick your brain into thinking you're eating real food. For a short time, you do feel full, but because your body isn't getting the nutrients and calories that should coincide with a satisfied tummy, your hunger returns with a vengeance. So you eat more. And more…

❯ Red Flags on Fad Diets

It's all but impossible to resist a plan that promises to produce quick weight loss and an instant boost to your health. Unfortunately, these easy-way-out slenderizing schemes rarely, if ever,

---

Fountain of Youth

TRIUMPHANT TRIAD TONIC

Studies show that this simple mixture can help you overcome obesity and a whole lot of other health woes besides.

> 1 cup of raw honey
> 1 cup of unfiltered apple cider vinegar
> 8 peeled garlic cloves
> Water or fruit juice

Mix the first three ingredients in a blender on high speed for 60 seconds. Pour the blend into a glass jar with a tight-fitting lid, and refrigerate for five days. Then every day before breakfast, take 2 teaspoons of the tonic stirred into a glass of water or fruit juice. Researchers recommend using fresh orange or 100 percent grape juice. **Note:** *This has also been shown to cure or prevent almost every ailment under the sun, including Alzheimer's disease, arthritis, asthma, high blood pressure, and ulcers, as well as muscle aches and colds.*

help you achieve your optimum weight and stay there. What's more, they can hand you more health problems than you had to begin with. In particular, turn two thumbs down on diets that meet any one of the following descriptions:

They confine the menu largely to one food or type of food. Examples are the Atkins Diet and similar low-carb, high-protein diets. They are not nutritionally sound, they have little scientific evidence to back them up, and they can even lead to serious problems such as loss of muscle density, enlarged kidneys, and renal failure.

They promise fast weight loss. On plans guaranteeing a loss of 2 pounds a week or more, you probably will drop weight quickly in the beginning, but most of it will be in the form of water, not fat. After the initial week, the pounds will come off more slowly. Plus, as soon as you stray from the diet, you'll rapidly return to your original weight. Even worse, though, is if you stay on the diet for any length of time, you could deprive your body of enough vital nutrients to severely damage your health.

They rely on "chemical reactions" to make the pounds flow off. They may also refer to "scientific proof," but have no evidence to back up their claims. One infamous example is the diet that has you start each meal with half a grapefruit on the premise that it contains fat-burning enzymes. (Actually, it doesn't.)

❯ To Get—and Stay—Slim, Don't Diet

Instead, take a tip from healthy, happy centenarians the world over: Develop sensible eating habits and make moderate exercise a part of your daily routine. The specific foods vary from one region to the next, but the basic principles are set forth in the famous Mediterranean diet, which, of course, isn't a diet at all. That is, it's not one of those regimens forcing you to count every calorie that goes into your mouth and swear off all the foods you love most. Rather, it's a way of life that emphasizes healthy foods and minimizes (but does not make you give up) the ones that are not so good for you. Here's a quick overview of the life-extending recommendations:

- Heaping helpings of fruits, vegetables, whole grains, nuts, and seeds
- A variety of foods—fresh, in-season, and locally grown whenever possible—to help ensure the maximum delivery of health-giving micronutrients and antioxidants
- Plenty of extra virgin olive oil
- Moderate amounts of cheese, milk, yogurt, fish, poultry, and eggs
- Minimal amounts of sugar, saturated fat, and red meat
- Moderate consumption of red wine (optional)
- Regular physical activity to promote a healthy weight, muscle tone, and overall well-being (more about that coming up in Chapter 7)

❯ Banish Banned Food

The surest route to a failed diet is to go cold turkey on any particular kinds of food or drink. Forbidding yourself to ever eat (let's say) a few French fries or a slice of cake inevitably leads to cravings for the "no-no" treat. More often than not, the longing for the food results in binges that cause you to gain weight rather than lose it, and your stress level

---

12 Steps to a Slimmer, Healthier You

For some folks, overeating is much more than a bad habit—it's a genuine addiction, akin to alcoholism or drug abuse (see "Addiction Alert: 7 Signs You May Be Hooked" on page 33). If you recognize any behavior patterns in that rundown, do yourself a favor and give Overeaters Anonymous a try. To find a chapter near you, visit www.oa.org. The group's 12-step process may not be up your alley...but if you do stick with the program, you could find that for the first time in your life, you're the one calling the shots—instead of the slave-driving food that's constantly at the forefront of your mind.

Tick-Tock TURN BACK the CLOCK

will soar when you bash yourself for going off the wagon. Despite what the promoters of certain diets may tell you, there's no "good" or "bad" foods. There are just good and bad eating habits. The only way to lose weight and keep it off permanently is to change the way you think about food, so you can alter your eating habits for the better.

❯ Keep Your Mind on Your Plate

According to a study published in *The American Journal of Clinical Nutrition*, distracted eaters whose minds are focused elsewhere are likely to consume up to 50 percent more calories than folks who devote their full attention to the matter at hand. In fact, they also eat more at the next meal or snack because their minds never fully registered what they consumed on the previous occasion.

> "
> The secret of staying young is to live honestly, eat slowly, and lie about your age.
>
> —Lucille Ball
> (1911–1989)
> "

The good news: If you routinely gobble lunch at your desk or eat dinner parked in front of the TV, you can cut your calorie consumption in a big way simply by kicking that habit. At home, turn off the television, computer, cell phone, and any other electronic devices. At work, flee your cubicle for the quietest space you can find. Then sit down and concentrate on enjoying your food. Take small bites, chew slowly, and savor the flavor of every mouthful. That way, both your body and your brain will be satisfied—with a lot less intake than you probably thought possible.

❯ 3 Ways to Outwit the Clean Plate Club

There are scads of reasons why so many people in our country are overweight, but one of the most common lies in three little words: "Clean your plate." If you grew up hearing that command around the family dinner table, it's a good bet your subconscious mind still hears it loud and clear every time you sit down to eat. The solution: Trick your inner eight-year-old into pleasing Mom *and* eating sensibly with these three simple strategies:

1. When you place your order in a restaurant, ask the waiter to put half of your serving in a doggie bag *before* it's brought to your table.

2. Whenever possible, shun buffets (including salad bars). The enticing goodies make it all but impossible to resist putting one of everything on your plate until you've got a mound the size of Mount McKinley.

3. At must-attend business or social events that serve food buffet-style, choose the smallest plate offered. Then plant your attention firmly on your fellow attendees and the action at hand so you'll be less tempted to go back for seconds.

> ## A Hot Tip for Weight Loss
>
> Recent studies have shown that adding just a few dashes of hot-pepper sauce to your daily diet not only reduces your levels of ghrelin, a hunger-causing compound, but also raises your level of GLP-1, a hormone that naturally suppresses your appetite. One of the tastiest ways to put this firepower to work is to add it to tomato juice (attention, Bloody Mary lovers!).

❯ To Shrink Your Belly, Shrink Your Plate

Waistlines aren't the only things that have expanded over the past 40 years. Since the 1970s, the typical dinner plate has grown in size from 10 inches in diameter to 12 inches or more (in some cases, a *lot* more). And that gives you an absolutely effortless way to drop your unwanted pounds. Simply by trading in your oversize plates for versions that are 2 inches smaller, you'll serve yourself 22 percent fewer calories per meal. That act alone can make you lose 2 pounds in 30 days—and most likely, you won't even notice the difference.

❯ Can Fiber Help You Win at Losing?

YES! It's ironic that many trendy diets severely restrict one of the most powerful weight-loss aids of all: fiber. If you're fighting a never-ending battle of the bulge, consider this amazing fact: Simply by eating more whole grains, nuts, fruits, and vegetables (including root veggies

AVOCADO-MANGO SALAD

Besides burning prodigious amounts of fat, avocados deliver a dynamic load of age-defying nutrients that not only keep your internal processes running smoothly, but also help your skin maintain its good health and good looks.

2 large avocados, halved, peeled, pitted, and chilled

2 large mangoes, halved, peeled, pitted, and chilled

Cayenne pepper to taste

Salt to taste

¾ cup of plain yogurt

Juice of 2 large limes

3 tbsp. of honey

4 mint sprigs for garnish

Cut the fruits lengthwise into ½-inch slices. Arrange them on plates, alternating colors. Mix equal parts of cayenne pepper and salt, and lightly sprinkle it over the slices. Stir the yogurt, lime juice, and honey in a bowl. Spoon 2 to 3 tablespoons of dressing over each salad, and garnish with the mint.

Yield: *4 servings*

with their skins), you could lose a couple of pounds a month without cutting a single calorie. That's because fiber pulls off a trio of fabulous fat-fighting feats:

It tricks your tummy. Many of the calories contained in fiber-rich foods can't be digested, but they do fill you up. So you feel full with fewer calories than you would normally eat.

It puts an end to hunger pangs. Water-soluble fiber absorbs water in your stomach and swells up to form a thick gel. This, in turn, alerts your brain that you're full. It also slows down the flow of food out of your stomach, which keeps you satisfied longer and releases a steady, prolonged supply of energy. Then you can go about your business without the constant need to nibble.

It empowers your slimming hormones. The fiber in fruits and vegetables raises the levels of GLP-1, a hormone in your gastrointestinal tract that—like the tummy gel—slows down your digestion, makes you feel full longer, and helps you lose weight.

Note: *Up your fiber intake gradually. A sudden surge of it won't hurt you, but it can trigger uncomfortable gas and bloating.*

❯ It's True: Fat Burns Fat

That is, if you choose the right kinds. Studies show that two dynamic dietary fats can increase your body's ability to burn fat, and also help fend off food cravings. These hot superstars can light a fat-shredding fire in your inner furnace:

Conjugated linoleic acid (CLA). The most powerful pyrotechnic performers are beef, full-fat dairy products, and egg yolks—ideally produced by grass-fed critters. When beef cattle, dairy cows, and chickens are fed genetically modified (GMO) grain or other processed feed, their CLA output plummets. There is also one potent vegetarian source of this ferocious fuel: white button mushrooms, like the ones you'll find in your local supermarket.

Monounsaturated fat. Avocados, flaxseed oil, nuts, and olive oil are all high in this ultra-healthy weight-loss helper!

❯ Don't Let Exercise Blow Your Diet

While it is true that the only way to lose weight is to burn more calories than you take in, trying too hard to keep the "fire" going could sabotage your efforts. That's because when a lot of folks embark on an intensive exercise program, they start eating more than they did before. In some cases, they think they're burning more calories than they really are, then rationalize that it's okay to toss back (for instance) an after-workout candy bar or two. But many exercisers don't even realize that they're upping their food intake. Whichever of those categories you fall into, these three tricks will help you stay on track:

Eat sooner. Studies have shown that if you eat meals within 15 to 30 minutes

Centenarian SECRETS 100

If your chosen form of exercise—whether it's working out, running, or swimming—leaves you too hungry to eat sensibly, give it up. Instead, find ways to move your body more without actually exercising. Puttering in your garden, walking your dog, sweeping the floor, and washing your car all burn calories. But because your mind doesn't count everyday activities as "real exercise," they're unlikely to set off your starvation alarm (see "Don't Let Exercise Blow Your Diet," at left). In Chapter 7, you'll find more ways to work rejuvenating movement into your life without a formal workout regimen.

MIND OVER MYTH

MYTH: Your excess pounds will slide right off if you confine the bulk of your intake to negative-calorie (a.k.a. catabolic) foods that have fewer calories than your body uses to digest them.

REALITY: While it's true that a few edibles, like celery, do require more energy to metabolize compared with the number of calories they provide, no scientific study has demonstrated the catabolic prowess of any particular food. That being said, nutritional scientists tell us that, in general, your body uses about 10 calories for every 100 calories it breaks down—which means there are plenty of ultra-nutritious metabolic champs that can help you slim down while keeping (or getting) your health in tip-top shape (see "Eat Your Way Thin," at right).

after exercising, you are much less likely to gain back the "fuel" you just burned than you will be if you wait until later.

Guzzle water. It's often easy to mistake thirst for hunger. So if you find yourself eating more than you should on workout days, try drinking more water than you normally do. That could solve the problem quick as a wink.

Give yourself a treat that you can't eat. If you think you deserve a prize for your physical labor, by all means go for it. Just make sure it's something inedible. (Habitually thinking of food as a reward for good behavior is a big part of what got you to an over-weight state in the first place!)

❯ A Berry Weird Way to Lose Weight

We all know that our sense of smell is the one most closely tied to our memories. But scents do a whole lot more than just carry our minds back to bygone days. They also stimulate all sorts of mental and physical functions. For instance, studies show that smelling strawberries before you exercise causes you to burn more calories. So before you head off on your next power walk, hit the tread-mill at the gym—or even haul your lawn mower out of the shed—pull some berries out of the fridge, and take a good, long whiff!

Strawberry isn't the only aroma that can help you slim down. In a study by the Smell & Taste Treatment and Research Foundation, 3,193 volunteers who frequently sniffed the scents of peppermint, green apples, or bananas throughout the day lost an average of 30 pounds in six months!

❯ Eat Your Way Thin

While the legend of the negative calorie has been debunked (see Mind Over Myth, at left), all of these fruits and vegetables deliver super health benefits with very few calories:

- Asparagus
- Berries
- Broccoli
- Citrus fruits
- Eggplant
- Lettuce
- Melons
- Pears
- Peppers
- Pineapple
- Sweet potatoes
- Zucchini

❯❯❯ WACKY WAYS TO PACK ON POUNDS

You say you're putting on weight, even though you don't think you're eating any more than usual? I'm not surprised. A whole lot of factors, from the decor in your kitchen to the pals you hang around with, can make you shovel in more food without even realizing it. And a few physical conditions cause pounds to pile up, regardless of how many calories you're taking in. The good news is, once you know the nature of the problem, it's easy to alter your routine and get your fat-burning engine back on track.

❯ Your Kitchen Could Broaden Your Belly

If your house is like most, the kitchen is action central—which may be partly to blame for your weight problem. If that statement sounds way-out wacko, consider this fact: On average, kitchens are 50 percent larger than they were 35 years ago, and in most households they've become the location of choice for activities such as paying bills, watching television, or cruising the Web, all of which provide snacking opportunities galore. Studies show that folks who routinely eat while doing something else consume more food and eat more frequently—devouring about the equivalent of an entire extra meal per day. Your pound-dropping mission: Move the computer and TV out of the kitchen. Shift bill paying and other paperwork chores to the den or family room. And when you talk on the phone, do it someplace where there's no food in sight!

❯ Your Lighting Invites Overeating

As bizarre as it may sound, the lighting in your kitchen and dining room may be hampering your weight-loss labors. It works in two ways: Bright lights raise your stress level, which stimulates your appetite and causes you to eat more than usual. On the flip side, low lighting lowers your inhibitions, causing you to eat more. Just about every restaurant uses one of these two tricks to up your consumption. The solution: When you're preparing meals, crank up the wattage as high as you'd like, but when it's time to eat, dim the scene to a comfortable, midlevel range. And between meals, keep kitchen lights off. That will send a clear message to your subconscious mind that the "restaurant" is closed!

Obesity Is Contagious

No, fat "germs" don't fly through the air in the same way cold and flu viruses do. Rather, obesity tends to get passed along because people within social networks often share many of the same behavioral traits—including eating and other lifestyle habits. For example, one study found that your likelihood of being obese is 57 percent greater if one or more close friends are obese, 40 percent greater if a sibling is obese, and 37 percent greater if your spouse is obese. Don't get me wrong—I'm not suggesting that you drop your nearest and dearest like hot potatoes! Instead try:

- Asking friends or family to join in adopting healthier behaviors
- Joining a weight-loss support group or activity-oriented group, such as a hiking, biking, or skating club, where you'll meet folks who share your desire to be healthy, active, and youthful

Tick-Tock
TURN
BACK the
CLOCK

❯ Rethink Your Glasses

Here's a piece of dietary trivia for you: Research shows that people serve themselves more of a beverage when they're using short, wide glasses than they do when the vessel is tall and thin. That's because when you pour yourself a drink, you unconsciously focus on the height of the container rather than the width. Try instead to use skinny glasses for soda pop, juice, and other caloric drinks, and chubbier ones for water and unsweetened iced tea. Chances are you won't even notice the difference—until you read the lowered numbers on your bathroom scale.

❯ Beware of Bulk Shopping

Yes, it can help cut food bills, but if you store that grub in its original, supersize packages, you're more likely to eat more. One study found that people prepared 23 percent more food at mealtimes when they took the ingredients from large containers. An even more dramatic example: Study subjects ate twice as many candies from big bags as they did from smaller ones. Researchers reckon that large packages don't have a natural stopping point, so the cook or snacker just keeps going. Your two-part action plan:

- Repackage cooking ingredients, such as flour, rice, and pasta, into smaller containers. (They'll also keep the contents fresh longer.)

- Divide cookies, candies, and other treats into single-serving portions.

Clear the Decks!

Kitchen counters attract all kinds of stuff, from baseball caps to supermarket receipts and week-old newspapers. If you think those littered surfaces are merely an aesthetic issue, think again. Not only does clutter lead to appetite-boosting stress, but it also makes it harder to maintain healthy eating habits. That's because it's a whole lot easier to grab a fattening frozen dinner from the freezer or order a pizza than it is to dig through the mess to clear a cooking surface. So get that stuff outta there now! Toss the obvious junk. Then gather up everything you don't routinely use in the kitchen, and take it elsewhere. Finally, round up the things that do belong in the kitchen, like culinary magazines or cooking gadgets that have migrated to the countertops, and tuck them away in designated drawers or cabinets.

❯ Your Computer Can Make You Fat!

Even if it's not in the kitchen—and not only because the time you spend in front of it keeps you from exercising. In this case, I'm talking about all those enticing pictures of beautifully prepared food that are shown on culinary websites and Pinterest pinboards. Research has shown that people who struggle most with their weight are more susceptible than their slender counterparts to stimuli in their environment—like those images on a computer screen. All the scrumptious-looking goodies can prompt these folks to eat even when they're not hungry. Here's an idea: If whittling your waistline has become a never-ending battle, sweep your screen of tempting edibles. Then replace those pics with images that relax you, make you laugh, or inspire you to keep the pounds flowing off.

❯ 2 Household Allies Just May Be Backstabbers

You say you're eating less and exercising more, but the pounds still aren't flowing off as they should? Well, if your home is like most, it's filled with a couple of hormone-disrupting "miracle" substances that have been strongly linked to obesity. These are the treacherous twins you'll want to dodge as much as possible:

1. Slick-surface treatments. Nonstick cookware, greaseproof food wrappers, and microwavable popcorn bags, as well as stain-proof and waterproof fabrics, all get their super shedding power from a chemical called perfluorooctanoic acid (PFOA). As long as your nonstick kitchenware is

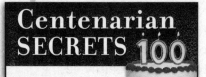

Centenarian SECRETS

Believe it or not, scads of scientific studies have shown that spending either too little or too much quality time between the sheets can make you gain weight. For most adults, the optimum is seven to nine hours of shut-eye a night. If you're heftier than you should be and you routinely sleep longer than that, see your doctor to rule out any underlying health conditions or drug-related causes. On the other hand, if you're neglecting snooze time in favor of more "productive" endeavors, set your priorities straight right now. (For the lowdown on slumber, see "Good Health—Sleep on It!" on page 20.)

in good shape, it's safe to use, but if the surfaces become scratched, cracked, or chipped, replace your gear with cast-iron or untreated stainless steel versions.

2. Vinyl products. The trouble-causing chemicals in polyvinyl chloride (PVC) are organotins and phthalates. And the worst part is that over time, PVC breaks down into tiny particles, so most likely the dust in your home is full of the stuff. Your best defense: Vacuum and clean thoroughly, and when it's time to replace vinyl flooring, look for friendlier options, such as wood, ceramic tile, cork, or rubber.

❯ Your Bulging Belt Line May Not Be Your Fault

If you've gained a lot of extra weight lately, even though your eating habits and activity level haven't changed, there's a good chance you can pin the blame on your underachieving thyroid gland. Have your doctor test you for hypothyroidism if your sudden weight gain is accompanied by any of these other symptoms:

- Achy muscles and joints, for no apparent reason
- Almost constant tiredness and trouble falling asleep
- Forgetfulness and an inability to concentrate
- Anxiety and depression
- Chronic constipation
- A vanishing sex drive
- Cold feet
- Extremely dry hair and skin

❯ Cool Down to Slim Down

In a study published in *The Journal of Clinical Investigation*, researchers exposed a group of men to 66°F temperatures for two hours a day for six weeks. Meanwhile, a control group went about life as usual in their normal living temperatures. The results: PET scans showed that the guys exposed to the lower

> **My secret for staying young is good food, plenty of rest, and a makeup man with a spray gun.**
>
> —Bob Hope (1903–2003)

temps had increased levels of brown-fat activity, and they burned 200 extra calories per day. They also had 5 percent less body fat mass. On the other hand, fat levels and calorie-burning action of the comfortably warm bunch remained unchanged.

❯ The Fattening Fungus among Us

The *Candida albicans* fungus is best known for causing agonizingly itchy genital infections, but according to natural health pros, an overgrowth of this yeast in your gut can also cause fluid retention and weight gain or the inability to lose weight. This fungus is always present in your digestive tract, but two common elements of modern life—overuse of antibiotics and a diet that's too high in sugar—can kick it into serious overdrive. *Candida* symptoms vary widely from one person to another and may or may not include the classic itch, as well as all the signs of hypothyroidism. But two sure indicators that you should see your doctor for a diagnosis and treatment are oral thrush (a white film on your tongue or in your mouth) and a constant craving for sweet treats.

❯❯❯ GOOD HEALTH—SLEEP ON IT!

A sleepless night every now and then won't do anyone any long-term harm. If it did, few parents would survive their children's infancies, much less live to see them graduate from college! But study after study has shown that consistently poor sleep can reduce your life span by (are you ready for this?) as much as 8 to 10 years. So don't just sit there—get ready to start doing some serious snoozing!

❯ 3 Deadly Dangers of Too Little Shut-Eye

According to the National Sleep Foundation, at least 7 out of 10 Americans have frequent sleeping problems. If you're one of those folks, you're at increased risk for shortening your life in a trio of ways, namely these:

1. Colon cancer. A recent study published in the journal *Cancer* found that people who sleep less than six hours a night on average were 50 percent more likely to fall victim to colorectal adenomas than folks who got at least seven hours of sleep each night.

2. Diabetes. Researchers at Harvard Medical School found that women who get fewer than five hours of sleep each night are one-third more likely to develop diabetes than their well-rested counterparts are.

3. Heart disease. Studies at both Harvard and the University of Chicago have found a direct correlation between too little sleep and a higher risk of heart disease—possibly because sleep deprivation can raise both blood pressure and blood sugar levels and pump extra stress hormones into the bloodstream.

❯ Beyond the Big 3

When it comes to negative effects of sleep deprivation, colon cancer, diabetes, and heart disease are only the beginning. Spending too little quality time between the sheets can also lead to or worsen a host of other physical and mental problems, including age-related disorders, depression, obesity, stroke, a weakened immune system, decreased memory retention, and impaired decision-making abilities.

Rejuvenating Recipe
SNOOZEFEST PUNCH

Whether you suffer from chronic insomnia or simply have trouble falling asleep once in a while, treat yourself to this delicious drink about half an hour before bedtime. Then when your head hits the pillow, you'll be in the Land of Nod before you know it.

- **8 oz. of milk**
- **2 tsp.–1 tbsp. of raw honey to taste**
- **⅛–¼ tsp. of ground nutmeg to taste**

Warm up the milk until it's hot, but not boiling, and pour it into a mug. Stir in the honey, and sprinkle the nutmeg on top. Let the potion cool to a drinkable warmth, and sip it slowly while you ease into sleepy-time mode.
Yield: *1 serving*

Get Your Beauty Sleep

No, that's not just a euphemism. Cutting enough quality z's each night is essential to retaining your youthful appearance. There are two reasons:

- It's only during deep, a.k.a. slow-wave, sleep that your body releases sufficient human growth hormone. Contrary to its name, this hormone is on the job throughout your life, increasing muscle mass, thickening your skin, strengthening your bones, and playing a role in normal tissue repair—patching up the daily wear and tear on your body.

- Failure to get enough sleep causes your body to release more of the stress hormone cortisol. That, in turn, can break down your skin's collagen, which is the protein that keeps your skin smooth, supple, and young-looking.

Tick-Tock **TURN BACK** the **CLOCK**

❯ 6 Signs That You Need More (or Better) Sleep

Here are a half-dozen hints that tell you you're sleeping either too little or not soundly enough:

- You've become accident-prone.

- You're often grumpy and irritable.

- You doze off while watching TV or reading.

- You fall asleep in public places, such as church, movie theaters, or waiting rooms.

- You get drowsy in a car, whether you're the driver or a passenger.

- You can't remember the last time you woke up without the aid of an alarm clock.

❯ How Much Is Enough?

Doctors who specialize in sleep disorders tell us that getting the right amount of sound, restful sleep has been scientifically proven to be the most important factor in predicting a person's longevity—even more than diet, exercise, or heredity. Yet, in our round-the-clock, squeeze-it-all-in society, sleep is often viewed as a waste of time. In fact, some famous motivational authors actually advise readers to shave hours of shut-eye time from their schedules in the interest of working more "accomplishments" into their days. The amount of sleep necessary to ensure peak health and performance varies from one person to the next, but the average adult needs seven to nine hours of good z's each night. So, if you haven't been getting your full allotment, now's the time to start!

> Too Much of a Good Thing

Craving excessive amounts of shut-eye can be a side effect of a medication you're taking, it could mean that you're depressed, or it might be that you simply enjoy sleeping. Or it may indicate an underlying health condition. Whatever the reason, sleeping too much can result in many of the same issues as snoozing too little. If you average more than seven to nine hours of sleep a night, ask your doctor about changing or eliminating the problem-causing meds. Or, if you're not taking any drugs, have a thorough checkup to determine the cause of your problem.

> 2 Basic Slumber Blunders

Occasional failure to get a good night's sleep may be caused by factors beyond your control, like a backache, a nagging cold, or a loud party next door. But if you suffer from ongoing sleeping difficulties, the problem—and, therefore, the solution—may lie with your own routine. Here are two ways you may be keeping yourself awake when you should be snoozing soundly:

MIND OVER MYTH

MYTH: Watching television in bed is a dandy way to lull yourself to sleep at night.

REALITY: While it's true that staring at the boob tube may cause you to conk out quickly, it's all but guaranteed that you'll wake up later on. What you're doing is establishing a pattern of poor sleep that can easily lead to chronic insomnia. The simple solution: Get the TV out of the bedroom—now! If you absolutely must watch TV in bed, make sure the set has a sleep timer so that you're not wakened during the wee hours by a loud commercial, the light from the screen, or both.

Blunder #1: Keeping an erratic schedule

The human body thrives on regularity. If, like many folks, you either stay up late on holidays and weekends, or use those mornings to catch up on the sleep you lost during the workweek, then you're throwing your internal clock out of whack.

Solution: Establish a routine and stick to it as best you can. By going to bed and rising at roughly the same times, day in and day out, you'll develop a consistent rhythm that tells your brain when to release the hormones that alternately play taps and reveille.

Blunder #2: Grinding to a screeching halt

Asking your body to go abruptly from full steam ahead to blissful slumber is a formula for failure. Your system needs time to produce enough neurotransmitters so that your brain knows when the hour has come to haul out the old bedroll and lay down for the night.

Solution: Let yourself gear down. Turn off the television set, talk radio, and all electronic devices at least two hours before bedtime. Otherwise, the potent load of stimuli they send to your brain may keep it in fast-action mode for hours after you hit the hay. An hour or so before bedtime, start setting your mind and body at ease by dimming the lights and doing whatever activities you find most relaxing, whether it's taking a warm bath, listening to calming music, or reading (but, please, no work stuff, action-packed thrillers, iPads, or newspapers!).

A Feet-On Cure for Chronic Insomnia

Lots of former insomniacs swear by this kooky-sounding, but effective trick: Lay a wooden rolling pin on the floor in front of your favorite chair, sit back, and take off your shoes (remove your socks, too, if you like, but it's not necessary). Put both feet on the pin, applying as much pressure as you can, and roll your tootsies back and forth for three minutes. Repeat this procedure each evening, an hour or two before bedtime, and within a week you should be getting a solid eight hours of shut-eye every night.

> Lights Out!

Believe it or not, that bedside alarm clock that wakes you up in the morning could also be keeping you from getting the deep, healthful sleep you need at night. That's because, in order to ensure the necessary quantity *and* quality of sleep, your body needs a steady supply of the hormone melatonin, which your pineal gland only produces sufficiently in intense darkness. Even the glowing numbers on your clock and the tiny lights on your cell-phone charger or cordless telephone disrupt melatonin production and disturb your sleep cycle. Your action plan: Remove all electronic devices from view or mask their lights, and install light-blocking window coverings. If those measures are not possible, wear an eye mask. **Note:** *If you wake up to go to the bathroom or get a drink, keep the lights as dim as safe navigation allows. Otherwise, you could have a dickens of a time falling back to sleep.*

❯ Decorate for Your Health

As wacky as this may sound, the design and decor of your sleeping quarters may also be hindering your ability to get an effective 40 winks each night. That's because, regardless of personal taste, there are some hard-and-fast rules of physics that influence the way your eyes, and therefore your mind, perceive your surroundings. Here's a duo of handy hints that can make your bedroom more conducive to rejuvenating downtime:

Color it restful. Get rid of any bedding, curtains, or wallpaper in bold colors or busy prints. No matter how much they appeal to you aesthetically, they deliver

Centenarian SECRETS 100

For centuries, the soothing scent of lavender has been helping people drift off to dreamland, with none of the toxic side effects of commercial sleep aids. Whether you're a genuine insomniac, or you only have occasional nights when you just can't fall asleep, try one of these fragrant options:

- Keep a vase of fresh or dried lavender on your bedside table.

- Fill a small fabric pouch with dried lavender, and tuck it under your pillow.

- On laundry day, put some dried lavender into a small zippered pillowcase or tightly closed cheesecloth bag, and toss it into the dryer with your bed linens. They'll emerge with a delicate, sleep-inducing aroma.

- Pour cooled lavender tea into a spray bottle, and spritz your pillowcase. (Give it time to dry before you hit the sack.)

a resounding wake-up call to your brain just when it needs to gear down. Replace the visual chaos with solid colors in soft, soothing tones. If you absolutely must have some pattern, make it very muted, and confine it to one element, like the curtains, bedcover, or a couple of decorative pillows.

Can the clutter. Keep stuff—especially small furnishings and tiny trinkets—to an absolute minimum in your sleeping area. As psychologists know, a space containing just a few large objects looks and feels more serene and restful than one filled with scads of little things, no matter how beautiful or treasured they may be.

❯ 6 Slick Signals That'll Summon the Sandman

It's probably safe to say that there's no one on the planet who doesn't have trouble falling asleep once in a while. So it's no surprise that there are more sleep-inducing methods than you can shake a pillow at. Here's a handy half dozen of the most effective:

1. Just before you hit the sack, mix 1 teaspoon of honey in a glass of warm milk, and drink it down. It's one of the oldest tricks in the book—and still one of the best!

2. Rub a little castor oil over your eyelids at bedtime. It sounds too simple to be true, but it works.

3. Cut a yellow onion into chunks, put the pieces in a glass jar with a tight-fitting lid, and keep it on your

---

Fountain of Youth

SWEET DREAMS PILLOW

Here's a project that'll send you off to dreamland in a flash.

- Dried catnip
- Dried rabbit tobacco, a.k.a. sweet everlasting (*Pseudognaphalium obtusifolium*)
- Mint
- Sage
- 2 washcloths or similar-size fabric squares

Sew the fabric together on three sides, front to front. Flip the pouch inside out, and stuff it full with equal amounts of the dried herbs. Sew the fourth side shut, and lay this pillow beside your head at night. **Note:** *Tip for traveling insomniacs: Make an extra pillow and put it into your suitcase, so you won't forget it on your next trip.*

bedside table. Then when you can't doze off, or you wake up and can't get back to sleep, open the jar and take a nice big whiff. Put the lid back on the jar, close your eyes, and you'll soon head back to dreamland.

4. Curl your toes up tightly, hold them for a count of seven, then relax them. Continue the tighten-hold-relax routine for every muscle group in your body, from your feet to your neck (in the unlikely event that you're still awake by the time you get that far).

5. Sing a lullaby. The soothing sound lulled your babies off to sleep, and it'll do the job for you, too. If you share the room with your spouse, croon the tune in your head—not out loud!

6. Silently repeat a word or phrase over and over as you breathe deeply from your diaphragm. Just be sure to use a made-up word or meaningless phrase. Otherwise, it could trigger associations that jolt you wide awake. For instance, let's say you choose "milk"—and then suddenly realize you forgot to buy some on the way home.

⟩⟩⟩ CUTTING BACK ON BOOZE

While it is true that moderate consumption of alcohol isn't likely to hurt you, and can even be beneficial to your health, overdoing it can be a first-class ticket on the aging express—or worse. If you automatically reach for an alcoholic beverage whenever you need to calm down, relax, sleep better at night, or summon up courage to tackle an unpleasant task, then it's time to either decrease your consumption or quit cold turkey.

⟩ The Cons and Pros of Alcohol

Hitting the bottle too hard too often (as one in three Americans do) can lead to increased risk for life-threatening problems, ranging from cancer and liver damage to obesity, an impaired immune system, and just about every infectious disease under the sun. On the other hand, drinking in moderation—especially when your beverage of choice is wine—has been shown to reap major benefits. For example:

Better mental, psychological, and emotional health. When consumed in reasonable quantities, alcohol can reduce stress, ease anxiety, and relieve tension. Studies also show that small amounts of alcohol can slow age-related decline in brain function and decrease your chances of developing dementia.

Fewer physical health woes. Worldwide scientific studies show that moderate drinkers are less likely than nondrinkers to develop any of these serious conditions: cardiovascular disease, cataracts, colon cancer, common colds, gallstones, heart attack, stroke, and type 2 diabetes.

Longer life. According to scientific research, hordes of centenarians, and eyewitnesses living in regions where folks routinely reach the century mark, people who enjoy alcoholic beverages in moderation tend to live longer (in some cases much longer) than either teetotalers or folks who drink in excess.

> How Much Is Too Much?

For many of us, alcohol, in one form or another, is such an integral part of our cultural and family traditions that it can be hard to know when we may

---

MIND OVER MYTH

MYTH: Having a glass of wine or a cocktail before bed will make you sleep better.

REALITY: Every once in a while, a bedtime toddy won't hurt (especially if it's a hot drink when you're battling a bad cold or flu). But if you make it a habit, you can seriously damage your health and decrease your longevity. Drinking even a little alcohol within three hours of bedtime can disrupt your most restful period of sleep, the rapid eye movement (REM) stage. As I explained in the previous section, an ongoing failure to get enough sound, soothing sleep is one of the surest routes to an early grave. Conversely, making quality snooze time part of your daily routine is a key to retaining—or regaining—your good health and youthful appearance.

be lifting the glass too often. Medical gurus suggest cutting back if you fall into one of these two categories:

- A woman who routinely has more than four drinks at one time or more than eight drinks per week

- A man who routinely has more than five drinks at one time or more than 15 drinks a week

Note: *In medical terminology, a "standard drink" is defined as one can or bottle of beer, one glass of wine, or one mixed cocktail.*

❯ Don't Be the Death of the Party

Whenever your plans involve alcohol—whether you're a host, a guest, or part of a happy-hour gathering—plan ahead. These three commonsense precautions could save lives. For example:

Before you head out with a group, assign a designated driver, or have a taxi or Uber driver drop you off and pick you up.

Anytime you've been drinking, snag a ride home from a friend or call a taxi, even if you have to go back the next day to retrieve your car.

When you're throwing a party, have nonalcoholic beverages available. Make sure everyone leaves with

---

Rejuvenating Recipe
ONE FOR THE ROAD

Wish your guests "safe home" (as the Irish like to say) by ending the evening with booze-free beverages, like this delicious, energizing cocktail.

> 3 ½ oz. of apple juice
> 1 ¾ oz. of pear juice
> ⅔ oz. of lemon juice
> Small chunk of fresh ginger
> Crushed ice
> Ginger ale
> Apple wedge (optional)
> Maraschino cherry (optional)

Fill a cocktail shaker with ice, and add the apple, pear, and lemon juices. Grate the ginger to taste into the shaker. Shake it vigorously so the juices soak up the ginger flavor. Strain the mixture into a highball glass filled with crushed ice. Fill the rest of the glass with ginger ale. If desired, garnish with the apple and cherry on a toothpick, and serve with a straw.

Note: *To serve a crowd, multiply the recipe as needed, and stir the ingredients in a pitcher.*

Yield: *1 cocktail*

a sober driver. And just to cover all bases, be prepared to have guests bunk down overnight if they don't have safe travel plans.

❯ Beware of Interactions

Alcohol has adverse interactions with hundreds of prescription drugs, over-the-counter medications, and even some natural and herbal remedies. The nature and severity of the interactions vary, depending on the meds in question and the amount of alcohol consumed, but here's the gist of it:

Problematic prescriptions. Dozens—if not hundreds—of alcohol-med combos can cause relatively mild reactions, such as nausea, headaches, and drowsiness. But when you combine alcohol with any of these widely used prescription drugs, you're asking for serious trouble:

- Blood-thinning medications can lead to internal bleeding.

- Heart meds can cause rapid heartbeat and sudden changes in blood pressure.

- Nonsteroidal anti-inflammatory drugs (NSAIDs) increase the risk of ulcers and abdominal bleeding.

- Sleep preparations can result in impaired breathing, decreased motor control, and unusual behavior.

Centenarian SECRETS 100

If you're trying to cut back on drinking, keep simple carbs, like refined sugar and processed food, to an absolute minimum. Aside from providing lots of empty calories, they cause your blood sugar to rise quickly, then plummet—and that can trigger alcohol cravings. Instead, eat plenty of complex carbohydrates such as whole-grain breads and cereals, legumes, and fresh fruits and vegetables. Because your body digests these fiber-rich foods more slowly, your blood sugar level remains steady, which helps keep alcohol cravings under control.

Over-the-counter catastrophes. Combining alcohol with the popular pain reliever acetaminophen (a.k.a. Tylenol®) ranks among the most common causes of severe liver damage. Some cases even require a liver transplant. OTC antihistamines, such as Benadryl® (known generically as diphenhydramine), and herbal remedies, like chamomile, kava kava, lavender, St. John's wort, and valerian, are also hazardous partners for booze.

The bottom line: Read and heed all warning labels, and always ask your doctor, pharmacist, or natural health practitioner whether it's safe to drink alcohol with the remedies you're taking. Safer yet, don't drink and dose!

❯ Curbing Your Consumption

A genuine addiction to alcohol demands serious help (see "Addiction Alert: 7 Signs You May Be Hooked" on page 33). But if you're simply imbibing more than you should, more often than you should, there's a good chance that with a little bit of willpower and a few timely tricks, trimming your intake can be a pretty straightforward project. The first step is to pinpoint the circumstances, times, and places in which you automatically reach for a drink whether you really want one or not (or where you're tempted to have more than you should!). After that, your best plan of action depends on the nature of those triggers (see "Get Booked Up" on page 32).

Head Off Trouble

A hangover may not be a life-threatening condition, but it can feel like one. There are ways to avoid that "I just want to die—now!" feeling. Here's a trio of the very best:

Before you leave for an event where you know that you'll be drinking, swallow a tablespoon of olive oil. It'll help prevent an upset stomach.

Alternate a glass of water with every cocktail or glass of vino. In addition to keeping you well hydrated, the H_2O will fill you up, so you'll drink less alcohol.

As soon as you get home, drink at least 8 ounces of Gatorade® or a similar sports drink. It'll replace the electrolytes the alcohol depleted from your system.

12 Steps to Broken Habits

Since 1935, Alcoholics Anonymous (AA) has helped many problem drinkers overcome their addiction. Now people with just about every unhealthy behavior you can name have adopted AA's famous 12-step approach to cleaning up their acts. This system is not for everyone, but if you're battling an obsession of any kind, or have a loved one who is, it's well worth investigating. You'll find a complete listing of programs at www.12step.org, but here are some of the most popular:

Alcoholics Anonymous® (AA): www.aa.org
Marijuana Anonymous (MA): www.marijuana-anonymous.org
Narcotics Anonymous (NA): www.na.org
Nicotine Anonymous® (NicA): www.nicotine-anonymous.org
Overeaters Anonymous® (OA): www.oa.org

Tick-Tock **TURN BACK** the **CLOCK**

❯ Get Booked Up

Until you've got your demons under control, do your best to avoid situations that could cause you to drink beyond your self-imposed limit. When you're invited to a social gathering where you know the drinks will be flowing freely, decline with regret, saying you have previous plans.

In the case of a recurring event, like your weekly poker game or the gang's after-work happy hour, establish another firm commitment to fill that time period. Your choices are all but limitless. Just make sure it's something you enjoy so much that you won't be tempted to play hooky (see "The Power of Positive Addiction" on page 39).

❯ 3 Cures for the Morning-After Miseries

Almost everyone who drinks at all gets a little carried away once in a while. For that reason, there are more hangover remedies than there were "champagne" bubbles on Lawrence Welk's TV stage set. But not to worry: Any of these winners should put you back in the land of the living in no time at all.

1. Mix 1 teaspoon of freshly squeezed lime juice and a pinch of cumin in a glass of freshly squeezed orange juice, and drink up.

2. Eat 1 teaspoon of raw honey every hour until you feel better. You can eat it any way that suits you: straight from the spoon, stirred into milk or tea, spread on toast or English muffins, or mixed with yogurt.

3. Drink a nice tall, cold glass of buttermilk.

❯ Addiction Alert: 7 Signs You May Be Hooked

Here are a Baker's half-dozen clues that your drinking habit may have crossed the line from social pastime, with perhaps an occasional overindulgence, to full-blown addiction:

Increased tolerance. You have to continuously drink more and more to produce the same effects.

Having more than you intended—more often. You often start out vowing to have only one cocktail, but then wind up having a whole lot more.

Inability to cut down. You've tried and tried to decrease your alcohol consumption, but you just can't.

Becoming dependent on it for relaxation. You simply can't chill out and relax unless you've got a drink in your hand.

Curtailed agenda. You no longer take part in activities you once enjoyed because you're too busy catering to your alcohol habit.

Trouble at work. The effects of your drinking "hobby" are definitely having an impact on your job performance.

Failure to learn from experience. You've harmed your health or you've suffered other consequences, such as damaged relationships or an arrest for driving under the influence, but you still can't stop or cut back.

Note: *These indicators can also apply to potentially obsessive behaviors like texting or talking on your cell phone, watching television, playing cyber games, and even compulsive eating, shopping, and gambling.*

>>> KICKING THE NASTIEST HABIT OF ALL

Smoking rates are in steady decline throughout the United States. Yet, despite the fact that more and more people are swearing off cigarettes, tobacco use remains the single largest preventable cause of death and disability in the country. In addition to raising your risk for just about every physical and mental ailment under the sun, smoking deprives your skin of oxygen and nutrients—thereby adding years, or even decades, to your appearance. And unlike alcohol, which in moderation won't hurt you, the same is not true of tobacco. It's toxic—period. On the bright side, if you quit cold turkey at any age, you can usually reverse much of the damage you've suffered, or at least halt its progress.

> Why Women Definitely Need to Quit

Although smokers of both sexes are at equal risk for most of the physical and mental problems caused by the noxious weed, the harmful effects of smoking on feminine hormones invariably lead to one or more of these three catastrophic consequences for women:

- Female smokers, especially those who started as teenagers, tend to reach menopause two to three years earlier than their nonsmoking counterparts do, and experience more severe side effects.

- Because smoking reduces estrogen levels, it leads to premature bone loss and, in turn, to the early onset of osteoporosis.

- Postmenopausal women who smoke, or used to smoke, have a higher risk of breast cancer than nonsmokers.

> On Your Mark, Get Set...

There's no getting around it: If you're like the vast majority of smokers, giving up the habit will be the hardest thing you've ever done or ever try to do. Nothing can make it easy, but this quartet of stage-setting steps can help ensure that you'll achieve your goal.

Mark your calendar. Get ready by choosing the day you will quit smoking. Many ex-smokers found that making the date meaningful, such as their or a loved one's birthday or anniversary, helped them take this first big step.

Set up a smoke-free environment. Get rid of all ashtrays, and clean your home and car(s) from top to bottom—or treat yourself to a professional cleaning service. Then declare a strict no-smoking policy for family members, visitors, and vehicle passengers. When your surroundings are spic-and-span, you'll be less tempted to sully the air.

Pinpoint your personal craving times and triggers. Often, the urge to light up is strongest first thing in the morning, after your body has been without nicotine for many hours. As for triggers, for most smokers, picking up the phone, sitting down with a cup of coffee, or being in a stressful situation may all scream, "I need a cigarette really bad—NOW!"

Establish a support system. Especially if your smoking habit is deeply entrenched, consider joining a formal support group (see "12 Steps to Broken Habits" on page 32). And line up a smoking cessation hotline that you can call in a pinch (you'll find dozens of them on the Internet).

❯ Go!

Once you're rarin' to go, get your habit-kicking "trip" under way with these proven success-boosting ploys:

Declare your intentions. Tell family and friends that you're quitting. They'll be delighted to join your booster squad and offer support—guaranteed!

Make it a team effort. Find one or more friends or coworkers who also want to kick the habit, and tackle the project

Centenarian SECRETS 100

It's no secret that a happy, secure marriage is one key to a longer life. Well, as wacky as this may sound, giving up smoking could actually prevent your home from breaking apart. Research has shown that marriages in which one or both partners smoke cigarettes have a 53 percent higher divorce rate than that of nonsmoking couples.

together. Better yet, challenge fellow smoker(s) to join you in a quitting competition, with the one who crosses the finish line first claiming the agreed-upon stakes.

Dangle a prize ahead of you. Make a promise that when you quit for good, you'll do something special—maybe take an exotic vacation or spend a week at a fancy spa. For best results, plan on family or friends joining you—you won't want to disappoint them!

Plan for hands-on success. Find a cigarette stand-in to occupy your hands. For example, keep pads and pencils handy so you can doodle. Or take up needlepoint, knitting, or cross-stitch, and stash your gear within quick and easy reach.

❯ Fill a Quitter's Cookie Jar

No, I'm not talking about sweet treats here. Rather, this is a slick trick to keep you motivated during your quit-smoking campaign. First, round up some slips of paper. On each one, write down a health problem that can be caused or worsened by smoking. Toss all of the strips into a big jar or basket. Then, every time you feel the urge to light up, reach in and pull out a reminder of the price you could pay for resuming your "hobby."

Instant Gratification?

Believe it or not, just 20 minutes after you snuff out your last cigarette, your blood pressure and heart rate should return to normal, or nearly so. That major bodily feat triggers a steady stream of other health benefits: Within 24 hours, your risk of a heart attack starts dropping. During the first few weeks after you quit, tiny, hair-like cilia in your lungs come out of their smoking-induced "retirement" and start sweeping disease-causing irritants away. Within a year, your chance of developing heart disease falls to half that of active smokers. And if you can remain smoke-free for 10 years, you will be no more likely to die of lung cancer than someone who has never smoked at all!

Tick-Tock- **TURN BACK** the **CLOCK**

As for what to write on your "price tags," here's a starter list: asthma, aneurysms, bronchitis, emphysema, pneumonia, cancer, cardiovascular disease, cataracts, macular degeneration, cognitive impairment, dementia, gum disease, tooth loss, impaired immune system, osteoporosis, and sexual impotence.

❯ Auxiliary Help

When you declare war on cancer sticks, don't simply rely on DIY tricks or your army of loved ones. Instead, up your odds of winning by opting for one of these proven helpers:

> A diplomat is a man who always remembers a woman's birthday, but never her age.
>
> —Zsa Zsa Gabor (1917–2016)

Acupuncture. Studies show that nearly 80 percent of people who try the narrow-needle treatment are able to quit.

Counseling. The American Cancer Society and the American Lung Association can direct you to smoking cessation counselors in your area, and the cost may be covered by your insurance.

Nicotine replacement aids. Patches, gum, inhalers, and sprays ease withdrawal symptoms and, when used in conjunction with behavioral changes, can double your chances of quitting. Ask your doctor or counselor which product should work best for you.

❯ 4 Reasons Why Former Smokers Gain Weight

Unfortunately, when you quit smoking, you're likely to gain some weight—although not nearly as much as some folks would have you believe (see Mind Over Myth on page 38). If you want to pack on as few surplus pounds as possible, it helps if you understand the four-pronged connection between smoking cessation and weight gain.

1. Nicotine helps keep your weight down in two ways: by acting as an appetite suppressant and revving up your metabolism. When it's gone from your system (surprise!), your desire for food increases, and your body burns calories less efficiently.

2. Once the aromas of tobacco and smoke are no longer all around you, food smells and tastes a whole lot better—so, of course, eating becomes a whole lot more enjoyable.

3. Most folks who give up cigarettes miss the hand-to-mouth gratification they provide. Food makes a dandy substitute.

4. Ex-smokers who routinely used to reach for a cigarette in stressful situations frequently turn to food instead.

❯ Simple Strategies for Staying Slim...

Or, at the very least, as slim as possible.

Aim for the status quo. Even if you're already overweight, don't embark on a weight-loss diet and a quit-smoking program at the same time. That's a recipe for disaster! Instead, strive to maintain your current weight while managing nicotine withdrawal. Once you're comfortable with your smoke-free status, focus your attention on shedding the extra pounds. Tackling these goals separately will be much easier— and less stressful—to accomplish.

Ditch temptation. Toss out all the junk food in your house, and keep your fridge full of nutritious, low-calorie—but delicious—snacks like apples, carrots, and sweet-pepper sticks. This way, when you feel the need for oral gratification, you can combat your cravings and give your health a big boost at the same time. (For more on foods that can help you quit smoking, check out "Terrific Tricks for Tossing Cancer Sticks" on page 172.

MIND OVER MYTH

MYTH: Quit smoking, and your weight will start to automatically skyrocket.

REALITY: While it is true that people who give up smoking tend to put on weight, the average gain is 5 to 15 pounds, and many folks lose it within 6 months to a year or so after quitting. Furthermore, you'll be a darn sight healthier toting a little extra baggage and not smoking than the other way around. So if you're using the thought of a ballooning waistline as an excuse to keep on puffing, forget it!

❯ The Power of Positive Addiction

Giving up a long-standing habit is hard for anyone, but mental health pros tell us that for folks with obsessive personalities, it's essentially impossible to shed one fixation without latching on to another one. If you even suspect that you have obsessive tendencies, get counseling help for your withdrawal process, and also choose a healthier focus to replace the one you're dropping. The right choice depends upon your interests and physical condition, but here are some helpful suggestions:

- Plunge into a sport, like tennis or golf, or another physical pastime, such as bicycling, dancing, hiking, pickleball, or yoga.

- Go back to school and study a subject that fascinates you.

- Take up painting, gardening, woodworking, or quilting.

- Become an active volunteer in your community, perhaps at the local zoo, animal shelter, museum, or hospital.

- Join Big Brothers Big Sisters of America (www.bbbs.org). Becoming a role model for a youngster should offer major encouragement to shape up your act.

Note: *This ploy applies just as much to excessive drinking and other compulsive behaviors as it does to smoking.*

Fountain of Youth
CRAVIN'-KICKIN' OIL MIX

This triple-oil blend will not only help you stop cigarette cravings cold, but will also help detoxify your system and heal the premature aging and other damage smoking has done to your body.

3 parts lemon oil

2 parts geranium oil

1 part *Helichrysum* (a.k.a. immortelle or everlast) oil

Mix the three oils in a small bottle, and carry it in your pocket, purse, or briefcase. Then, whenever you crave a smoke, open the bottle and take a deep sniff. Or, if you prefer, use a spray bottle and spritz the blend into the air around you. **Note:** *All of these essential oils are available in health-food stores, herbal-supply stores, and online.*

8 Quirky Hints from Successful Quitters

There is no single best way to quit smoking. A strategy that works like a charm for one person may be a total dud for someone else. But here's a smorgasbord of tips, tricks, carrots, and sticks that have helped legions of folks over the years ditch the horrible habit.

1. Count on cloves. Throughout the day, suck on a whole clove for a couple hours, then toss it out and put in a fresh one. They'll neutralize the taste of nicotine in your mouth, which, according to the experts, is a major reason that a smoker wants a steady stream of cigarettes.

2. Get a job where you can't smoke. Many companies have really strict no-smoking rules. A give-it-up-or-get-fired policy can be a mighty powerful incentive to puff no more.

3. Frequent no-smoking zones. In your free time, hang out in places where smoking is not allowed, like theaters, museums, libraries, and churches.

4. Reward yourself—frequently. Collect your former smoking money in a container. At the end of the week, month, or whatever deadline you choose, spend your "winnings" on a special treat.

5. Camp out with your cigarettes left behind. Exploring the great outdoors for a few days, smoke-free, is liberating and should make you realize how much better you feel without them.

6. Gross yourself out. Cruise the Internet for pictures of longtime, heavy smokers and cancer-infested body organs, so you'll have clear visual proof of the damage smoking is doing to your body. (Relevant factoid: In Australia, cigarette packages are required to sport photos showing smoke-damaged body parts.)

7. Brush, brush, brush your teeth. When you feel the urge to light up, reach for your toothbrush or swish with some mouthwash instead. And for good measure, have your teeth cleaned frequently.

8. Try, try again. If at first you don't succeed, don't give up—and don't be surprised. Most smokers quit as many as five times before they're finally able to swear off the cancer sticks for good.

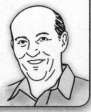

CHAPTER 2

Living Well with Chronic Pain

Pain that's caused by arthritis, back problems, migraines, and other agonizing ailments can make you age quickly and grow older before your time. On the upside, managing the pain that's plaguing you will help you stay healthier, more active, and younger—physically, mentally, and emotionally. Unfortunately, though, many pain-relieving medications—both prescription and over-the-counter types—can deliver side effects that cause more harm than the discomfort you're suffering. In this chapter, I'll share a treasure trove of safe, natural ways to relieve your pain so you can regain your youthful mobility and live a long, active life.

>>> ARTHRITIS

Arthritis is the number one cause of disability in the United States, and it's on a fast upward track across our land. There are two major reasons. One is our ever-growing girth (obesity is the leading cause of arthritis). The other is simply that more Americans are living longer. It's a basic law of physics that the more time passes, the more wear and tear we put on our joints—even if we're in tip-top shape. But that doesn't mean you have to just grin and bear any related pain. Read on for surefire strategies to ease and avoid the condition altogether.

> 2 Major Misunderstandings about Arthritis

With so many suffering from arthritis, it's no wonder a mountain of misinformation is floating around about what causes it and how to cope with it. These are the two most prevalent misconceptions:

Misconception #1: All joint pain is arthritis.

Fact: Tendinitis, bursitis, and soft-tissue injuries can also cause joint pain. So before you try any do-it-yourself remedies, get a diagnosis from a rheumatologist.

Misconception #2: Arthritis is arthritis—period.

Fact: There are more than 100 forms of arthritis. They operate in slightly different ways, and some are more debilitating than others. Again, a rheumatologist can tell you which kind (if any) you've got and the best ways to treat it.

❯ A Trio of Joint-Troubling Terrors

Out of the hundreds of forms of arthritis, these are the three that are the most commonly diagnosed:

Osteoarthritis (OA). This is the most prevalent kind, and it results from injury or from wear and tear on your joints. If your hips or knees ache when you climb out of bed in the morning, and you were a jock or a dancer in high school or college, it's all but guaranteed that OA is the culprit.

Rheumatoid arthritis (RA). This autoimmune disease occurs when your immune system malfunctions and attacks your body.

Lose Weight and Lose Arthritis Pain...

Or at least delay its onset and lessen its severity. The reason: According to the Centers for Disease Control and Prevention (CDC), obesity is the single leading cause of osteoarthritis. The more you weigh, the sooner this type of arthritis is likely to set in, and the more severe your symptoms will be. That's because as any human body grows older, its cartilage slowly starts to wear out, and the fluid between the joints begins to dry up. When you put a bigger load on those joints than they were made to handle, the wearing-out and drying-up processes happen a whole lot faster.

Tick-Tock **TURN BACK** the **CLOCK**

Over time, the resulting inflammation can cause severe joint damage and deformities. This serious condition demands top-notch (and consistent) medical care, but many of the same pain-relieving and mobility-enhancing tricks that work for OA can also work wonders for RA sufferers.

Gout. Contrary to folklore, gout is not limited to old men who eat too much rich food. Rather, it can strike anyone whose body can't eliminate uric acid effectively. The excess acid settles in your joints, where it forms needle-like crystals, which in turn cause swelling and severe pain. (You'll find more grist on gout beginning on page 62.)

❯ Nix the Nightshades

If you suffer from arthritis and you love spuds and tomatoes, this news will not be music to your ears, but it could be a sweet lullaby for your aching joints: For some people, vegetables in the tomato (a.k.a. nightshade or *Solanaceae)* family can intensify arthritic pain. To find out whether you're sensitive to these foods, either get an allergy test or—simpler and a whole lot cheaper—go cold turkey on the entire clan for a month or so, and see if you feel any relief. These are the suspects in question:

- Eggplant
- Peppers (both sweet and hot)
- Potatoes (sweet potatoes are okay)
- Tomatoes

MIND OVER MYTH

MYTH: Habitually cracking your knuckles puts you on a fast track to arthritis.

REALITY: According to numerous studies, as well as the orthopedic experts at Harvard Medical School, it does no such thing. But there are plenty of other reasons to kick the habit. Aside from annoying the daylights out of people around you, repeatedly cracking your knuckles can spur the development of skin pads or calluses over your joints, weaken your grip, cause your hands to swell up, and even damage the ligaments in your fingers. So stop it already!

> Arthritis-Relief Rub

Here's another effective alternative to commercial pain-relief creams: Mix equal parts of sesame oil and ginger juice, and massage the rub into the painful areas. If the burning sensation produced by the ginger feels too strong, add more sesame oil to bring the heat down to a tolerable level. **Note:** *To produce ginger juice, grate fresh ginger, and squeeze the gratings through cheesecloth to extract the liquid.*

Fountain of Youth
HOT HEALING LINIMENT

This dandy DIY potion brings warm relief to your aching joints—and muscles, too!

> 1 cup of grated fresh ginger
> 1 tsp. of cayenne pepper
> 1 tsp. of vegetable glycerin
> 2½ cups of unflavored vodka

Combine the first three ingredients in a large jar with a tight-fitting lid. Pour in the vodka, and shake vigorously for 30 seconds to blend. Put it in a cool, dark place and shake it for 20 seconds every day. After four weeks, pour it through a strainer lined with a paper coffee filter, pressing all of the fluid out of the herbs. Funnel the liniment into a clean bottle, cap it tightly, and store in a dark, room-temperature cabinet, where it'll keep for about two years.

> Don't Horse Around with Arthritis

You can make the pain gallop away with this terrific trick: Boil ½ cup of milk, and mix 3 tablespoons of grated horseradish into it. Pour the mixture onto a piece of cheesecloth, and lay it on your aching joint. By the time the poultice cools off, you should feel like hopping on your pony and headin' down the trail!

> Pack Away Your Problems

A castor oil pack is just what the doctor ordered for relieving the pain of arthritis—and bursitis, too. To make this magic bullet, follow this five-step procedure:

Pour some castor oil into a bowl, and add a soft, clean cloth that's big enough to cover the problem area. (A towel, piece of wool, or cotton flannel rag is perfect.)

Lay the oil-soaked fabric on your bare skin, and add a sheet of plastic wrap over it. Make sure you've got complete coverage—you don't want castor oil stains on your clothes, bedsheets, or upholstery fabric!

Top the plastic wrap with a heating pad set on "low." Or, if you prefer, use an old-fashioned hot-water bottle wrapped in a towel.

Leave the pack in place for 60 minutes. Repeat as needed once a day.

Tuck the pack into a plastic bag and store it in the refrigerator. Then, before the next healing session, warm it up slightly in the microwave, or simply let it come to room temperature on the counter.

❯ Roses to the Rescue!

No, not because their beautiful scent can take your mind off your aching joints. Believe it or not, those pretty petals are packed with plenty of healing power that can ease the pain of arthritis and other joint woes, too. And here's more good news: The petals' medicinal power increases as the flowers fade, so you can make your "medicine" from blooms that you'd otherwise toss in the compost bin. Here's all you need to do:

Pull the petals from four over-the-hill roses, toss them into a bath full of water (the temperature is your call), and settle in for a good soak. Just be sure to put a piece of cheesecloth or old panty hose over the drain so you don't wind up with clogged plumbing!

For OA Relief, Count to TENS

If you have osteoarthritis, you could join the legions of sufferers who have opted for acupuncture. It's been proven to relieve pain and improve mobility for weeks after treatment. You say you don't fancy having needles stuck in your knees or elbows? Not to worry! Transcutaneous electrical nerve stimulation (TENS) can work just as well, with no poking required. A TENS unit is a battery-powered device, smaller than a deck of cards, that you attach to your belt or waistband. It delivers electrical impulses (painlessly!) through your skin, which increases endorphins—i.e., naturally occurring narcotics in your body—that inhibit pain impulses arising from the spinal cord. Although TENS won't cure your arthritis, it may greatly ease the aches in your joints. Ask your doctor if TENS is for you!

❯ Beware of Topical Pain Creams

Pain-relieving ointments and creams can soothe your achy joints and muscles every bit as well as aspirin does. And there's a good reason: Many of them contain salicylates, the main ingredient in aspirin. That could translate into big trouble in two ways:

- Salicylates interact with many kinds of drugs, so if you're on any other medication—either prescription or OTC—check with your doctor before using a topical rub.

- If you happen to be allergic to aspirin, you could have a reaction when the medicine is absorbed into your body. If you know that you're allergic to aspirin, read the package labels carefully and (of course!) bypass any product that contains salicylates.

Your best bet: Forget about commercial pain creams, and use the ultra-safe natural alternatives in this chapter.

❯ 5 Safe Supplements to Soothe Sore Joints

Aspirin and other nonsteroidal anti-inflammatory drugs (NSAIDs) are renowned for their ability to ease the discomfort of arthritis and many other aches and pains. But when NSAIDs are used continuously, they can deliver serious side effects. Fortunately, a handful of supplements can help ease your pain without the risks associated with common pain-relieving meds. You can find these winners in health-food stores and online at sites that carry natural health and nutrition products:

- Chondroitin sulfate
- Glucosamine sulfate (generally used in conjunction with chondroitin sulfate)
- L-glutamine
- Methylsulfonylmethane (MSM)
- S-adenosylmethionine (SAMe)

Note: *Before you start taking these or any other supplements, check with your doctor to find out which one(s) and the dosage that will work best for you.*

Draw Out the Ouch

Long before commercial pain relievers came along, folks swore by hot, dry salt for treating the agony of arthritis. It works its wonders by drawing out pain quickly, safely, and inexpensively. So give it a try! Just heat a few tablespoons of kosher salt in a dry frying pan until the grains are hot, but not too hot to touch. Either pour the stuff into a clean cotton sock or wrap it up in a clean, dry dish towel. Then lay it on your aching joint until you feel relief. To keep the salt comfortably warm, put a hot-water bottle or heating pad on top of it.

Toss Tater Chips and Ease Your Joint Pain

How so? Because they, and scads of other processed foods, are commonly made with vegetable oils high in omega-6 fatty acids, which increase inflammation in your body, thereby intensifying arthritis pain (or any other kind). Your best feel-better policy: Whenever you're shopping for processed foods—especially snacks or baked goods—read the labels carefully, and steer clear of anything that contains more than trace amounts of corn, safflower, soybean, or sunflower oil. And for cooking purposes, go with avocado oil, olive oil, or nut oils like almond, coconut, or peanut. They're all rich in unsaturated fats, which, aside from not worsening your misery, actually enhance the health of your joints.

> " You know you're getting old when you stoop to tie your shoelaces and wonder what else you could do while you're down there.
> —George Burns (1896–1996) "

Flaxseed Fights Arthritis

Flaxseed contains compounds that reduce the inflammation associated with rheumatoid arthritis and osteoarthritis. All it takes is 1 tablespoon of seeds per day, and you can meet your quota in a couple of ways:

Grind the tasty seeds in a coffee grinder or food processor, and add the powder to a smoothie, mix it into yogurt or cottage cheese, or sprinkle it onto whatever you're having for breakfast, lunch, or dinner.

Take 1 teaspoon of flaxseed oil (available in health-food stores) three times a day. Either sip it straight from the spoon, or mix it into food or beverages. Keep the oil refrigerated to prolong its shelf life.

Note: *Like all natural remedies that go to the root of a problem, this one will take a little time to work. You can expect to wait at least a month for it to perform its pain-relieving magic.*

❯ Eat to Beat RA Pain

For years, medical pros have been singing the praises of the Mediterranean diet for its ability to prevent or treat conditions ranging from heart disease, diabetes, and stroke to poor vision, osteoporosis, and excess weight— as well as to increase your life span. Now, it turns out that it can also reduce inflammation caused by rheumatoid arthritis and help stop flare-ups in their tracks. For the full scoop on this medical marvel, see "To Get—and Stay—Slim, Don't Diet" on page 8.

❯ A Grape Way to Ease Arthritis Pain

The skin of grapes contains resveratrol, a natural compound that helps reduce inflammation caused by an injury or disease. A study published in *The Journal of Biological Chemistry* confirmed that eating 1 cup of either white or red grapes each day will increase your comfort level considerably. Drinking 100 percent purple grape juice does the trick, too. The recommended dose is one 8-ounce glass per day.

4 Winning Ways to Outwit Osteoarthritis

You don't have to be a gung-ho athlete to put yourself at high risk for developing OA. There could be potent dangers lurking in your everyday routine. Like these, for instance:

1. The shoes you wear. If you opt for high heels day in and day out—whether they're pencil-thin stilettos or chunkier versions—you're all but begging for OA in your knees. Plus, high-heeled shoes (or boots) that are pointy or tight can also lead to arthritis of the toes. Wearing dress-up pumps only on special occasions won't cause any damage, but for daily wear, choose footgear with ample toe room and sturdy heels no more than 1 to 2 inches high to avoid unnecessary strain on your joints.

2. The loads you tote. Walking with heavy bags (or any other weighty objects) in your hands, with your arms stretched downward, puts undue strain on your shoulders, elbows, wrists, and fingers. When your shopping haul weighs any more than a couple of pounds, cradle the bag in both arms, or use one or two long-handled canvas sacks slung over your shoulder(s). If you routinely carry a heavy briefcase to work or school, consider trading it for a wheeled model or one with a shoulder strap.

3. The pounds you pack. Obesity is the leading cause of osteoarthritis because excess weight puts enormous stress on your knees and hips. Need more incentive to drop your excess baggage? Then consider this fact: If you shed just 10 pounds, you'll reduce the stress on each knee by a full 40 pounds!

4. The moves you don't make. Couch potatoes are prime targets for OA. Conversely, as the Arthritis Foundation reminds us, "Moving is the best medicine." Even if you're not overweight, regular physical activity is a must for strengthening the muscles that support your joints—and keeping the joints themselves flexible. But there is one caveat: Running, especially on hard pavement, is murder on your knees. So opt for more easygoing activities, such as walking, yoga, or even bowling. Better yet, sign up for an aquatic exercise class, like the ones conducted by the Arthritis Foundation. To find a location near you, visit www.arthritis.org and get started today.

This sweet and spicy salsa is one of the most delicious, and versatile, ways to enjoy these fabulous anti-aging fruits.

- 2¼ cups (about ¾ lb.) of pitted sour cherries, chopped (fresh or thawed)
- 1 tbsp. of sugar
- ½ small red onion, finely chopped (about 3 tbsp.)
- ¼ cup of chopped fresh cilantro
- 1 large fresh jalapeño pepper, finely chopped, including seeds*
- 2 tbsp. of freshly squeezed lime juice

Stir the cherries and their juices with the sugar in a small bowl. Then mix in the remaining ingredients, and let the blend stand at room temperature for 30 minutes or so to let the flavors develop fully. Serve it as a dip for your favorite corn chips or as an ultra-tasty accompaniment to grilled chicken or pork.

* Or substitute diced canned chiles.

Yield: *About 2 cups*

❯ Honey, Pass the Pain Relief

Honey is renowned for its prodigious health-giving powers—including its ability to help relieve arthritis pain. Here's a trio of ways to use it:

- Mix equal parts of apple cider vinegar and raw honey, and store it in a lidded glass jar at room temperature. Once a day, stir 1 teaspoon of the combo and 1 teaspoon of Knox® orange-flavored gelatin powder (not sweetened Jell-O®) into 6 ounces of water, and drink. Your joints should soon be jumpin'!

- Every morning before breakfast, take 1 tablespoon of honey with ½ teaspoon of ground cinnamon mixed into it. According to a study done at the University of Copenhagen, arthritis sufferers who faithfully swallowed this tasty medicine reported noticeable relief within the first week. By the end of one month, they were even walking with no pain at all.

- Each morning and evening, take 1 teaspoon of honey mixed with 1 teaspoon of apple cider vinegar.

Note: *For each of these remedies, always use pure, raw (unprocessed) honey, not the brands you find next to the jelly in most supermarkets. The common commercial types of honey have been put through a* *heating and filtering process that kills off the health-giving enzymes and nutrients. Also (unless otherwise noted), use only raw, organic, unfiltered apple cider vinegar for health and beauty purposes.*

❯ A Jolting Java Joint Cure

This quirky arthritis remedy has proven successful for many folks: First thing each morning, drink a cup of hot black coffee with the freshly squeezed juice of a large lime mixed into it. It may get rid of your aches for good. But don't try it if you have a sensitive stomach!

❯ Drink Your Woes Away

Easing your arthritis woes could be as simple as drinking eight or more 8-ounce glasses of water or other unsweetened, nonalcoholic beverages a day. That's because H_2O is a key ingredient in cartilage and may help rebuild that damaged tissue. Water also helps cushion and lubricate your joints, making them less painful and easier to bend and move around.

❯❯ BACK & NECK PAIN

Just about every adult on the planet has had a backache at one time or other. If there is any doubt in your mind about how widespread the problem is, consider this fact: Back pain is the second leading cause of lost work time (the common cold is number one). Chronic back and neck pain is also the most common reason that people undergo a surgical procedure. So if you want to grow younger, not older, do yourself a favor: Before you take that dire (and often unsuccessful) step, give the tips, tricks, and tonics in this section a try.

❯ 3 Crazy Co-Conspirators

Health-care statisticians tell us that at least 8 out of every 10 people experience disabling back pain at some point in their lives. While all backaches have physical origins, a trio of other factors can play a huge role in how severe the pain is and how long it lasts. Here's the terrible triad:

Depression or anxiety. Either one—or worse, a combination of the two—greatly intensifies your discomfort.

Insomnia. Getting too little shut-eye, for whatever reason, can contribute mightily to back pain.

Stress. It causes your muscles to tense up, thereby increasing your misery.

Your pain-relieving R$_X$: Cheer up, relax, and do your best to get a good 40 winks each night! You will find a ton of terrific sleep-tight tips in Chapter 1, and Chapter 4 is chock-full of proven ways to boost your mood and ease anxiety and stress.

❯ 2 Sneaky Spinal Self-Deceptions

Optimism is a wonderful trait—but not when it morphs into denial about a potentially dangerous condition. Here are a couple of fibs your subconscious mind may use to convince you that, barring unforeseen injuries, you're safe from back problems:

Fib #1: Only folks who are out of shape get back trouble, and I'm active and as fit as a fiddle.

The truth: Physical exercise can go a long way toward preventing back injury. But if you tend to focus on one activity that uses a particular set of muscles—say, bowling, tennis, or dancing—you're actually increasing the likelihood of developing back pain. That's because you build up tension in one area that causes weakness in other places. The key to fending off trouble is to design an exercise program to strengthen and stretch all of your muscle groups.

Fib #2: I know that fat people are prone to backaches, but I'm positively skinny, so I don't have to worry.

The truth: Although being overweight is a major cause of back problems, they can strike anyone. Furthermore, if you're too thin, whether the cause is a naturally tiny appetite or an eating disorder, you're a prime candidate for bone loss, which could easily result in fractured or crushed vertebrae. The bottom line: Try to maintain the optimum weight for your height and bone structure.

❯ Yet Another Reason to Quit Smoking

Some folks who suffer from chronic pain—in their backs or anyplace else in their bodies—find that a quick smoke gives them blessed, albeit temporary, relief. Well, if you're in that unfortunate crowd, I have news for you: Smoking will actually make your pain worse in the long run (if you don't puff your way into a disease that kills you first). In addition to its other vile deeds, puffing the wicked weed slows healing, hinders circulation, and triples the risk of spinal degeneration.

❯ Banish Extra Pounds and Save Your Back

Besides putting you at risk for such life-threatening conditions as heart disease, diabetes, and stroke, being overweight also makes you prone to spinal problems. Carrying excess fat around your belly can make you a prime target for lower-back pain. To relieve current back pain and prevent future trouble, try dropping to within 10 pounds of your ideal weight. See Chapter 1 for tried-and-true tips on shedding your excess baggage—and keeping it off.

When to Dial a Doc

While it is true that in most cases a backache is a straight-forward problem, it can be a warning sign of a potentially life-threatening condition. If any of the situations below apply to you, get medical help immediately.

- Back pain is accompanied by either bladder or bowel incontinence or progressive weakness in your legs.
- Fever
- Unexplained weight loss
- Pain occurs after a fall, car accident, or other mishap.
- You suffer from osteoporosis or multiple myeloma.
- You have a history of breast, lung, or prostate cancer, all of which can spread to the spine.

❯ Dodge the Worst Hazard on the Golf Course

If you're thinking of taking up golf, or you're new to the game, here's a dirty little secret you should know: This seemingly benign pastime can be big trouble for your spine. Nearly all golfers develop backaches or suffer from injuries, ranging from twisted muscles and pinched nerves to ruptured disks, spinal stenosis, and sciatica. But you don't have to join the crowd. Just take this handful of simple precautions to keep yourself safe on the links.

Make sure your clubs fit you perfectly. If the shafts are either too long or too short, you're asking for trouble from the get-go.

Start slow. If you're a beginner, or you haven't played for a while, spend some quality time on the driving range before tackling the full course.

Condition your body. Focus on exercises that incorporate rotation, as well as strengthen the muscles in your back, abdomen, pelvis, and buttocks.

Stretch your muscles. Do this before, during, and after each round.

Rest between rounds. Swinging a golf club is not a natural human movement. If you play day after day, you put more strain on your body than it was designed to handle.

> " We don't stop playing because we grow old; we grow old because we stop playing.
> —George Bernard Shaw (1856–1950) "

❯ Baby Your Feet to Save Your Back

If your feet aren't comfortable, your back will suffer. So wear footgear that's suitable for whatever you're doing—whether it's strolling along city sidewalks, hiking mountain trails, or playing a cutthroat game of badminton in the backyard. And, ladies, be especially wary of high heels because they throw your center of gravity out of whack, which wreaks havoc on your back. Except perhaps for very special occasions, opt for heels no higher than 2 inches.

Back Safety at Work

Conventional wisdom holds that to protect your back, you should always sit up straight in your chair. Not so. While it is true that slouching is bad for your back, sitting up too straight for long periods of time can do even more damage. If your work keeps you largely office-bound, stay on the move with these three spine-saving tricks:

- Several times a day, for a few minutes, lean back in your chair with your feet on the floor and your back slightly curved.

- Work standing up, or even walking around your cubicle when you can—for instance, while you're reading or talking on the phone.

- Whenever it's feasible, instead of phoning or e-mailing a coworker, stroll down the hall for a personal conversation.

3 Simple Secrets for Soothing a Sore Back

Back-relief remedies don't come any simpler than this highly effective trio:

1. Soak for 20 to 30 minutes in a bathtub of hot (but not burning hot!) water with a handful each of sea salt and dry mustard mixed in.

2. Fill a basin with hot, but not

Fountain of Youth

SOOTHING MASSAGE OIL

When a round of golf—or any other strenuous work or play—leaves your back so stiff and sore that you can hardly move, a massage with this potent herbal blend is just what the doctor ordered. It's also highly effective at relaxing tight, painful muscles in any part of your body.

> **10 drops of rosemary oil**
> **5 drops of lavender oil**
> **5 drops of lemon oil**
> **5 drops of peppermint oil**
> **5 drops of Roman chamomile oil**
> **1 oz. of sweet almond oil**

Drip the first five oils into a glass bottle with a tight-fitting cap. Then add the sweet almond oil, screw on the top, and shake well. Massage the blend into any strained, painful areas for deep-down relief. For a more effective treatment, book an appointment with a professional massage therapist, and take the potion with you to the spa.

scalding, water, and for every quart of H_2O, stir in 5 to 10 drops of lavender oil. Settle into a comfy chair, put your tootsies in the tub, and relax for at least 10 minutes. The fluid will get your blood flowing all through your system, just like an internal hot compress—and that's exactly what your muscles need for quick healing.

3. Take a nice, gentle stroll whenever your back feels stiff, sore, and cranky. The movement will send blood flowing to your achy muscles and help relieve the pain lickety-split.

Note: *If these DIY efforts don't alleviate your pain after three or four days, especially if you don't know the cause, see your doctor to rule out a serious illness.*

❯ A Sensational Sciatica Solution

Your sciatic nerve is your body's biggest nerve, and it can also produce one of its biggest pains. But—as unlikely as it may seem when that "fire" is shooting down your leg—you can relieve the discomfort. Just mix equal parts of castor oil, arnica oil, and St. John's wort oil, and gently massage the mixture onto the nerve track. Begin at your buttocks, and go down the back of your leg. If you have a disk problem, massage the oil into that area, too. Repeat as needed for soothing relief.

❯ Just Say "Om"

Yoga can be an effective treatment for chronic back pain—but only if you keep these two pointers in mind:

- Opt for hatha yoga, which features gentle stretching, deep breathing, and relaxing poses. Avoid the trendy, action-packed styles that could actually cause more harm.

Exceptions to the Rule

While it is true that most neck pain is the direct result of stress and muscle tension, it can also be a sign of far more serious trouble. Make a mad dash for the ER in any of these four instances:

- The problem was caused by a fall or other accident.
- The pain radiates down your arms and legs.
- Your neck discomfort is accompanied by a headache, numbness, tingling, or weakness.
- Your vision is disturbed in any way, shape, or form.

- Find a highly skilled instructor who has experience working with back pain sufferers and who promotes a noncompetitive, stress-free atmosphere in class.

❯ Sweep Your Spasms Away

Believe it or not, a plain old broom is one of the best friends an aching back could ever ask for. To tap into its soothing prowess, first remove the broom handle from its head. Next, roll a thick towel around the handle to pad it. Then lie on your back on top of it, with your spine lined up vertically with the broomstick. Stay there for five minutes. Gravity will pull your shoulders down and stretch out the muscles around your spine and you'll feel a whole lot better!

❯ Back Pain Panacea

Even if it's not the result of a serious condition, back pain can still be so crippling that it can ruin your entire day. Relieve the agony with this terrific tea that's tailor-made for those times when your schedule needs to keep running smoothly. To start, mix equal parts of dried chamomile flowers, dried peppermint leaves, and grated fresh ginger, and put 1 to 2 teaspoons of the mixture in a mug or teapot. Pour in 1 cup of boiling water, cover, and steep for 10 minutes. Store any remaining herbal blend in a container with a tight-fitting lid. Drink 1 cup of the tea three or four times a day to ease your pain and keep your plans on track.

❯ Tennis, Anyone?

Tennis balls, rather. As crazy as it may sound, these ordinary orbs can ease your, or someone else's, achin' back. Just stuff three or four balls into a kneesock, and knot or stitch the end closed. Then lie facedown or, if that's not possible, sit upright in a chair, relax as much as you can, and have a pal roll the ball-filled sock over your back. You'll feel your sore muscles heave a sigh of relief.

❯ Your Job Can Be a Pain in the Neck

Literally—and no matter how much you may love your work. How so? Because the vast majority of neck pain is caused by muscle tension. Leaning over a work surface, hunching in front of a computer screen, and slouching at the wheel of your car all make your neck muscles tighten up. So can emotional stress generated by constant deadlines, testy meetings, and clogged highways. That's when a vicious circle begins: When your muscles tense up, the blood flow to them decreases, thereby triggering pain, which, in turn, increases your tension. The good news is that this cause-and-effect scenario makes neck trouble a prime candidate for successful DIY treatment. The challenge lies in carrying out three critical missions at the same time:

Eliminate as much emotional stress as possible, and learn to deal with the rest in a healthy manner (see "Relieving Stress," starting on page 129).

Resolve the ergonomic issues— that is, the physical positions in which you work, sit, and sleep.

Get—and stay—in shape because the stronger and more flexible you are, the less likely you will suffer from neck pain. In particular, well-toned stomach muscles are a must for keeping your whole spine in good working order.

❯ 3 Slick Tricks for Pulverizing Neck Pain

This trio of simple actions will put you on the fast track to freedom from distress:

1. Practice the Complete Breath. This classic yoga exercise opens up your airways and is a surefire way to relax and soothe achy muscles in your neck—or anyplace else in your body. For the complete how-to, see "A Breathtaking Breath-Giving Fix" on page 88.

2. Keep your work at eye level. Looking down or reaching up for long periods of time is guaranteed to give you a sore neck. Adjust the height of your desk, chair, or computer monitor so that you're looking straight at the screen. If you do a lot of reaching up—for instance, to pull supplies from shelves—use a stool, stepladder, or elevated platform to bring you even with your targets.

Boomeritis: First Response

So many baby boomers are injuring themselves trying to get back in shape at the gym, overdoing it on the tennis court, or launching an impromptu game of hoops with their grandkids that boomeritis has since become an emergency room byword. Fortunately, Epsom salts can relieve the pain of almost any sports injury. The exact R_X depends on the nature of the problem.

- When you're having muscle spasms that make you feel like you're being stabbed in the back over and over again, pour 2 cups of Epsom salts in a tub filled with hot water, ease yourself in, and have a good soak. You'll start to feel relief almost instantly. Afterward, lie down for 30 minutes or so with an ice pack on your back.

- For overall aches and pains, use a more concentrated solution: Add 1 to 2 pounds of Epsom salts to a tub of warm water, and soak your woes away.

Tick-Tock
TURN BACK the **CLOCK**

3. Change your habits. Poor posture puts a huge strain on your neck muscles. So do seemingly innocent activities, such as washing your hair in the sink, cradling a phone receiver between your ear and shoulder, or falling asleep in a chair and winding up with your head at an awkward angle. Identify and change behavior patterns that keep your neck in unnatural positions for any length of time. And for Pete's sake, do what your mother (or your drill sergeant) always told you: Stand—and sit—up straight!

MIND OVER MYTH

MYTH: To accurately pinpoint the source of your back or neck pain, you need to get an MRI or a CT scan.

REALITY: In all but a tiny percentage of cases, a health-care professional can successfully diagnose and treat your problem based on your medical history and a thorough physical exam. What's more, these expensive tests often reveal common abnormalities, such as a degenerated disk, that cause no trouble at all and probably never will. Yet they can fail to show any problems in a person who is suffering great pain. The bottom line: Unless you're prepping for surgery, ask your doc if you can skip the scans.

❯ Sleep Better, Hurt Less

For years, experts on spinal health have advised us that sleeping in the wrong position and using the wrong bedding can cause chronic neck pain. (The recommendation: Sleep on your back or side on a firm mattress, using a pillow that is neither too high nor too stiff.) Now it appears that sleep itself also plays a major role in neck pain. In a study at the Harvard Medical School, researchers compared musculoskeletal pain in more than 4,000 volunteers with and without sleep problems, including difficulty falling asleep, trouble staying asleep, waking prematurely in the morning, and nonrestorative sleep. The result: People who reported difficulty in at least three of the four categories were significantly more likely to develop chronic pain than those who reported little or no trouble in the snooze department. (If you're not sleeping as long or as well as you should be, see "Good Health—Sleep on It!" on page 20.)

Carpal Tunnel Syndrome

Spending hours on end in front of a computer is not the only way to get carpal tunnel syndrome (CTS). This painful and often debilitating condition occurs when your tendons swell up and compress the median nerve inside your wrist's carpal tunnel canal. Usually, it's caused by the continuous, rapid use of your fingers, wrists, and/or arms. It can strike hairstylists, supermarket checkout clerks, tailors, truck drivers, musicians, or anyone else whose work entails repetitive motion of the hands and arms.

SORRY, LADIES! CTS strikes women more often than men for one reason: The hormonal fluctuations caused by the menstrual cycle, pregnancy, and menopause all contribute to the swelling of tissues surrounding the carpal tunnel. This is most dangerous for women who are either pregnant or taking birth control pills.

3 EQUAL-OPPORTUNITY RISK FACTORS. Three other factors paint a CTS target on men's and women's backs. Fortunately, you can eliminate this trio:

Smoking reduces the blood flow to your tissues in two ways: Nicotine constricts your blood vessels, and carbon monoxide shoves out the oxygen in your bloodstream.

Excess weight reduces blood flow to your tissues. Plus, the more you weigh, the harder your muscles have to work to move your hands and arms.

A sedentary lifestyle decreases the flow of oxygenated blood to your hands, thereby hindering the removal of inflammation-causing waste products from your tissues. Conversely, the more you move, the more efficiently your system can get rid of the toxic stuff.

WACKY WAYS TO TOSS CARPAL TUNNEL. No matter what's caused your CTS, any of these tricks will ease the pain:

- Mix 1 teaspoon of cayenne pepper into ¼ cup of skin lotion, and rub 1 teaspoon of the mixture (no more!) on the sore area. Don't get it on broken skin or near your eyes!

- Drink several cups of chamomile tea each day.

- Soak a soft cotton cloth in castor oil, and heat it in the microwave until it's warm (not hot). Wrap it around your wrist, cover it with plastic wrap, and leave it in place for several hours.

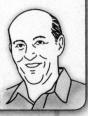

>>> GOUT

The prevalence of gout in the United States has more than doubled over the past 20 years. And, in fact, its meteoric rise exactly parallels the dramatic increase in obesity over that same time period. (Are you beginning to see a pattern here, folks?) Fortunately, there are simple ways to relieve the excruciating pain of gout—and a whole lot you can do to avoid it in the first place.

> Have You Got Gout?

While gout is a form of arthritis, the causes—and the symptoms—are very different from those of either OA or RA (see "A Trio of Joint-Troubling Terrors" on page 42). Most often, gout announces itself in the form of a nighttime attack on one of your big toes. You'll be awakened by sudden, severe pain in that digit. Upon examination, you will find that it is swollen, tender, red or purple, and warm to the touch. Later, gout may also rear its ugly head in other leg joints or (less often) in your arms and hands.

> " Growing old is no more than a bad habit, which a busy man has no time to form.
> —André Maurois (1885–1967) "

Another major distinction: Unlike OA and RA, which serve up ongoing agony, gout is likely to torment you for a few days or weeks and then vanish for months—even years—before it strikes again.

Note: *Even after your pain is gone, the buildup of uric acid that led to your gout attack can still harm your joints—and can return with a vengeance. So after an initial episode, see your doctor and also heed the DIY advice in these pages.*

> Curious Causes of Gout

This painful, sometimes debilitating condition results from too much uric acid in your joints. But what causes the buildup? Frequently, it's an overload of purines, which are compounds found in many fatty foods, such as organ meats, sardines, anchovies, and (attention, heavy beer drinkers!) yeast. But the following handful of triggers can also launch a gout attack: crash dieting; dehydration, excessive use of aspirin, diuretics, levodopa, or cyclosporine; injury to a joint; and stress.

▶ A Gout Reality Check: Good News and Bad News

First the bad news:

- There is no cure for gout.

- The condition can run in families (about 20 percent of cases are hereditary).

- About 62 percent of people who have a gout attack for the first time will suffer a repeat performance within a year, and 95 percent will be clobbered again within five years.

Now the good news:

- Contrary to rumors that you've heard, gout is not contagious.

- It does not spread from one joint to another.

- Even if your genes predispose you to the Big G, there is plenty you can do to help prevent trouble (see "Bar the Gate on Gout" on page 64).

MIND OVER MYTH

MYTH: Men are far more likely than women to suffer from gout.

REALITY: Yes and no. Here's the gist of the matter:

- Men aged 40 to 60 are 10 times more likely than premenopausal women to develop gout.

- Women become a bit more vulnerable after menopause.

- Between the ages of 60 and 80, the disease targets both genders equally.

- A woman is actually more gout-prone than a man after her 80th birthday.

▶ Don't Let a Good Thing Hurt Bad

Vitamin B$_3$ (a.k.a. niacin) is an absolute must for good health. In addition to being one of your body's major energy sources and a key player in your metabolic processes, niacin may help prevent heart problems and Alzheimer's disease. But a steady oversupply of this nutritional hero can give you gout—big-time—along with even more serious problems, such as liver damage. So do yourself a favor: Unless your doc has prescribed supplemental doses to treat high cholesterol or another specific condition, get your daily quota from niacin-rich foods like avocados, eggs, legumes, milk, and whole grains instead of from pills. That way, there's no chance of an overdose.

❯ Bar the Gate on Gout

Just because you have a family history of gout doesn't guarantee you'll get it—but it does mean you had dang well take some commonsense precautions to head off trouble and woe. Here's your to-do list:

Control your weight. In addition to all the other health hazards of weighing more than you should, it makes you a prime candidate for gout. And the more excess baggage you pack, the more likely you are to be "elected." Numerous studies show that achieving the obesity category quadruples your risk of developing gout.

Exercise with caution. Although regular exercise is essential for

---

Watch Out for Trouble-Packin' Purines

Although both organ meats and beer are two of the most potent sources of purines, some other highly common—and otherwise ultra-healthy—foods harbor the joint-provoking substances. If you're gout-prone, avoid, or at least minimize, your intake of these menu items:

• Fatty fish and shellfish, including herring, mackerel, anchovies, sardines, crabs, and shrimp

• Some vegetables, such as asparagus, cauliflower, mushrooms, and spinach

• Red meat, including gravies and extracts

Note: *Nutritionists recommend consuming no more than 4 to 6 ounces per day of fatty fish, red meat, or any other animal proteins.*

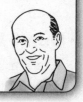

good health, if you're at high risk for gout or already have it, you need to choose your activities with care. For example, running and jogging can easily put enough strain on your joints to spur an attack. And any kind of strenuous exercise carries the potential for dehydration, which increases the concentration of uric acid in your blood. So play it safe: Opt for milder pastimes, like walking, swimming, or biking.

Watch your diet. Even if your scale shows exactly the right numbers, beware of overeating. If you're predisposed to gout, shoveling in too much food at once—especially those that are high in purines—can easily launch an attack (see "Watch Out for Trouble-Packin' Purines," at left).

❯ 2 Fruity Gout Fighters

As strange as it may seem, a couple of delicious—and all-around healthy—fruits have been proven to rank among the most effective remedies for gout. That's because compounds in the fruits neutralize the uric acid that causes the misery in your joints. Here's how to put this dynamic duo to work:

1. Cherries. Either drink a cup or two (or more) of 100 percent cherry juice each day, eat 4 ounces of cherries a day (preferably fresh,

---

Fountain of Youth
GOUT-PAIN-BEGONE PASTE

Whenever gout pain "bites," this variation of the old-time mustard plaster can mitigate your misery.

1 part dry mustard*

1 part whole-wheat flour

Water

Petroleum jelly or vegetable shortening

Combine the mustard and flour in a bowl, and mix in just enough water to form a thick paste. Cover your achy joint with the petroleum jelly or shortening. Then spread a generous layer of the paste onto a piece of gauze or soft cotton fabric, lay it over the lubricated area, and secure it with adhesive tape. Leave the poultice in place overnight or for at least several hours. Then remove the covering, gently wash off the grease, and heave a sigh of relief. Repeat as needed whenever a flare-up flashes.

* Or substitute crushed mustard seeds.

but canned or frozen versions will also work), or take 1 tablespoon of cherry juice concentrate (available in health-food stores) three times a day.

2. Strawberries. For three or four days, eat almost nothing but strawberries. Voilà—that's all there is to it! The 18th-century botanist Carl Linnaeus, who devised our modern plant-classification system, came up with this "strawberry fast" solution.

❯ An Amazing Apple Remedy

Cherries and strawberries aren't the only gout fighters on the fruit stand. Apples can also relieve your pain and swelling by neutralizing the uric acid in your blood. Here's one of the easiest—and tastiest—ways to put apple power to work:

- Peel, core, and slice four apples (any kind will do fine), put them in a pan, and add just enough water to cover the slices.

- Simmer for three hours or more, until the apples turn thick, brown, and sweet, adding more water as necessary. Store the mixture in a lidded container in the refrigerator.

- Spread the preserves on toast or bagels, use it as a condiment with chicken or pork—or put it in a bowl and dig in with a spoon.

❯❯❯ CHRONIC HEADACHES

Anything from a skipped meal to a stressful day at work or a sudden weather change can make your head hurt. But if the same triggers start the nasty throbbing time and time again, it's likely that the problem is in your genes. According to headache specialists, about 90 percent of people who get chronic cluster headaches have a family history of them. Fortunately, while you can't change your genealogy, there is plenty you can do to ease your torment—and regain the youthful zip in your step.

8 Freaky Headache Triggers

The vast majority of headaches—both chronic and occasional—are brought on by stress or nervous tension. So before you start popping pain relievers or searching for crazy remedies, try to pinpoint the reason that your head hurts. That should help you find the most effective solution. Ponder the past 24 hours, and ask yourself these questions:

- Are you facing a pressing work deadline?
- Did you get a good night's sleep?
- Have you moved your bowels?
- Have you eaten well?
- Have there been changes (for better or worse) at home or work?
- Is there something you're dreading (like dental work or a job interview)?
- Have you had a frightening experience (like a near-miss accident, on foot or in your car)?
- Have you experienced an unpredictable event, like uninvited houseguests, or an invitation to chat with the IRS?

> " The age of a woman doesn't mean a thing. The best tunes are played on the oldest fiddles.
>
> —Ralph Waldo Emerson (1803–1882) "

3 Common Headache Beliefs Busted

People have been suffering from headaches since the dawn of time. So it's no wonder that many theories have sprung up about what causes the annoying pain. These are three of the most common:

Belief #1: Pollen allergies cause headaches.
Fact: Not so. Your allergy may clog your sinuses, thereby leading to head pain, but the pollen itself is not the culprit—and, therefore, any allergy medication you're taking will not relieve the ache in your head. You need to treat the two conditions separately.

Belief #2: Food sensitivities cause chronic headaches.
Fact: Sometimes yes, but more often not. According to specialists

in the field, food affects only one in three chronic headache sufferers. Very often, people mistake a food allergy for a highly common pain trigger: low blood sugar. You can solve that problem by making sure you eat at least three meals a day, every day, to keep your glucose levels on an even keel.

Belief #3: If you have a chronic headache, there's a good chance you have a brain tumor.

Fact: Not by a long shot. Rarely does a headache—no matter how agonizing or long-lived—signify a brain tumor. Long-lasting head pain could indicate other serious conditions, so play it safe and see your doctor to be sure.

❯ The Curious Coffee Connection

An overload of caffeine can cause a headache—but so can abruptly swearing off the stuff. If you routinely drink four to six cups of coffee a day, and then suddenly stop, it's all but certain that your head will hurt like the dickens. If you want to break the coffee habit, then reduce your intake slowly over a month or so. Trust me, you'll be glad you did!

❯ Don't Let Painkillers Bite Back

If you routinely take either OTC or prescription medications of any kind to treat chronic headaches, don't be surprised if your pain returns with a vengeance. Scientists don't know exactly why these so-called rebound headaches occur, but most likely it's because repeated use of the drugs changes the way certain pain pathways and receptors work in your brain. Anything from aspirin, Tylenol®, and Excedrin® to potent narcotics can cause problems. Taken in the prescribed amounts every now and then, the meds are generally safe and effective, but if you reach for them too often, or exceed the normal dosage, you could find yourself with a low-grade headache that just won't say "Uncle!"

The simple solution: When that old familiar ache arrives, try one of the "10 Wacky Ways to Cure a Headache" on page 137. Whichever one you choose, it'll pulverize your pain without risk of a rebound.

❯ An Angelic Headache Remedy

As soon as that familiar devilish throbbing starts, mix ½ teaspoon of angelica tincture in ¾ cup of hot water, and drink it down. Not only will it ease the pain in your head, but it will also lift your spirits—and maybe a case of the blahs that caused your headache in the first place.

❯ When to Act Fast

If a severe headache comes on suddenly—especially if you're over age 50—or if you also lose consciousness, your speech becomes slurred, or you experience partial paralysis, nausea, vomiting, and/or a fever, get help immediately! You may have suffered a stroke or have a potentially deadly aneurysm or brain tumor.

A Simple Solution for High-Tech Headaches

Tick-Tock TURN BACK the CLOCK

One of the most common causes of headaches is staring at a computer for hours on end. The easy good-riddance routine: Leave your desk every now and then, or at least shift your eyes away from the screen and focus them on a point as far away as possible. That should nix your noggin pain for good!

>>> MIGRAINES

If you're among the millions of Americans who suffer from migraines, you know the upheaval and turmoil these often days-long episodes can cause in your life. But before we move on to some helpful hints on how to conquer, or at least coexist with, the enemy in your brain, you might take comfort in a bit of historical trivia: Lewis Carroll, Charles Darwin, Thomas Jefferson, Robert E. Lee, and Vincent van Gogh (to name just a handful of rather successful folks) battled severe migraines throughout their lives, but they still managed to accomplish a thing or three along the way—and you can, too!

> 2 Migraine Misunderstandings

More than 37 million Americans suffer from migraines. As common as the condition is, it still remains a mystery to a lot of folks—including many doctors. Here are a few of the misconceptions that are floating around out there:

Misunderstanding #1: A migraine is just a bad headache.
The truth: A migraine is a neurological disease characterized by flare-ups that may not even include a headache. For an accurate diagnosis of a migraine attack, there must be symptoms other than headache (see "Sinister Signs of a Migraine," at right).

Misunderstanding #2: Women are the only ones who get migraines.
The truth: Although the disease is most prevalent in women, it can attack both males and females of any age.

Misunderstanding #3: Migraines are not life-threatening, just annoying.

Keep on Track

Believe it or not, there is no specific medical test for a migraine. To ensure accurate diagnosis, you must track your own symptoms and confer with a doctor who is an expert in migraine treatment (see "The Keys to Coexisting with Migraines," at right). What's more, several migraine symptoms mimic those of other illnesses. If you experience a pain or odd sensation that you've never felt before, hightail it to the ER!

The truth: The attack itself may not be life-threatening, but the associated complications and risk factors can be. Studies have shown a link between migraines and cardiovascular diseases, including stroke. Other research has confirmed a strong connection between migraines and suicide, even when major depression is not present.

› Sinister Signs of a Migraine

Unlike your garden-variety headache, a migraine attack presents an agonizing assortment of symptoms that may include any or all of these:

- Blurred vision

- Light sensitivity

- Nausea

- Sound sensitivity

- Throbbing, pulsating pain on one side of your head

- Vomiting

> " When you're younger, you get blamed for crimes you never committed, and when you're older, you begin to get credit for virtues you never possessed. It evens itself out.
>
> —Casey Stengel (1890–1975) "

› The Keys to Coexisting with Migraines

There is no cure for migraines. The secret to living a normal life is to take charge of your treatment. Here's how to put yourself in the pilot house:

Write all about it. Record the circumstances surrounding each attack, including your sleeping patterns, activities, mood, and everything you've eaten.

Team up with the right doctor. Not all neurologists are migraine specialists, and not all migraine specialists are neurologists. So to manage your condition and the recurring attacks, find a qualified physician who understands your symptoms and will work with you to formulate the best treatment option(s) to keep things under control.

Speak up. Tell your doctor everything about your symptoms and how they affect your activities. That way, the two of you can come up with a plan to keep your life on a steady course.

❯ The Awful Aura

More than a third of migraine attacks begin with an aura. Not the kind where you can predict the future or see into other realms. This aura can present itself in a number of weird and wacky ways. You could see a show of lights or spots dancing before your eyes, experience a tingling sensation in your body, or suddenly find yourself craving a particular food. Other common "auratic" features include sudden bursts of energy; frequent yawning (even when you're not sleepy); and abrupt, unexplained mood changes.

❯ To Halt Migraines, Toss the Tyramine

Tyramine is an amino acid that occurs naturally in your body and helps to regulate blood pressure. It's also found in a great many foods. For most, that poses no problem, but for many who suffer from migraines, it brings on major episodes. To find out if tyramine is triggering your torment, try eliminating these sources from your diet:

Aged cheeses, including blue, Brie, cheddar, Swiss, Parmesan, Gouda, and feta. Cottage and ricotta cheeses are okay.

Say "Nuts!" to Your Migraine

As strange as this remedy may sound, it's powerfully effective at relieving the agony of a migraine attack. Put 2 tablespoons of pecans and 2 tablespoons of walnuts in a blender, and mix them with just enough water to make a thick puree. (Add the water a teaspoon at a time until you get the right consistency.) Spread the mixture on two squares of gauze, and tape one to each of your temples. Then lie down in a comfy spot for a few hours, or until the throbbing stops.

Tick-Tock
**TURN
BACK** the
CLOCK

Aged or processed meats, like bacon, corned beef, hot dogs, salami, pepperoni, and sausage. Fresh meats and fish are fine as long as they're eaten within a few days or frozen.

Dried fruits and fermented foods, like sauerkraut and condiments such as soy sauce and Asian fish sauces. Fresh, frozen, and canned fruits and vegetables contain little tyramine, but the content in fresh produce increases if it's stored for more than 48 hours.

Homemade yeast breads, sourdough bread, and yeast extracts. All commercially baked breads are safe, as are rice, pasta, and cereals (both hot and cold).

▶ Don't Drink to Your Migraine Misery

If, like many folks, you're a fan of draft beer, I have some sorry news for you: Hoisting a pint of your favorite brew might be giving you a monstrous migraine. That's because, like many types of food, beer on tap contains tons of tyramine. So do unpasteurized (home-brewed) beers and ales. You wine lovers need to exercise caution, too, because both red and white versions can cause trouble. The tyramine content in vino varies greatly, though, so check with your doctor to pinpoint the safest kinds.

Fountain of Youth

MIGRAINE-MASHING TEA

This triple-threat herbal blend just might be the ticket you need to stop migraine attacks in their tracks.

1 part dried feverfew*

1 part dried lemon balm (Melissa officinalis)*

1 part ground ginger

Combine all of the ingredients, and store the mixture in a container with a tight-fitting lid away from light and heat. As soon as you feel a migraine coming on, steep 1 teaspoon of the mixture in 1 cup of just-boiled water for 10 minutes. Strain out the solids, and sip the tea slowly. Drink up to 3 cups a day, as needed.

* *Available in health-food and herbal-supply stores, and online.*

❯ 6 Far-Fetched Migraine Relievers

A migraine treatment that works like a charm for one person may be a total dud for another. But legions of sufferers have found relief with some mighty kooky-sounding tricks. At the first hint of symptoms, try one of these remedies:

1. Boil a handful of cabbage leaves until they're soft. When they've cooled to a comfortable temperature, place them on your forehead and the back of your neck, and secure them with bandages. Then relax while the leaves draw out the pain.

2. Mix a few drops of lavender oil with a dab of moisturizer, and massage it into each temple.

3. Soak your feet in a basin of ultra-strong, warm black coffee until you feel relief.

4. Stir ¼ teaspoon of ground ginger into a glass of water, and drink up.

5. Take a tablespoon of raw honey. If you don't feel better within 30 minutes, repeat the dose, and chase it down with three glasses of water.

6. Brew an extra-strong cup of black tea (two bags per cup of boiling water, steeped for five to six minutes), and drink it while it's still very warm but not hot enough to burn you.

❯ Call on Pepper Power

Legions of migraine sufferers swear by this old-time remedy: At the first sign of symptoms, dip a flat-ended toothpick into a jar of cayenne pepper, and sniff a teeny-tiny bit into each nostril. This classic remedy works well because of two compounds contained in hot pepper. The ingredients in question are magnesium, which helps ward off migraines, and capsaicin, which blocks pain impulses from traveling to your brain. But remember to use only a few grains of cayenne—even a midsize dash of pepper in your nose will deliver a very HOT surprise!

FIBROMYALGIA & CHRONIC FATIGUE

Not long ago, these two mysterious but agonizing, youth-destroying conditions were considered to be entirely separate disorders. Now, though, the medical community generally views them as essentially two faces of the same coin. While it is possible to have one without the other, most people who suffer from fibromyalgia (FM) are also clobbered with chronic fatigue syndrome (CFS)—hence, the widely used moniker CFS/FM.

> An Odious Energy Crisis

The scientific jury is still out on the precise cause, or causes, of CFS/FM. But it most often sets in during, or following, a long illness or prolonged period of physical or mental stress, when your body uses so much energy that it overloads the generating powers of your hypothalamus. This is the part of your brain governing such crucial functions as sleep, blood flow, blood pressure, body temperature, sex drive, mood, hunger, and thirst. This cerebral dynamo also regulates your pituitary gland and its production of hormones that control metabolism, energy, and immune function. CFS/FM can rear its ugly head in one of two forms:

FM-dominant. Your major symptoms are insomnia and intense muscle pain. At first it may be intermittent or affect only specific parts of your body, but in most cases the pain expands and, before long, you're aching all over, all the time.

CFS-dominant. In this case, your insomnia is accompanied by debilitating fatigue that just won't go away no matter what you do.

> " Men are like wine—some turn to vinegar, but the best improve with age.
> —Pope John XXIII (1881–1963) "

Look for a Lyme Link

Studies have confirmed that Lyme disease can trigger CFS/FM, and the two conditions share many of the same symptoms. If you suspect that you may have CFS/FM, have yourself tested for Lyme disease as well, even if you don't think you've been targeted by a tick. The menaces spreading this and many other infections are so tiny (about the size of a period at the end of a sentence) that many people don't even realize they've been bitten. Plus, only 40 to 50 percent of victims develop the infamous bull's-eye rash commonly associated with a Lyme infection.

❯ 10 Hints That You May Have CFS/FM

Regardless of whether your condition leans toward CFS or FM, these are 10 of the most common symptoms:

- Achiness
- Brain fog or an inability to concentrate
- Digestive or bowel disorders
- Exhaustion following even mild exertion
- Forgetfulness
- Increased thirst
- Low or nonexistent sex drive
- Recurring infections or chronic low-grade fever
- Sleep disturbances
- Weight gain

❯ Dodge Dr. Denial

Although there is no actual cure for CFS/FM (not yet anyway), it is possible to recover from the debilitating symptoms. The key to success lies in finding a doctor who will work with you to find the most effective treatments—natural, conventional, or (more likely) a combination of both. But be forewarned: While the top players in the medical world now recognize both CFS and FM as real and highly common diseases, most physicians still are not trained in diagnosing and treating them. Some docs will tell you that your symptoms are "all in your head" or attribute them to a hard-charging, overachieving lifestyle. So take the time to seek out a partner who is keeping up with all the cutting-edge research and will help you tap into the latest and greatest. Several online sources provide searchable databases that can get you started. Look for "CFS/FM trained physicians."

❯ 5 Daily Dietary Dynamos

A great many CFS/FM sufferers see one of the most horrifying results of the disease on their bathroom scales: weight gain of 30 pounds or more. But, as distressing as that baggage may be, specialists advise patients not to launch any weight-loss efforts until other symptoms are under control. Instead, you should focus on filling your plate with nutrients that can help put your system back on track—namely, this heroic handful:

B vitamins. The whole clan helps improve your energy level, immune function, and mental sharpness, but B_1 (a.k.a. thiamine) and B_{12} are especially important in that regard. Seafood, beef, lamb, and yogurt contain big supplies of B_{12}. Wheat germ, rice bran, peanuts, pecans, and walnuts are all excellent sources of B_1. **Note:** *Too much thiamine can cause nerve damage, so steer clear of high-dose supplements.*

Calcium. If nighttime muscle cramps prevent you from sleeping deeply, it's a sure bet that you're deficient in this important mineral. The simple solution: Get milk, and guzzle a glass of it every day.

Wake Up and Smell the Rosemary

When your energy flags and your brain begins to fog over, don't reach for a jolt of java—reach for rosemary instead. According to studies conducted by the Smell & Taste Treatment and Research Foundation, the herb's pungent aroma triggers your trigeminal nerve, which jump-starts beta brain waves that boost alertness and concentration. Put this "scent"-sational power to work in two ways: Either set a potted rosemary plant on your desk and rub its leaves to help you focus on the task at hand, or dab rosemary oil on the pages of a report or other paperwork that you need to concentrate on.

Tick-Tock **TURN BACK the CLOCK**

Magnesium. It's a must for boosting your energy and relieving muscle pain. Prime sources include avocados, cornmeal, dried beans, lentils, spinach, and other fresh, leafy greens.

Malic acid. It jump-starts the production of adenosine triphosphate (ATP), your body's energy-storage molecules, and it's most effective when you team it up with magnesium. Apples are the most abundant source of malic acid, but it's also found in tomatoes and most fruits, including apricots, berries, mangoes, pineapple, and watermelon.

Vitamin C. Citrus fruits and C-rich vegetables, such as broccoli and red peppers, spur your body's production of glutathione, a powerful antioxidant that CFS/FM drains from your system. Doctors often prescribe glutathione supplements, but some studies have questioned their ability to work effectively on their own.

❯ Your Fabulous 5-Point Action Plan

Natural health pros who specialize in treating CFS/FM recommend a five-part regimen to conquer the malevolent miseries:

- Treat any underlying infections.
- Get your hormones back in balance.
- Restore your healthy sleep patterns.
- Correct nutritional deficiencies that contribute to the problem

(see "5 Daily Dietary Dynamos" on page 77).

- Begin getting regular exercise—but very gradually.

While it is crucial to carry out this strategy under expert medical direction, you can make plenty of effective changes in your daily routine to help get the parade under way.

▶ The Gluten as Gremlin Theory

Some folks insist that simply swearing off gluten will cure your CFS/FM. Are they right? Maybe yes and maybe no. Some sufferers have reported remarkable results when they eliminated gluten from their diets, while others have found it made no difference in their condition whatsoever. Experts speculate that when going cold turkey on the Big G is effective, it's usually because the patient has undiagnosed celiac disease or a gluten sensitivity, both of which can mimic or intensify the symptoms of CFS/FM. The bottom line: If you want to try it, by all means, go ahead and give it a shot—but don't expect miracles. If this doesn't work for you, try some of the tips in this chapter instead.

Rejuvenating Recipe

SPINACH-APPLE SALAD

The synergistic combo of spinach and apples helps ease your pain and delivers a delicious energizing jolt to your inner engine.

- 2 apples, cored and diced
- 4 tbsp. of freshly squeezed lemon juice
- 3 tbsp. of extra virgin olive oil
- 2 tbsp. of raw honey
- 1 tbsp. of unfiltered apple cider vinegar
- Salt and pepper to taste
- 8 cups of baby spinach leaves, washed
- 2/3 cup of crumbled goat cheese
- 1/2 cup of walnuts

Toss the diced apples with 2 tablespoons of the lemon juice. Whisk remaining juice with the olive oil, honey, and vinegar, and season with salt and pepper if desired. Combine the spinach, apples, and dressing, and divide into four bowls. Top with the cheese and nuts, and dig in!

Yield: *4 servings*

A Couple of Classic Colossal Afflictions

While earaches and toothaches rarely pose serious health problems, either one can deliver a load of agony! For that reason, folks have created a gazillion down-home remedies to ease woes and help regain their youthful exuberance. These are some of the best we've found.

2 EXCELLENT EARACHE ERADICATORS

Many factors, from wax buildup and altitude changes to food allergies and secondhand smoke, can bring on an ear infection. Here are a couple of ways to punt the pain:

- Heat half an onion in the oven or the microwave until it's warm (not hot). Wrap it in cheesecloth, and hold it against your sore ear. The chemicals in the onion will help increase blood circulation and flush away the infection.

- Spread castor oil on a piece of soft, clean cotton, and sprinkle it with black pepper. Hold the cloth over your ear—don't put it into the ear canal.

3 TERRIFIC TOOTHACHE-TOSSING TECHNIQUES

Only your dentist can solve the problem for good. But in the meantime, any of these tricks can ease your discomfort temporarily:

- Mix 3 drops of olive oil with 1 drop of clove oil, and dab the mixture onto your aching tooth with a cotton ball. Leave it in place until the pain is gone, and then rinse your mouth with clear water.

- Put a sliver of pork fat between your gum and cheek, directly over the sore spot. You should feel almost instant relief.

- Saturate a white washcloth with strong chamomile tea, wring it out, and press it against your outer cheek. When the cloth cools off, soak it again and reapply. Your pain should be gone!

CAUTION: DANGER AHEAD

Sometimes, ear or tooth discomfort can indicate a bigger problem. Get help quickly in either of these instances:

- You feel numbness or tingling in your teeth or gums (a possible symptom of oral cancer) or a neurological problem such as atypical facial pain (ATF) or trigeminal neuralgia. In both cases, your dentist can recommend an appropriate specialist for treatment.

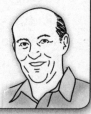

- Your ear is discharging liquid from the canal. If that happens, don't put anything in it, but do head for the ER. Your eardrum may have ruptured, or you may have a serious infection.

CHAPTER 3

Conquer Chronic Conditions

A lot of folks would have you believe that chronic, debilitating diseases are part and parcel of aging. Hogwash! Every day, medical science is learning that simply by adopting sensible eating habits, moving your body around as Mother Nature intended you to do, and keeping toxic crud to a minimum in your daily environment, you stand a very good chance of avoiding trouble. Plus, if you do come down with a serious condition, those same maneuvers—along with appropriate medical care—can help you alleviate or cure the problem, so you can grow younger, not older.

>>> ASTHMA—BREATHE EASIER!

Breathing is something that most of us take for granted. But for folks with asthma, the simple act of inhaling life-giving air is a constant struggle. And the ranks of those who wage battle are on the rise—big-time. Over the past 25 years, asthma rates have quadrupled and the number of deaths from asthma attacks has doubled. Whether you're included in those statistics—or you simply want to avoid making the list—the tips, tricks, and tonics in this section can help.

> Controllable Asthma Triggers

About three-fifths of all asthma cases are hereditary, according to medical statisticians. No one knows for sure what launches attacks in folks whose genes don't predispose them to the condition, but natural health practitioners point their fingers at four factors—all of which have surged to near-epidemic proportions during the period that asthma rates have soared. The good news is that you can alleviate every single one of these and greatly diminish your chances of developing the Big A. These are the un-fab four:

The modern American diet (MAD) and its two ugly offspring: chronic inflammation that causes your airways to swell up and become clogged with mucus, and nutritional deficiencies that make you more prone to diseases of all kinds, including asthma (see Chapter 5 and also "The Easiest Toxin to Toss" on page 112).

An overload of chemicals in our food, water, and air—indoors and out—that weaken your immune system and throw hormones out of balance.

Increasing levels of allergens (such as mold, mildew, and toxin-bearing dust mites) in our homes and offices.

A tidal wave of tension, anxiety, and stress, all of which contribute to or worsen every health problem under the sun—and all of which you can overcome using the timely tips in Chapter 4.

❯ Slim Down, Breathe Easier

Harvard researchers have found that women who are 30 percent over their normal weight for their height are more than twice as likely to develop adult

MIND OVER MYTH

MYTH: People with asthma shouldn't exercise.

REALITY: In most cases, nothing could be further from the truth. Regular exercise not only improves your lung function but also helps you maintain a healthy weight. One of the best exercises for asthma sufferers is swimming because it builds up the muscles used for breathing. Plus (provided you take your dips in a heated indoor pool), it exposes your lungs to plenty of warm, moist air, which is less likely to trigger asthma symptoms. **Note:** *Check with your doctor before you begin any exercise program. Also, beware of exercising vigorously in cold, dry air because it can trigger attacks in some people.*

asthma than ladies who are not packing extra pounds. So if you're bearing a bulge, and you want to keep—or start—breathing freely, your mission is clear: Strive to lose weight at a sustainable rate of about one pound a week through regular exercise and healthful eating (*not* a crazy quack diet!). Within four months or so, you should drop enough weight to greatly lessen the chance that your bronchial tubes will betray you. If you already have asthma, your inhaler should start seeing a lot less action.

› Avoid Asthma, Shun HRT

For years, the media has reported studies showing that hormone replacement therapy (HRT) can increase a woman's risk for heart attack, stroke, and breast cancer. But here's a stunner that hasn't gotten as much airplay: Thanks to its load of supplemental estrogen, HRT can double your risk of developing asthma. Especially if this bronchial nightmare runs in your family, ask your doctor about a friendlier, over-the-counter alternative to HRT called Promensil®.

Its key ingredient, red clover, delivers herbal estrogen that may help reduce hot flashes and other menopausal discomforts without the dangers of the heavy hitters in traditional HRT meds.

Fountain of Youth
ANTI-ASTHMA MASSAGE OIL

Legions of asthma sufferers have found relief with this airway-opening, aromatic rub.

4 parts eucalyptus oil

3 parts Roman chamomile oil

2 parts lavender oil

2 parts myrrh oil

1 tsp. of olive oil

Mix together the essential oils,* and store the blend in a dark bottle with a tight-fitting cap. At bedtime, mix 10 drops of the oil combo with the olive oil, and massage the potion onto your chest. Then, before you hit the sack, put on an expendable T-shirt or old pajamas to protect your bed linens!

* *Available in health-food stores, herbal-supply stores, and online.*

❯ A Cough-Canceling Kitchen Caper

Breathing in steam laced with lavender can help stop an asthma attack in its tracks. At the first sign of symptoms, fill a pot with water, and for each quart, add 2 tablespoons of either fresh or dried lavender flowers. Boil the water, and inhale the rising steam, being careful not to burn yourself. It will open your respiratory passages and relax your facial muscles in no time. Before you know it, you should be breathing freely again. **Note:** *You can find dried lavender flowers in herbal-supply stores and on many websites. Just be sure to specify organic food-grade lavender for this or any other health-related purpose.*

❯ 5 Simple Steps to Clog-Free Airways

Since as far back as the 1600s, medical gurus have been touting garlic's miraculous lung-clearing prowess. Taking this potent syrup consistently may just keep you free of asthma symptoms and prolong your health and longevity. Here's your five-step game plan:

1. Separate and peel the cloves of three garlic bulbs.

2. Put them in a non-aluminum pan with 2 cups of water, and simmer until the garlic cloves are soft and about 1 cup of water is left in the pan.

3. Using a slotted spoon, transfer the garlic to a lidded jar.

4. Add 1 cup of unfiltered apple cider vinegar and ½ cup of organic raw honey to the water in the pan, and then boil the mixture until it's syrupy.

5. Pour the syrup over the garlic in the jar, put the lid on, and let it sit overnight, or for at least eight hours.

Every morning on an empty stomach, swallow one or two garlic cloves along with 1 teaspoon of the syrup.

❯ Asthma-Bashing Beverages

A couple of common—and ultra-healthy—drinks can often stop asthmatic episodes cold turkey, or at least lessen their severity.

Cranberry juice. Take 2 tablespoons of pure, unsweetened cranberry juice 30 minutes before each meal and at the onset of an attack. Just be sure to use 100 percent cranberry juice (not juice combos), with no sugar or preservatives added.

Garlic milk. As soon as you feel an attack coming on, stir 5 teaspoons of minced garlic into ¼ cup of milk and heat in the microwave until just boiling. Strain out the garlic, let the milky "tea" cool to a comfortable temperature, and drink it down. (Keep a jar of minced garlic in the fridge so you can whip up this drink in no time.)

❯ That Old Cliché about Apples...

Is worth taking to heart if you've got asthma. A recent study at the University of Nottingham in England found that asthmatics who ate more than five apples a week really did keep the doctor away. The volunteer subjects had less wheeziness and other symptoms, as well

---

Centenarian SECRETS 100

One of the best anti-asthma meds you could ever ask for is in the produce aisle of your local supermarket—or may even be growing in your own garden. What is it? Onions. The pungent bulbs are rich in compounds that reduce inflammation and help stave off spasms like nobody's business. Eat 'em raw in salads, stir-fry them with other veggies, or make yourself a big bowl of onion soup. No matter how you eat them you should soon feel your airways opening up.

---

as improved overall lung function. But wait—there's more! The nutrients, enzymes, and biochemical compounds in Eve's favorite fruit have also been proven to help lower high blood pressure and cholesterol; prevent or dissolve gallstones; keep blood sugar under control; and fend off or relieve scads of other potentially deadly conditions, including cardiovascular disease, colon cancer, stroke, and coronary heart disease.

And here's more good news: Apples pack the same healthy wallop whether you eat them fresh, dried, frozen, or cooked—or drink them in the form of 100 percent apple juice or cider.

❯ An Asthma Antidote: Sunny and Sweet

Legions of chronic asthma sufferers swear by this classic preventive potion: Put 4 cups of shelled sunflower seeds in a pan with 2 quarts of water, and boil until the water is reduced by half. Strain out the solids, add 8 cups of raw honey to the liquid, and boil again until it becomes syrupy. Pour into a sterilized glass jar with a tight-fitting lid (a canning jar is perfect), and store at room temperature. Then take 1 teaspoon of the syrup half an hour before each meal. **Note:** *To sterilize jars (for this or any other health or beauty concoction), fill them with boiling water, and let* *them sit for 10 minutes. Then empty the water, and let the jars cool down to room temperature before filling them with the potion. Likewise, soak any lids or caps in boiling water for 10 minutes.*

❯ The Hidden Healing Secrets of Citrus Peels

Studies have found that a chemical called limonene, which is found in the rinds of all citrus fruits, can provide potent protection against obstructions in your bronchial tubes. But that's not all! In addition to easing your wheezing woes, limonene may help prevent breast, colon, and prostate cancers. Put this "a-peeling," life-extending healer to work in one of three ways:

Sniff it. Fold a piece of peel between your fingers, and squeeze it. Then slowly inhale the refreshing aroma.

Eat it. Add freshly grated lemon, lime, orange, grapefruit, or tangerine peels to stir-fries, salad dressings, baked goods, and rice. Or top your toast, bagels, and muffins with marmalade.

Bathe in it. Stuff cheesecloth bags or panty hose feet with crushed citrus peels, and toss them into your bathwater. Whatever you do, though, never put loose rinds—or any other solid material—in the tub, or your cleared-up windpipes will come at the expense of clogged-up drainpipes!

A Calming, Curative Facial Splash

This aromatic oil potion is the thing to reach for whenever an acute asthma attack hits. To make it, mix 7 drops of lavender oil, 5 drops of cedarwood oil, and 2 drops of marjoram oil in a dark bottle with a dropper top. At the onset of an attack, fill a sink or basin with cold water, add 2 drops of the oil blend, and stir it in thoroughly with your hand. Then splash your face with the mixture, keeping your eyes tightly closed, until you feel calm and your spasms have subsided. Repeat as needed until you're breathing easy again.

Tick-Tock TURN BACK the CLOCK

❯ A Breathtaking Breath-Giving Fix

A breathing technique used in yoga, called the Complete Breath, both relaxes and strengthens the muscles that you use to breathe, thereby reducing the nerve activity in your airways and helping them constrict less during an asthma attack. Here's the simple six-step process:

- Sit in a comfortable chair, or lie on your back on the floor.

- Put one hand on either side of your lower rib cage, with your fingertips touching lightly.

- Breathe in through your nose, letting the air fill your lower lungs and the lower part of your chest.

- Concentrate on making your ribs expand sideways as your lungs fill. You should feel your fingers draw apart as your chest expands.

- Continue inhaling for about 10 seconds, but go gently; you should feel no strain in your stomach or chest muscles.

- Exhale as slowly as you can—through your nose—for 10 seconds.

The more experienced you become at this technique, the longer you'll be able to stretch out the exhalation part. Perform the Complete Breath for at least five minutes whenever you feel your stress level rising, or as often as you like throughout the day.

❯❯❯ DIABETES—GET IT OUTTA DODGE!

Hand in glove with the obesity epidemic, diabetes rates have sky-rocketed in recent decades. But, although being over your fighting weight makes you a prime candidate for what old-timers called "sugar," there are plenty of other risk factors that may be painting a big D target on your back. Some of these conditions you bring on yourself; others are passed down through your genes. But none of them guarantees that you will get diabetes. If you make some major lifestyle changes—fast—you may be able to dodge a bullet and sail on to a healthy, active old age.

> Diabetes Demystified...

And remystified. "Huh?" I hear you saying. Here's the deal: Historically, there have been two main types of this dastardly disease:

Type 1, a.k.a. juvenile or insulin-dependent diabetes, is one classic example of an autoimmune disease in which the body mistakenly identifies normal cell tissue (in this case, insulin-generating cells produced by the pancreas) as outside invaders and attacks them. Type 1 most commonly strikes during childhood or adolescence, and its victims can survive only with the help of frequent insulin injections. About 5 percent of diabetics fall into this category (see "Juvenile Diabetes: It's Not Just Kid Stuff" on page 94).

> " Middle age is the awkward period when Father Time finally starts catching up with Mother Nature.
> —Harold Coffin (1905–1981) "

Type 2, a.k.a. adult diabetes, is a metabolic condition in which the pancreas either stops producing insulin or loses the ability to use it effectively enough to control blood sugar levels. It accounts for about 95 percent of cases. While some folks in this classification may need insulin injections, very often the disease can be controlled with oral medications, or simply by weight loss, exercise, and healthier eating habits. **Note:** *A variant of type 2, called gestational diabetes, sometimes occurs in pregnant women and then vanishes after the baby is born.*

Here's the fly in the ointment: In recent years, doctors have been diagnosing more and more adults who have what's called latent autoimmune diabetes in adults (LADA), sometimes referred to as type 1.5. These people test positive for the antibodies that attack the pancreatic cells, but they may or may not develop the full-blown autoimmune disease. The medical community has no idea why this "cross-pollination" is occurring, but researchers at the country's top medical schools are hard at work looking for answers.

Knowledge Is Power

One out of every three Americans has prediabetes, with higher blood sugar levels than normal, putting them at a higher risk of type 2 diabetes. Here's the lowdown:

- Without proper treatment, prediabetes could morph into the real deal within 10 years.

- Long-term effects, such as damage to your heart and circulatory system, may already be under way.

- In many cases, prediabetes won't produce classic type 2 symptoms and you won't have a clue that anything's gone awry.

Now for the good news! If the condition is diagnosed early, you can bring your blood sugar level down to normal before major trouble sets in. The American Diabetes Association recommends getting a periodic blood glucose screening beginning at age 45, or sooner if you have any of the risk factors for type 2 diabetes (see "6 Risk Factors for Diabetes," at right).

> Diabetes Is a Stealthy Stalker

One of the most frightening facts about type 2 diabetes is that you can have it for years before any symptoms appear. Plus, when they first show up, they may be so mild that you don't even notice them—or simply fail to recognize them as signs of a serious problem. If you experience any of the danger signals listed below, hightail it to your doctor for a blood glucose test.

- Areas of darkened, often velvety skin on your neck, armpits, or joints

- Blurred vision

- Constant fatigue

- Increased hunger accompanied by weight loss

- Increased thirst and frequent urination

- Numbness or tingling in your hands or feet

- Slow-healing wounds or frequent infections

- Unexplained itching

> 6 Risk Factors for Diabetes

No one knows exactly why some people develop type 2 diabetes while others don't, but there are certain factors that have been proven to put you at greater risk. If one or more of the items in the list below hit home, get a blood glucose screening to rule out either active diabetes or prediabetes.

The trio you're stuck with:

1. Gestational diabetes. If you had it during a pregnancy, you are more likely to get type 2 later in life.

2. Your genes. If a parent or sibling has type 2 diabetes, your chance of getting it escalates.

3. Your race. For reasons unknown, diabetes is more prevalent among African Americans, Asian Americans, Hispanics, American Indians, and Pacific Islanders than it is among Caucasians of European descent.

The trio you can triumph over:

1. Your weight. Both obesity and lesser degrees of overweight pose major risks. But belly fat is particularly apt to send your glucose into the stratosphere because the bigger your spare tire is, the more resistant your cells become to insulin. See Chapter 1 for surefire ways to deflate that tire and slim down all over.

2. Couch potatohood. The less you move your body, the more you up the odds that you'll get the Big D. And this danger applies even if you're pencil thin. In Chapter 7, you'll find hordes of hints for making movement a bigger part of your daily life.

3. Your overall health. High blood pressure, high levels of triglycerides in your blood, and low levels of HDL (good) cholesterol all contribute to insulin resistance. And when you combine those conditions with the two factors mentioned above, you're begging for big-time trouble.

Another Risk Factor You Can Toss

Numerous studies show that exposure to phthalates—chemicals used in synthetic fragrances, as well as in many plastics—can actually double your risk for contracting diabetes. The jury is still out on exactly how the process works, but scientists reckon that phthalates disrupt your hormones, hindering your body's ability to metabolize and regulate fat. Even at low levels, these substances promote weight gain, thereby making you a prime candidate for trouble. Your mission: Do your best to keep the sinister stuff out of your life!

Tick-Tock
TURN BACK the CLOCK

To Beat the Big D, Cut Z's

If you're among the many folks who don't get enough quality sleep—whether the reason is clinical insomnia or the desire to pack more into your day—here's a tidbit you need to know: After just one night of poor sleep, your body can show signs of insulin resistance, which is a major risk factor for diabetes. Routinely sleeping less than six hours makes the danger skyrocket (also, consistent lack of sleep makes you look years older). If you already have diabetes, sleep deprivation can undermine your efforts to control your blood sugar. For the whole nine yards on getting 40 winks, see "Good Health—Sleep on It!" beginning on page 20.

Trick to Dodge Diabetes

Studies show that simply adding ½ to 1 teaspoon of cinnamon to your diet every day could be enough to help control your blood sugar levels and avoid diabetes. That's because it can improve the ability of your body's cells to recognize and respond to insulin. But if you already have either type 1 or type 2 diabetes, consult your doctor before you start dosing yourself with cinnamon.

Research also shows that consuming just ½ to 1 teaspoon each day can also lower your LDL (bad) cholesterol, lessen your risk for chronic diseases of all kinds, and may reduce the growth of leukemia and lymphoma cancer cells. To get your daily dose of cinnamon, just sprinkle it on cereal, toast, or English muffins; add it to coffee or tea; stir it into yogurt; or blend it into a drink like the Banana-Walnut Smoothie (at right).

Centenarian SECRETS 100

To scent the air in your home without the dangerous chemicals found in commercial products, whip up your own aromatic blend. Combine 13 cups of your favorite dried herbs and/or flowers with 1 ounce each of orrisroot and sweet flag powder (available in health-food or herbal-supply stores and online). Then fill bowls or baskets with the mixture, and set them wherever you like. Pour any extra blend into glass jars with tight-fitting lids, and store in a cool, dark place.

❯ Savvy Strategies for Deterring Diabetes

While phthalates floating in your household air may not directly cause diabetes (see "Another Risk Factor You Can Toss" on page 91), they dramatically increase the chance that you and your family will get the disease. So, especially if you have risk factors that can't be eliminated, strengthen your defenses with these four simple measures:

Burn candles made of beeswax to produce air-cleaning negative ions. Send air fresheners and scented candles packin'! If you like pleasant aromas drifting through the air, bring in fresh flowers, or make herbal potpourris (for a simple formula, see Centenarian Secrets, at left).

Carefully read the labels of personal-care products and cosmetics, and avoid anything that has the word *parfum* or *fragrance* on the ingredient list. To find safe, natural alternatives, check the Environmental Working Group's Skin Deep® Cosmetics Database at www.ewg.org. Or, see Chapter 6 for safe DIY versions.

Choose unscented versions of laundry detergents and household cleaning products. You'll find them in your local supermarket right next to the odiferous kinds.

Shun products that are made of flexible plastic and vinyl as much as possible. Phthalates are used in the manufacture of household staples ranging from shower curtains, wallpaper, and vinyl miniblinds to food packaging and plastic wrap, as well as pet toys and beds. (Yes, these hormone-disrupting demons are just as dangerous for pets as they are for you.)

Rejuvenating Recipe

BANANA-WALNUT SMOOTHIE

In addition to providing your daily dose of disease-fighting cinnamon, this delicious drink serves up a major load of vitamins, minerals, and protein. Whip it up and take it along as an on-the-go breakfast, or enjoy it as a healthful snack.

 1 ½ cups of milk

 1 banana, peeled and sliced

 ¼ cup of chopped walnuts

 2 tbsp. of honey

 ½ tsp. of cinnamon

Put the ingredients in a blender, puree until smooth, and enjoy.
Yield: *1 serving*

Juvenile Diabetes: It's Not Just Kid Stuff

This nightmare is now more often called by the problem it leads to: insulin-dependent diabetes. That's because more and more adults are being diagnosed with the type 1 form. Why? No one knows, but scientists are working round the clock to find the reasons, and they're constantly developing more effective ways to treat the condition and its many side effects.

If there is any consolation, unlike type 2 diabetes, which can perform its dastardly deeds in your body for years before the problem is diagnosed, type 1 strikes quickly, with its symptoms developing over a period of just weeks or months. And, unlike type 2 indicators, the clues are not subtle. These are the most common signs that you need to see your doctor—*fast*:

- Constant hunger, accompanied by weight loss
- Extreme thirst and dehydration and the need to urinate often
- Heavy, labored breathing
- Stupor or unconsciousness
- Weakness and loss of muscle power

THE NOSE KNOWS

If you're a diabetic, you know that your blood sugar can plummet to dangerous levels (a state called ketoacidosis) without your being aware of any change in your system. What you may not know is that when it happens, the odor of your breath changes. No human on earth can detect the subtle difference in aroma, but dogs can. That's because, depending on the breed, a pooch's sense of smell is anywhere from 1,000 to (yes, you're reading this right) 100 million times more sensitive than ours. For that reason, a number of nonprofit organizations around the country now train and supply companion canines to diabetics. Here are four of the finest outfits:

- National Institute for Diabetic Alert Dogs (www.nidad.com)
- Dogs Assisting Diabetics (www.dogsassistingdiabetics.com)
- Dogs 4 Diabetics (www.dogs4diabetics.com)
- Early Alert Canines (www.earlyalertcanines.org)

▶▶ GIVE HEART DISEASE THE HEAVE-HO

We all know that heart disease (a.k.a. cardiovascular disease, or CVD) is the number one killer in the United States. And even if it doesn't prove fatal, battling the condition can age you fast. But here's something you may not know: A full 99 percent of heart disease is preventable. So get with the program—*NOW!*

❯ You've Heard It Before...

And you're gonna hear it again: Quit smoking! Chances are you already know that smoking is one of a half-dozen risk factors for heart disease, but here's a shocking factoid you may not know: The *single biggest* risk factor for sudden death from a heart attack is cigarette smoking. To be precise, a smoker who has a heart attack is more likely to die within 60 minutes of the episode than a nonsmoker is. If that isn't enough to make you toss the sinister sticks in the trash, I don't know what is!

❯ The Cholesterol Connection

It's an almost universally known fact that high cholesterol puts you on the high road to heart trouble and premature aging. Yet despite all we've learned about heart health in recent years, a lot of folks still think that all cholesterol is bad cholesterol. Well, think again! Yes, it is true that the total amount of cholesterol in your system does matter—less than 200 milligrams per deciliter of blood (mg/dL) is considered healthy; any more than that indicates that you could be headed for heart problems. But there are two types of cholesterol, and how your blood stacks up in regard to each of them determines how close you are to major trouble.

> " I don't feel old. I don't feel anything till noon. Then it's time for my nap.
> —Bob Hope (1903–2003) "

Low-density (LDL) cholesterol is the villain

that causes plaque to build up in your arteries, and you want to keep it to a minimum.

High-density (HDL) cholesterol appears to actually help prevent arteriosclerosis, and the more of it you have, the merrier your heart will be.

The Other Heart-Hurtful Stuff in Your Blood

Although cholesterol gets most of the attention when the topic turns to heart health, a fat called triglycerides can also cause serious problems if the level in your blood rises to 150 mg/dL or above. Fortunately, you send your numbers downward-bound simply by losing weight, getting more exercise, and cutting back on sugar and processed foods—all of which can also make you feel like your young self again!

Preventing Cholesterol Catastrophes by...

Chilling out! What do I mean by that? Just this: Everybody talks about the effect of diet on cholesterol—both good and bad kinds. But more and more studies are showing how big a role stress plays in the DL drama. To be specific, stress raises your levels of villainous LDL cholesterol and lowers the amount of its good-guy counterpart, HDL. The good news is that when you cope with stressful, emotionally straining situations in a positive way, you increase the HDL crew. This lets it carry on one of its most important missions: mopping up excess LDL in your blood. For the full lowdown on stress and how to control it, see "Relieving Stress," starting on page 129.

❯ The Truth about Weight and Heart Disease

It's true that overweight and obese folks are most likely to get ticker trouble, but even those who are as slim as fashion models die of heart attacks. That's because a predisposition to the plaque that clogs coronary arteries can be passed along in your genes, and it carries no warning signs. So do yourself a favor: Make sure you know the levels of your dangerous (LDL) and good (HDL) cholesterol, as well as your triglycerides, and do all you can to keep those numbers within the heart-healthy range.

❯ Say "Cheers!" to a Healthy Heart

For years, health gurus have told us that drinking red wine in moderation can help keep our hearts in good working order. Well, it turns out that sipping a bit of the bubbly every day may be even more helpful in that regard. A study at the University of Reading in England found that drinking two glasses of champagne (or other sparkling wine) per day improves the functioning of blood

MIND OVER MYTH

MYTH: When you're having a heart attack and you've called 911, you can ensure your survival by coughing repeatedly and very vigorously until the EMT crew arrives.

REALITY: Although this logical-sounding advice repeatedly circulates in e-mail chains, it will do nothing to keep you in the land of the living. But these three steps might:

1. At your first inkling of a heart attack, chew—don't swallow—an aspirin (any strength you have on hand will do).

2. Unlock your door so the paramedics can get in quickly.

3. Until help arrives, repeatedly squeeze the end of the little finger on your left hand as hard as you can. This acupressure technique has been reported to do what the coughing gambit won't— namely, save your life.

vessels, and thereby reduces the risk of heart disease and stroke. In a study published in the *Journal of Agricultural and Food Chemistry*, researchers found that the same pleasant R_X also protects the brain from injuries that occur during a stroke, Alzheimer's disease, Parkinson's disease, and other illnesses.

According to scientists, the secret lies in vino's high concentration of particular kinds of polyphenols (powerful antioxidants) that are not found in nonsparkling wines. These potent substances help regulate cells' response to injury and clear out dangerous chemicals from your body. What's more, these astounding compounds can cross your body's blood-brain barrier and confer their good deeds on your entire central nervous system!

❯ The Doggone Purr-fect Secrets to a Healthy Heart

Over the years, a body of scientific research has shown that pet owners are happier and healthier than folks who do not share their homes with furry companions. After examining scads of studies, the American Heart Association (AHA) has issued a statement saying that owning a pet can reduce your danger of cardiovascular disease and improve your odds of surviving a heart attack. There are four reasons:

Increased movement. Dog owners who walk and play with their pets are 54 percent more likely to reach the daily level of physical activity recommended for good heart health. But having a cat in the household also demands that you get up off the couch and move your body around at least a few times a day—and (as you'll see in Chapter 7) every step helps.

Lower key numbers. Owning a pet, whether canine or feline, has been directly linked to lower blood pressure, reduced LDL (bad) cholesterol levels, and a lower likelihood of obesity—thereby mitigating three of the major risk factors for heart disease.

Reduced stress. Research shows that simply looking at a beloved pet calms you down in two ways: Your body releases a powerful feel-good chemical called oxytocin and, at the same time, decreases its output of the stress hormone, cortisol.

Social interaction. This is an especially important factor if you live alone because study after study has found that interacting with animals (just as with people) leads to better health—including a stronger heart—and a longer life. Plus, when you have a dog, in addition to benefiting from his companionship at home, you get daily opportunities to boost your social time by taking Fido out to mix and mingle with human neighbors and passersby.

Cats Are Medical Miracle Workers

Tick-Tock TURN BACK the CLOCK

Depending on which studies you read, cat owners have been found to have a 30 to 60 percent lower risk of heart attacks than folks who do not keep a feline in the household. Apparently, the secret lies in kitty's purr, which medical pros have termed a "natural healing mechanism." Purring emits low-frequency vibrations that, in addition to making you less prone to cardiovascular problems, may help strengthen and repair bones, relieve pain, and heal wounds.

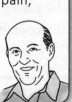
❯ Watch Less, Live Longer

A recent study found that adults who watched television for more than four hours a day were a whopping 80 percent more likely to die from cardiovascular disease than those who spent fewer than two hours in front of the boob tube. If that isn't enough to make you tuck your TV into a back room—or even boot it out the door—I don't know what is!

❯ Giving Blood Is an Act of Kindness...

And it's also one of the best things you can do for your health. How so? Studies show that donating blood on a regular basis can lower your risk of heart disease —and possibly cancer and Alzheimer's disease to boot. This generous gesture is especially helpful if you eat too much red meat, thereby consuming an over-load of iron, which can help trigger the formation of dangerous free radicals. But when your blood flows out of your body and into the hanging bag, it reduces the amount of troublemaking iron in your system. So don't count on blood-drive dates alone to keep your iron supply at a healthy level. Also go easy on beef and other red meats. Health-care experts recommend eating no more than two or three deck-of-card-size servings per week—and the less, the better.

❯ Get in Rhythm

Almost everyone experiences heart palpitations (a.k.a. arrhythmia) at one time or another. That's because, no matter how healthy you are, the electrical impulses that power your heart are not absolutely perfect. If you've received a clean bill of health from your doctor and still your heart starts thumping, or seems to skip a beat or two, try this old-time trick to calm it down: Make 2 cups of strong chamomile tea, and while it's brewing, shred three or four cabbage leaves and steam them. Combine the tea and the leaves in a bowl, and sip the soup. It won't be the tastiest dish you've ever had, but it should tune up your ticker in a hurry. **Note:** *If your palpitations persist, or if they're accompanied by chest pain, dizziness, or fainting spells, head to the ER!*

❯ A Heart-Healthy Handful

Nuts are packed with unsaturated fat that keeps your heart in good working order. In fact, studies at major medical schools have shown that people who eat a handful of nuts (especially walnuts, pecans, and almonds) five or more times a week cut their heart attack risk in half compared with folks who say, "No, thanks." How you eat your nut quota is up to you: You can snack on them; add them to salads, pasta, stir-fries, or smoothies; or use almond, peanut, and walnut oils for cooking and in salad dressings.

Rejuvenating Recipe
BRACING BLACK BEANS

One key to staying younger is eating a plant-based diet. That doesn't mean you have to give up meat entirely. It means getting more of your protein "fix" from other sources —like these delicious and heart-healthy black beans.

- ¼ cup of diced onion
- 2 garlic cloves, minced
- 1 tbsp. of extra virgin olive oil
- 1 can (15-oz.) of black beans, drained and rinsed
- ½ tsp. of dried oregano
- ½ tsp. of ground cumin
- ¼ tsp. of ground bay leaf
- Salt and pepper to taste
- 2 tbsp. of salsa

Sauté the onion and garlic in olive oil over medium heat until soft (about four minutes). Stir in the beans and cook for five minutes. If necessary, add more oil to keep the beans from sticking. Mash a few beans with the back of a spoon, and stir in the spices. Add the salsa before serving.
Yield: *4 servings*

❯ Avocados—Double-Barreled Heart Protection

Believe it or not, these creamy green treats contain larger supplies of two powerful heart-protecting compounds than you'll find in any other commonly eaten fruit—in some cases, up to seven times as much! These are the big guns:

Beta-sitosterol inhibits the absorption of cholesterol from your intestines into your bloodstream, thereby reducing your risk of heart disease. Research has also shown that beta-sitosterol reduces inflammation, boosts the immune system, and may hinder the growth of cancerous tumors.

Glutathione is a powerful antioxidant that not only helps prevent heart disease, but also boosts the immune system, encourages a healthy nervous system, slows the aging process, and may help fend off cancers of the mouth and pharynx.

Put 'em together, and you've got one whale of a life-saving combo!

❯ Make a Heart-Guarding Super Team

Medical science tells us that red wine and onions are both rich in compounds that help keep your heart in good working order. So why not combine those two powerful healers in one easy tonic? Simply add the juice of a medium-size onion (see "Onion Juicing 101," below, to make your own) to a 750-ml bottle of red wine, and shake it for a few minutes. (You may need to mix the two fluids in a slightly larger bottle or jar.) For maximum protection, take 1½ to 3 tablespoons of the potion each day.

❯ Onion Juicing 101

You can buy onion juice to make your red wine cocktail above, but the fresher it is, the better it will be for you. And it's a snap to make your own supply. Just grate a raw onion, or chop it finely in a food processor, and squeeze the pieces through cheesecloth to extract the juice. Voilà, that's all there is to it!

Don't Let Your Pills Kill You

According to an article in the *Journal of the American Medical Association*, each year 106,000 people die in American hospitals from "adverse drug reactions." Some natural health pros think the actual number of victims is at least double that figure. In large part, many hospital deaths attributed to various diseases are actually caused by the meds these patients were taking to treat the condition. The estimate also fails to include two huge categories:

- Drug-related deaths that occur at home.

- Deaths caused by over-the-counter products such as nonsteroidal anti-inflammatory drugs (NSAIDs). For example, each year, bleeding ulcers triggered by aspirin and related analgesics kill more than 16,000 people and send another 200,000 to the hospital.

OTHER UNINTENTIONAL CO-CONSPIRATORS

Overdose, allergies, and multiple medications reacting with one another rank high on the list of reasons for death by drugs. But even used as directed, a great many "miracle" medicines, both R_X and OTC varieties, deliver potentially fatal consequences, ranging from liver damage to nerve disorders, diabetes, kidney disease, and stroke—as well as insomnia and weight gain.

YOUR LIFE-SAVING ACTION PLAN

Don't get me wrong here, folks—modern drugs can (and do) save lives. But it does pay to take these precautions:

Find an MD who understands the benefits of natural remedies and can help you reduce your need for certain drugs, or decrease their side effects, by making lifestyle changes and upping your intake of natural remedies.

Whenever you see a doctor, take along a detailed list of everything you're taking, including prescription and OTC drugs, as well as herbal remedies, nutritional supplements, and even your daily multivitamin pill.

Ask the doc about possible food interactions with the drug(s) you're prescribed. For example, garlic has adverse reactions with blood-thinning meds.

Never talk to a nurse or pharmacist while they are getting medications ready for you. Even the most careful and highly trained professionals can make big mistakes when they're distracted.

⟫⟫ GET YOUR BLOOD PRESSURE DOWN

While high blood pressure itself is not a disease, it puts you at a greatly elevated risk for every heart problem under the sun—and packs the "feel-like" years on fast! What's even more sobering, though, is that your blood pressure can be sky high without your even knowing it. So use the tips in this section to lower those numbers and start growing younger.

⟩ Major Incentive to Ease the Pressure

It's probably safe to say that for most of us, the prospect of a stroke—either our own or one befalling someone we love—ranks right up there with cancer and Alzheimer's disease as a horrifying nightmare. Even if you manage a full recovery, the effort can age you fast. This devastating blow to the brain comes in two forms. The good news is that the vast majority of both kinds can be prevented—and keeping your blood pressure down is key to doing just that. Here's the gist of the matter:

Ischemic stroke is the most common type. It occurs when blood can't get to the brain, most often because a clot or fatty deposit is blocking a blood vessel. In addition to high blood pressure, high cholesterol levels, smoking, sleep apnea, and a family history of stroke all put you at high risk for this demon.

> " I don't know how you feel about old age...but in my case I didn't even see it coming. It hit me from the rear.
>
> —Phyllis Diller (1917–2013) "

Hemorrhagic stroke is directly tied to high blood pressure as well. It occurs when a blood vessel bursts in your brain.

The bottom line: Start getting those blood pressure numbers down now—and rest easier about your risk of stroke!

❯ Alarming Reasons to Turn Down the Volume!

For years, research has shown that noise can raise your stress and your blood pressure to highly unhealthy levels. Well, a growing body of evidence is now showing a direct correlation between noise and stroke. For example, one recent study in Denmark exposed 51,000 people to road-traffic sounds ranging from 40 to 82 decibels (dB). The results: For every 10-dB increase in volume, the risk of stroke grew by 14 percent in subjects 65 and younger, and (attention, baby boomers!) it rose 27 percent in folks over 65. Just to put those numbers in perspective, here are average ratings for some common sounds:

- Quiet room: 40 dB
- Vacuum cleaner: 70 dB
- Power mower: 107 dB
- Gunshot: 140 dB
- Normal conversation: 65 dB
- City street: 85 dB
- Amplified music or chain saw: 110 dB
- Jet aircraft at takeoff: 180 dB

Note: *For every 10-dB increase in volume, your perception of the loudness doubles—in addition to your increased risk of stroke!*

If You Think You're Having a Stroke...

Or you're with someone who may be having one, don't hesitate for a second—make a mad dash to the ER. The docs can sometimes stop an ischemic stroke in its tracks with an enzyme called tissue plasminogen activator (tPA), but it *must* be administered within three hours of the onset of symptoms—and the sooner, the better. These are the danger signals:

- Weakness or numbness in your face, arm, or leg on one side of your body
- Difficulty speaking or understanding others
- Dimness or impaired vision in one eye
- An unexplained dizzy spell
- A severe headache with no apparent cause

Even if the symptoms pass quickly, get immediate help because you may have had a transient ischemic attack (TIA), which means that the real deal could be barreling down the pike—fast!

❯ Don't Let Coasters Kill You

If you think that the worst trouble you can get from a super-colossal roller coaster is a queasy stomach (or tossed cookies), think again. In some cases, those twists, turns, and bone-jarring plunges can cause bleeding in your brain that could trigger a stroke. So do yourself a favor: If you suffer from frequent headaches; you have high blood pressure, arteriosclerosis, or cardiovascular problems of any kind; or you're on blood-thinning meds, stay off of those big mamas! Even if you aren't among the high-risk crowd (at least not to your knowledge), be alert for the major danger signal— a post-ride headache—and if one occurs, see a doctor immediately.

❯ Track Your Blood Pressure at Home ...

And set your mind at ease. A DIY blood pressure monitoring kit gives you a dandy way to keep tabs on your vital stats between doctor's appointments. But it can give you even more peace of mind *after* a visit with the doc. How so? Because of a common but little-known condition that medical pros call "white-coat hypertension." It's caused when a doctor or nurse walks into the examining room (wearing a white lab coat or not), and your anxiety level automatically leaps skyward—accompanied by your blood pressure. If going to the doctor makes you anxious, there is nothing you can do to lower your reading while you're in the office, but chances are your blood pressure will begin returning to normal once you get outta Dodge and head for home. When you arrive and settle in, you can confirm the good news by checking the numbers for yourself—and rest a whole lot easier afterward.

❯ To Lower Your BP, Up Your K and Mg

Adequate intake of both potassium and magnesium (which you may recall from high school chemistry are K and Mg on the periodic table of elements) is essential for maintaining proper blood pressure. So if you need to get your numbers down, or simply want to stay on an even keel, pack plenty of these health workers into your daily diet:

Potassium. Men and women both need at least 2,000 milligrams per day. You'll find it in avocados, baked potatoes, bananas, milk, cantaloupe, mushrooms, dried fruits, tomatoes, and yogurt.

Magnesium. The RDA is 350 milligrams for men and 280 milligrams for women. Good sources are baked potatoes, bananas, broccoli, dairy products, nuts, pumpkin seeds, spinach, and wheat germ.

Pets Can Make Blood Pressure Plummet

University of Buffalo scientists researched the connection between pet ownership and blood pressure using some of the most stressed folks on the planet: New York City stockbrokers. All 48 men and women had high blood pressure, were on medication to control it, lived alone for at least five years, and all were willing to adopt pets. Half, selected at random, were directed to acquire a cat or dog, while the other 24 subjects remained critter-free.

By the end of the six-month study, every pet "parent" had significantly more stable blood pressure than the nonadopters. As you might expect, when the brokers in the control group learned the results of the study, a lot of them got furry roommates of their own!

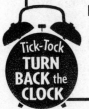

Tick-Tock
TURN BACK the **CLOCK**

➤ Celery Can Lower Your Blood Pressure?!

Yep. This underrated vegetable contains a plant chemical that can be one of your strongest allies in sending your numbers downward. It works by relaxing your artery walls, thereby increasing blood flow and reducing blood pressure. An added benefit is that celery contains fiber, magnesium, and potassium—all of which help regulate blood pressure. Research suggests that eating four ribs a day will do the trick.

➤ A Bedtime Boon for Blood Pressure

In a recent study, participants who took aspirin each night for three months registered a 5.4-point drop in their systolic blood pressure. But those who took the same dosage every morning saw no change at all. If your doctor has already prescribed aspirin to lower your blood pressure, ask whether you would be better served by taking it at night.

➤ 3 Funky Formulas to Foil High Blood Pressure

Our unhealthy 21st-century lifestyle has contributed to the soaring rates of high blood pressure, but the condition itself has been plaguing mankind since the dawn of time. Long before the arrival of sophisticated medicines—or nutritional supplements—folks had their own highly effective ways of solving the problem. Here's a trio of the best:

1. Scrub and peel five potatoes, then simmer the skins in 2 cups of water for 20 minutes. Drink 1 cup of the strained brew twice a day.

2. Three times a day, drink a potion made from ½ teaspoon of cream of tartar mixed with ½ teaspoon of lemon juice in 8 ounces of water. For the sake of convenience, you can multiply the recipe and store it in the refrigerator for up to 48 hours.

3. Steep 6 tablespoons of dried raspberry leaves in 4 cups of just-boiled water for 40 minutes, then strain. Either drink the tea hot, put it in the fridge to chill, or pour it into ice cube molds and freeze. Raspberry leaves are available in health-food and herbal-supply stores, and online. You can also harvest wild or cultivated raspberry leaves in spring or midsummer. Dry them indoors, away from light, before using.

>>> AUTOIMMUNE DISEASES

The human immune system is programmed to detect any substance that does not belong in your body—and then to whip the daylights out of it. Unfortunately, on occasion, your inner army mistakes your own tissue for an invading substance and attacks it. The result is an autoimmune disease. They've always been around, and there is no single factor that causes them. Today, though, the condition has turned into a spiraling epidemic, which most experts pin on the steady stream of toxins coming at us from every direction. Fortunately, while you can't stop the onslaught entirely, you can erect an inner fortress that will say a loud, clear "Keep out!" to a whole lot of the hellions.

❯ Don't Push the Panic Button

Our century's colossal chemical overload is as a leading cause of not only autoimmune diseases, but also just about every other chronic condition under the sun, not to mention making us old before our time. But don't get obsessed with "de-toxing" or "green living" and force yourself to rid your home of every synthetic chemical and scrap of plastic. Fear, anxiety, and stress are every bit as toxic as most of the unnatural nuggets you're fretting about. You also don't have to sit back and pretend that everything's fine. Just use this two-point commonsense strategy:

- Give the cold shoulder to as much toxic stuff as you can.

- Stay—or get—in good shape, because a healthy body is better able to fend off any kind of trouble that comes its way, from the common cold to an autoimmune disease to any other chronic condition. Your best plan here is to follow the advice in "10 Steps to a Stronger Immune System" on page 116.

> " A bad habit never disappears miraculously; it's an undo-it-yourself project.
> —Abigail Van Buren (1918–2013) "

❯ The Internal Battle: The Major Players

Researchers have identified more than 100 different autoimmune diseases—and every one of them can make the years pile on long before their time. A full-scale discussion of all the various autoimmune diseases is way beyond the scope of this chapter. Coming up, we'll talk about two of the most prevalent: inflammatory bowel disease and psoriasis. In the meantime, here's an overview of other common types:

Celiac disease occurs when the immune system overreacts to gluten, a protein found in barley, rye, and wheat. The reaction damages tiny, hair-like projections called villi that line your small intestine and prevents them from performing their normal function: absorbing the nutrients from the food you eat. The only way to avoid having your vital organs deprived of nourishment is to follow a strict gluten-free diet.

Graves' disease results from hyperthyroidism—an overproduction of thyroid hormones. Left untreated, it can result in problems ranging from glaucoma to heart disease.

Lupus can affect many different parts of the body, including your blood cells, brain, heart, lungs, and joints. It's tricky to diagnose because most of its symptoms mimic those of other ailments. But there is one distinct sign that appears in many cases of lupus: a facial rash that resembles the wings of a butterfly unfolding across both cheeks.

Multiple sclerosis (MS) strikes when the immune system attacks your body's myelin, the protective coating that covers your nerves. The resulting damage causes disrupted communication between your brain and the rest of your body, and your nerves may ultimately deteriorate. The

Get to the Point–*Fast!*

When you see a doctor these days—for whatever reason—you're likely to have his or her ear for about three minutes, max. So don't waste time chatting about your golf game or your new grandchild. Instead, after a polite hello, jump right into your most urgent health concern. The sooner you bring up troubling issues, the more likely you are to get effective solutions.

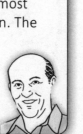

severity of MS varies greatly, depending on which nerves are affected and the degree of damage. Many victims enjoy long periods of remission between flare-ups. Skilled medical treatment is essential to help control the disease, manage symptoms, and speed up recovery from attacks.

Sjögren's syndrome (pronounced SHOW-grins) frequently accompanies other immune system disorders like lupus and rheumatoid arthritis. The initial targets are usually the glands that produce tears and saliva, so the first symptoms are likely to be dry eyes and a dry mouth. But the attack can include your skin, joints, kidneys, and other organs.

❯ 2 Terrible Types of IBD

Inflammatory bowel disease (IBD) occurs when your immune system mistakenly attacks your digestive tract. There are two major types:

1. Crohn's disease (CD) can affect any part of the gastrointestinal tract from the mouth to the anus, but most often it strikes the end of the small intestine (the ileum) and the beginning of the large intestine (the colon). The inflammation tends to appear in patches, with healthy bowel tissue in between.

2. Ulcerative colitis (UC) affects only the large intestine (which comprises the colon and the rectum). It appears as a continuous

MIND OVER MYTH

MYTH: Autoimmune disorders are all genetic in origin.

REALITY: Once upon a time, that was the common assumption in the medical community. And, yes, there is a genetic connection. But even if you have a family history of autoimmune disorders, it is not a slam dunk that one will befall you. Something in your environment must flick the switch to send your immune system into attack mode. Furthermore, the latest research indicates that more than 50 percent of autoimmune disorders have no genetic connection at all. The bottom line: By making wise dietary choices, reducing toxins in your body, and revving up your immune system, you stand a good chance of avoiding and (yes) possibly even reversing autoimmune diseases.

sheet of inflammation on the intestinal lining, generally beginning at the anus and reaching into the colon.

IBD does not limit its dirty work to your digestive tract. It can also cause a host of wide-ranging, youth-robbing problems such as arthritis, kidney stones, gallstones, inflammation of eyes or skin, and clubbing of your fingernails. What's even worse, over the long haul, it frequently results in osteoporosis and increases your risk for colon cancer.

❯ IBD vs. IBS: The Dramatic Difference

It's easy to assume that there is no difference between inflammatory bowel disease and irritable bowel syndrome (IBS), but there is. While IBS (a.k.a. spastic colon) can deliver agonizing symptoms, including abdominal pain, bloating, gas, and alternating bouts of constipation and diarrhea, it is not an actual disease—much less one that could threaten your life. Rather, IBS is a digestive problem with diagnosable, treatable causes. These are the most common:

The Easiest Toxin to Toss

Natural health gurus tell us that acid appears to trigger autoimmune disorders and the modern American diet (MAD) is chock-full of this toxin. Your simple acid-reduction plan:

- Cut back on such acidic edibles as processed foods, red meat, sugar, and other refined carbs, and watch your intake of alcohol and coffee.
- Up your intake of alkaline-rich fruits, vegetables, nuts, and seeds.

The healthiest pH balance is slightly on the alkaline side—just a shade above 7 on a scale of 1 to 14 (with 1 being completely acid and 14 being completely alkaline). If you want to see where your system ranks, pick up a supply of Hydrion® paper at your local drugstore, or order it on the Internet, then check your urine or saliva first thing in the morning, before you've had anything to eat or drink. The color of the paper will show your pH level. (Complete instructions and a color chart come with the paper.)

Tick-Tock
**TURN
BACK** the
CLOCK

- Bacterial, parasitic, or yeast (*Candida albicans*) infection

- Celiac disease

- Food allergies or sensitivities

- Underactive thyroid

Finally, according to both conventional and naturopathic doctors, it appears that (again unlike IBD) IBS can be—and very often is—caused by anxiety. So if intestinal cramps and spasms are getting you down, don't suffer silently. Get medical and, if necessary, psychological help ASAP! Coming up in Chapter 4, you'll find tons of DIY tips and tonics that'll help tame nervous tension.

❯ Psoriasis—the Painful Skin You're In

Psoriasis is a case of your immune system turning a simple bodily function into a speed demon. As we all learned back in high school biology class, our bodies are constantly growing new skin cells, and shedding the old ones. Normally, the process occurs in a smooth 28-day cycle, in which new cells gently shove the ones

above them to the surface of your skin, where they're sloughed off. But in people with psoriasis, the "assembly line" ramps up its production schedule to such an extent that cells begin to pile up, causing thick, red, scaly patches that are not only unsightly, but also itchy, and often excruciatingly painful. There is no cure, but trouble tends to occur in cycles, with flare-ups lasting for weeks or months, then going into remission for a time. One major difference between psoriasis and most other autoimmune disorders is that there are a myriad of effective ways

---

Centenarian SECRETS 100

Bathing in Dead Sea salt water is a slam-dunk way to heal psoriasis lesions, but it's not your only excellent option for soothing relief. Just pour any of these easy-to-come-by healers into a tub of warm water, and soak for 20 minutes or so. Repeat as often as needed to minimize your misery and feel better fast:

- ¼ cup of extra virgin olive oil mixed in 8 ounces of milk

- 2 to 4 cups of buttermilk

- 2 cups of raw, unfiltered apple cider vinegar

- 10 drops of either bergamot, cedarwood, or geranium oil

to help make those time-outs as long as possible, and to minimize the discomfort (see "Stop Psoriasis Dead in its Tracks," below).

❯ Stop Psoriasis Dead in its Tracks

Possibly the most potent psoriasis reliever of all is Dead Sea salt water. Scientific studies have shown that folks who took regular dips in the Dead Sea sent their excruciating scales packing within three to four weeks. If you can't jet off to Israel, just pick up some Dead Sea salt at an herbal-supply store, or order it online. Toss 2 pounds of the salt into a tub full of warm water. Soak for 20 minutes. Then rinse off, and wrap yourself up in a thick bathrobe or towel to intensify the healing power while you let your skin air-dry. Repeat the procedure three or four times a week, and your scales should soon hit the trail.

❯ Has Your Immune System Gone Haywire?

Once autoimmune diseases kick into high gear, their symptoms and the degree of danger involved can vary greatly. But in the early stages, they all tend to show similar warning signals. If you experience any of these symptoms—or, especially, a combination of them—see your doctor. And be quick about it. The sooner you get help, the more likely it is that you and your doc will be able to contain the collateral damage so you can stay young at heart—and body.

- Abdominal pain, diarrhea, or blood or mucus in your stool
- Blood clots or multiple miscarriages
- Constant tiredness or fatigue
- Dry eyes, mouth, or skin; hair loss
- Insomnia
- Intolerance to heat or cold
- Muscle tremors or rapid heartbeat
- Numbness or tingling in hands or feet
- Pain or weakness in joints or muscles
- Recurrent hives, rashes; sun sensitivity
- Trouble concentrating
- Unexplained weight gain or loss
- White patches or ulcers in your mouth

➤ 5 Sneaky Psoriasis Starters

While the underlying cause of psoriasis lies within your immune system, a number of factors can launch an attack or make symptoms worse when a flare-up is raging. Here's a handful of triggers to be aware of and avoid to the greatest extent possible:

1. Cold, dry weather. Conversely, sunny skies, hot temps, and high humidity appear to control psoriasis symptoms in many people.

2. Heavy alcohol consumption. Primarily men are affected; alcohol does not seem to cause problems for women. (I hasten to add, ladies, I am not implying that you should start hitting the bottle to nurse your sore skin!)

3. Infections, such as strep throat or tonsillitis. On the bright side, flare-ups often calm down once the infection has cleared up.

4. Various skin injuries, including cuts, bruises, bumps, burns, and bug bites.

5. Some medications used to control arthritis, heart disease, high blood pressure, malaria, and psychiatric conditions (in particular, lithium, a common treatment for bipolar disorder).

Rejuvenating Recipe
ALOE-BLUEBERRY SMOOTHIE

This delicious drink combines the potent healing power of aloe with the antioxidant-rich fruits to deliver a knockout punch to psoriasis woes.

- 1½ cups of fresh or frozen blueberries
- 1 large apple, peeled and chopped
- 1 medium banana, peeled
- 2 oz. of pure, food-grade aloe vera gel*
- 1 cup of water

Liquefy all of the ingredients in a blender, pour the potion into a glass, and drink to healthier skin!

* This is equivalent to 8 ounces of aloe vera juice. You can buy food-grade aloe vera gel online, as well as in herbal-supply stores and many supermarkets. Or, if you have an aloe vera plant, remove the spiky edges from a leaf, then slice it in half lengthwise and use a spoon to scrape out the gel. Repeat the process until you have about 4 tablespoons of gel.

10 Steps to a Stronger Immune System

A robust immune system is your best ally in fending off not only autoimmune diseases, but also both infectious diseases and chronic conditions of all kinds. It also ups your chances of making a complete and speedy recovery when you do fall sick with anything from a common cold to a strep throat, or even TB or hepatitis. Here's your 10-step to-do list (all backed up by extensive scientific research):

1. Stop smoking! Of all the ways to suppress your immune system, smoking tops the list. Just one everyday example: Smokers get the flu more often—and are more likely to die from it—than nonsmokers.

2. Lose weight! Carrying too many pounds is second only to smoking as the surest route to a shorter, sicker life.

3. Sleep tight. Too little, or poor-quality, sleep impairs overall immune system function and also reduces the number of specific germ-killing cells in your body.

4. De-stress. Chronic stress causes a measurable downturn in your system's ability to fight off or recover from diseases of all kinds.

5. Get happy. Even mild sadness can weaken your immune system, and the more negative and pessimistic you are, the more likely you are to get sick. On the other hand, cheerful, optimistic people have an army of infection-fighting T cells in their bodies.

6. Get a move on. Example: A recent four-month study compared people who took almost daily brisk walks with folks who were basically inactive. The result: The nonwalkers took twice as many sick days.

7. Pal around. The more human (and critter) connections you have, and the more you get out and about, the better you are at fighting off illnesses.

8. Eat well. The better nourished you are, the stronger your immune system will be. In particular, avoid refined sugar and polyunsaturated fats as much as possible because they are major immunity busters.

9. Yuck it up. Laughter decreases stress hormones and raises your supply of immune-boosting growth hormones and endorphins.

10. Limit antibiotics. While they are sometimes necessary, they can suppress your immune system and make you more likely to become sick again.

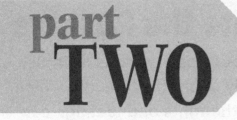

part TWO

$\mathscr{Live}$ SMARTER

What do I mean by "living smarter"? Simply this: By implementing a few savvy strategies, you can look and feel years—even decades—younger than your birth certificate says you are. In this section, you'll discover delicious superfoods and miraculous eating plans that can slow down, and even reverse, the aging process, in your mind as well as your body. You'll also learn tons of terrific tips for looking good from the top of your head to the tips of your toes, including remarkable anti-aging treatments for your skin, hair, and (yes) your wardrobe. And we'll start off in this chapter with what any healthy "old codger" (or codgerette) will tell you is the real key to longevity: maintaining a positive, upbeat attitude.

CHAPTER 4

Accentuate the Positive

Your brain and your body work as a single, intertwined, highly sophisticated unit, which means that your thoughts and feelings can literally make you sick and old before your time. On the other hand, if you play your cards right, your marvelous, miraculous mind can help you stay healthier, longer. In this chapter, you'll find tips, tricks, and tonics that'll help you get and stay happier, sack the seasonal blues known as SAD, and conquer two vile villains that can age you in a flash—namely, stress and anxiety. I'll also share effective, cutting-edge secrets for fending off the curses we all fear the most: Alzheimer's disease and other forms of dementia.

⟫⟫ THE MAGIC OF HAPPINESS

For decades, science has known that chronic unhappiness contributes to all forms of mental and physical illness. Now, medical research is finding that it's not simply the absence of negative emotions that helps keep us well. Happiness itself actually makes people stay healthier and live longer. Happy folks have stronger immune systems, which make them more resistant to ills ranging from life-threatening cardiac disease to the common cold. They handle stress better, and they're far less likely to suffer from anxiety or depression. What's more, they even have fewer accidents.

❯ Do You Need a Happiness Boost?

No one except a performer in an old MGM musical can possibly go around singing, dancing, and smiling *all* the time. But if you're constantly frowning, fretting, and complaining about everything from the potholes in the road to the papers in your in-box, the clouds in the sky, and the food on your plate, your grumpiness can't help but affect your health, your personal relationships—and, yes, your longevity. The good news is that, regardless of your age, you can lift yourself up by the bootstraps and hit the road to happiness. **Note:** *You might start the journey by popping your favorite comedy movie or TV sitcom into your DVD player or queuing up a funny video on YouTube.*

❯ Secrets of Happy People

Happiness cuts across all ages, occupations, geographic regions, and socioeconomic categories. But invariably, the folks who rank highest on happiness surveys and tests (including those conducted year after year by the famous Pew Research Center) share four common traits:

- They read newspapers (yes, actual printed newspapers!).

- They go to church regularly and are active in their congregations.

- They routinely socialize with family and friends (in person—not simply on Facebook or by e-mail).

- They accentuate the positive, habitually viewing their personal "glass" as half full rather than half empty.

❯ Go with the Flow

A great many happy, contented people have a major habit in common: They frequently flow. In psychological terms, "flow" is a state in which you're so focused on what you're

Centenarian SECRETS 100

The folks who keep such stats tell us that 1 in 26 baby boomers can expect to live to the century mark or beyond. And legions of their cohorts will reach their mid- to late 90s. So it's no wonder that every time you turn around there's another book, article, or survey exploring the lives of current centenarians. These folks come from all walks of life, they live all over the world, and they've pursued every career you can imagine, from goat herder to housewife and car mechanic to CEO. Well, guess what? Virtually across the board, when asked the most important factor in remaining youthful and living a long, productive life, the answer is the same: a positive, optimistic attitude.

MIND OVER MYTH

doing that you become one with the task. Nothing distracts you, and your emotions—whether anger, anxiety, fear, or sorrow—simply vanish. For many, running is a flow experience. For others, it may be bird-watching, painting a room, digging a garden bed, or working a jig-saw puzzle. Give it a try. Even if you're already as happy as a clam, flowing is a great way to get some deep-down relaxation after a long week at work or a traffic-clogged drive home!

> Turn Off the TV!

The same surveys that show what happy people do (see "Secrets of Happy People" on page 119) also name one thing they *don't* do—that is, watch very much television. Conversely, numerous scientific studies, including a recent one published in the *American Journal of Preventive Medicine*, reveal that the more time you spend in front of the boob tube—no matter what you are watching—the more depressed, anxious, and generally miserable you become. There is no guarantee that pulling your eyes away from the screen will lift your spirits, but given the fact that Americans spend almost 30 percent of their waking hours watching TV (an average of 142 hours a month), it can't hurt to give it a try!

> 4 Steps to Happiness

The first step to achieving real happiness is accepting the fact that no one else can make you happy. Only you can do it. Here's a primer to get you started on that DIY project.

1. Do the things you love—as often as you can. For example, throw dinner parties, plunk out your favorite tunes on the piano, putter in your garden, or simply chill out with a good book.

2. Hang around with happy people. Happiness is contagious. Seek out people who can "infect" you with their joyful outlook on life.

3. Have faith. And live it to the hilt, whether you practice the tenets of an organized religion or develop your own personal spirituality. Establishing a connection with the source of all creation can give you a deep sense of purpose, which is a hallmark of happy—and successful—people.

4. Laugh a lot. It releases torrents of feel-good brain chemicals that boost your spirits. Every day, make it a point to share jokes, watch a funny movie, read a funny story, or check out your favorite comic strips (in the newspaper or online).

❯ Money Can't Buy Happiness

We all know that (or should!). But it is true that certain kinds of expenditures can boost your mood more than others. To be specific, scientists have long known that spending money for a memorable experience, such as seeing a good show, taking a hot-air balloon ride, or going on a sightseeing tour, makes people happier—for much longer— than buying stuff like jewelry, cars, or a new lamp for the living room.

Researchers have discovered a sort of hybrid purchase that they've dubbed experiential, a.k.a. "to have in order to

Pleasant Aromas Make You Happy...

Or at least happier. In 17th-century Europe, soldiers used good-smelling spices to distract injured comrades from their pain. And, it still works. Only you don't have to be hurting to tap into the mood-boosting power of scent. Science has proven that pleasant smells lift your spirits—probably because they evoke subconscious memories of good times or favorite things. Conversely, unpleasant odors trigger feelings of unhappiness and disgust. The bottom line: Exposure to your favorite fragrances—whether it's cookies baking in the oven, a vase of red roses, or fresh-cut grass—is an easy trick sure to send your mood upward in no time.

do" products. Musical instruments, sporting gear, art supplies, and books all fall into this happiness-enhancing category. That's especially the case when they're helping you pursue a new second-prime venture like the ones we'll talk about in Chapter 9.

The bottom line: If you want to be happier—and younger—at any age, put your money where your passion is!

> " They say the seeds of what we will do are in all of us, but it has always seemed to me that in those who make jokes in life, the seeds are covered with better soil and with a higher grade of manure.
>
> —Ernest Hemingway (1899–1961) "

› Laughter Really *Is* the Best Medicine

No, laughing can't actually cure everything that might ail you. But data is mounting about the amazing things it can do for your physical as well as mental health—whether you're guffawing at Lucy and Ethel on a TV rerun or enjoying a quiet chuckle over a *Peanuts* comic strip.

In the short term:

• Laughing increases your intake of oxygen-rich air, which in turn stimulates your heart, lungs, and muscles, and also triggers your brain to release more health-enhancing endorphins.

• A hearty laugh stimulates your blood flow and relaxes your muscles. The result is that you feel good all over—fast!

For the long haul:

• Laughter boosts your immune system by releasing neuropeptides that fight stress and help fend off illnesses.

• It causes your body to produce its own natural painkillers.

• It helps lessen depression and anxiety—including the kinds people often experience in response to chronic illness.

• Laughing can shave years from your appearance. That's because the same revved-up blood flow that eases tense muscles also makes your skin more radiant and younger-looking.

❯ Shake for Joy

Believe it or not, a simple, firm handshake—whether it's with your best pal or a total stranger—can deliver a joyful jolt to your subconscious mind. That's because any friendly human touch activates the reward center in your central nervous system, automatically giving you a cheery lift. A quick hug, a pat on the back, or a kiss on the cheek can perform the same fabulous feat. And the more often you make physical contact with others, the happier you'll be.

❯ Boost Your Mood with Random Acts of Kindness

This idea was all the rage a few years ago, when bumper stickers, buttons, and posters urged us all to get out there and do nice things for strangers—for instance, put a quarter in an expired parking meter before a cop got there, pay a bridge toll for yourself and the car behind you, and so on. Well, guess what? It works just as well today as it did back then. Only now, the reason has been proven in scientific studies: Performing a kind act triggers your brain to release a joy-enhancing chemical called serotonin. But your good deeds don't have to be anonymous. Giving a gift, helping a neighbor, or simply offering someone a sincere compliment makes you *and* the recipient of your kindness happier. **Note:** *Recent studies have shown that anyone who even witnesses an act of kindness gets a jolt of serotonin. So there's no telling how far your simple gesture can ricochet!*

Forgive and Grow Younger

When hurtful or downright nasty things happen to happy people, they don't deny their hurt and anger. They feel it to the core—but then they find a way to release those emotions and feel compassion toward themselves and the perpetrator of the dirty deed. Don't get me wrong! Forgiving does not mean you condone or excuse the action in question. Nor is it easy. It takes time, honest reflection, and sincere effort. But it pays off in a big boost to your happy spirit and healthy body.

Tick-Tock
TURN BACK the CLOCK

❯ A No-Fail Formula for Nixing Negativity

Many moons ago, one of our most masterful songwriters, Johnny Mercer, offered up the surest route to a happy life when he advised us to "Accentuate the positive, eliminate the negative." Easier said than done, you say? Not necessarily. Simply follow this basic guideline: Never engage in a conversation that is neither pleasant nor productive. And how, you ask, can you pull *that* off without moving into a cave? Just use either of these two tactics:

Tactic #1: Let's say you're speaking with a neighbor who starts complaining about litter on the streets. Instead of joining in an "Ain't-it-awful?!" groan fest—or denying that a problem exists—take the comment as a call to action. Say something like, "Yes, it is mushrooming. Let's organize a neighborhood cleanup next weekend."

Tactic #2: In situations where nothing you say will steer the discussion in a more positive direction, glance at your watch and "remember" an urgent engagement elsewhere. Then hightail it outta there!

❯ Put on a Happy Face

Or, to put it another way, fake it till you make it. As showbiz pros have known since Will Shakespeare was a young lad—and behavioral scientists have confirmed—if you go around acting as if you're cheerful, positive, and joyful, before long you will be. So get out there and (as the old song goes) smile, darn ya, smile!

Centenarian SECRETS 100

Author Wilferd A. Peterson, who made it almost to the century mark (he died at age 95 in 1995), took the idea of gratitude to heart. He wrote about—and practiced—what he called "thanksliving." That means expressing thanks for good fortune with your actions, not merely with your words. For example:

- It is thanking God for all that has been done for you by doing things for others.

- It is thanking God for opportunities by accepting them as a challenge of achievement.

- It is thanking God for beauty by helping to make the world more beautiful.

- It is thanking God for health by the care you show your body.

> Numbers Talk...

And they tell us that happy folks live longer—and better, too. According to numerous scientific surveys:

- Happy people live 10 to 40 percent longer than less cheerful folks.

- Optimists have 19 percent longer life spans than pessimists.

- The risk for dementia is 30 percent higher in pessimists than in optimists.

> Just Say "Thanks!"

If you've spent your whole life gazing at clouds and ignoring silver linings—especially when you've reached a certain age—you're not likely to change that habit overnight. But there is one surefire way to get the ball rolling in a much more positive direction. What is it? Instead of fretting about what you *don't* have, be grateful for what you do have. Here's a foolproof four-part plan for cultivating an attitude of gratitude:

Count your blessings. Each evening, list (preferably in writing) five happenings from that day for which you're grateful. At first, it may take some stretching to fill your quota, but think back over the past 24 hours. Did you see a beautiful sunset or a patch of colorful flowers? Have a pleasant chat with a neighbor? Open your mailbox to find no bills inside? Or maybe, on the way to work, you had a fender bender that could have been a *whole* lot worse. You get the idea.

Say grace. Even if it's only a short, silent prayer when you're grabbing lunch on the run, giving thanks for abundant, healthy food is a powerful reminder of a blessing that most of us take for granted, except perhaps on Thanksgiving Day.

Your Fundamental Flax Fix

People who feel down in the dumps, for no apparent reason, often have low levels of essential fatty acids. One simple solution: Take 1 tablespoon of flaxseed oil once or twice a day until you feel chipper again. If you suffer from seasonal affective disorder, continue this R$_X$ right through the winter months (see "'Tis the Season to Be SAD" on page 149).

Send thank-you notes. And don't send them just to friends who've given you a gift or entertained you in their home. When people have helped or encouraged you in some way—even if they don't know it—write and mail them letters of gratitude. For example, maybe seeing an exhibition of a particular artist's paintings inspired you to take up the pastime. Your expression of thanks will benefit you as much as it pleases the recipient.

Express your appreciation—often. Make a point of saying a sincere "Thank you!" to everyone who gives you a compliment, does you a favor, or performs any service for you, even if it's part of his or her job. You'll feel good for acknowledging the kindness— and it just might make that person's day.

❯ 3 Nuts You Need

Feeling a bit blue? Then just say, "Nuts!" No matter what has you feeling down in the dumps, nuts can help. Best of all, nuts solve the problem at its root, rather than a prescription drug that only temporarily relieves your symptoms. These three types of nuts are all highly effective at beating the blues—and the only side effect you'll have will be better health!

1. Brazil nuts are one of Mother Nature's best sources of selenium, a mineral that is likely to be lacking in your system if you're feeling depressed, anxious, irritated, and tired for no apparent reason. (Studies show that most people today are deficient in selenium.) Simply eating three Brazil nuts a day will fulfill the recommended daily dose of this essential nutrient.

2. Cashews have been shown to work just as well as, if not better than, prescription antidepressants such as Prozac®. The secret lies in tryptophan, an amino acid that helps boost your mood, stabilize your thoughts, and produce a general mellow feeling. Just one large handful of cashews contains a whopping 1,000 to 2,000 milligrams of tryptophan. That will sure put the pep back in your step in no time!

3. Walnuts are high in serotonin, which can help to lift your spirits when you're suffering from seasonal affective disorder (SAD) or wallowing in a general funk. The easy fix: Enjoy a handful in your morning cereal or oatmeal, blended into an afternoon smoothie, or sprinkled over a scoop of your favorite ice cream. Just a few walnuts every day or so during your next blue phase will have you feeling better fast.

A MENTAL HEALTH FIRST-AID KIT

With this magical bath time mixture at your beck and call, you can use the power of aromatherapy to lift your sagging spirits, lower anxiety, reduce stress, or simply relax your racing mind. Start by mixing 1 cup each of Epsom salts, sea salt or kosher salt, and baking soda, and store the blend in an airtight container. To use it, add about 2 tablespoons of the mixture to your bathwater, along with a few drops of essential oil as the tub fills. As for which oil you want, here's the rundown:

Essential Oil	What It Does for You
Chamomile	Soothes and relaxes
Cinnamon	Energizes and stimulates
Geranium	Helps balance mind and body
Grapefruit	Lifts spirits
Lavender	Relaxes and rejuvenates; pairs well with chamomile in a nighttime bath
Peppermint	Cools you off and refreshes mind and body

▶ Avocados Get an A+ for Happiness

That's because they contain potent supplies of serotonin and tryptophan, two compounds that boost your brain's natural mood-lifting chemicals. So whenever you're feeling down, whether the cause is your monthly bout with PMS, a wintertime SAD attack, or a simple case of the blahs, avocados can cheer you up fast. So eat 'em up in whatever form you choose, whether it's sliced and added to a salad, blended into guacamole, or whipped up into the Tasty Avocado Spread (below). **Note:** *If you're battling prolonged depression, rather than just a short period of the gloomy-doomies, don't fuss with dietary or any other DIY remedies—get professional help pronto!*

▶ Hooray for Hugs!

Looking for a really simple way to make your spirits soar and stay young at heart? Then start giving bushels of big bear hugs to all your favorite people. The simple act of hugging, or being hugged by, someone close to you (or hugging a beloved pet) triggers the pituitary gland to release a hormone called oxytocin, a.k.a. the "cuddle chemical," which automatically elevates mood. Engaging in sex with your spouse also sends heaping happy helpings of oxytocin into the bloodstream. But wait—there's more! In addition to cheering you up, this heroic hormone also enhances the ability to handle stress, lessens addictive cravings for drugs and alcohol, and even reduces inflammation and speeds up wound healing.

Rejuvenating Recipe

TASTY AVOCADO SPREAD

You couldn't ask for a more delicious way to boost your mood and your health, too!

- **1 avocado, peeled and pitted**
- **2 tbsp. of chopped fresh basil***
- **2 tbsp. of lemon or lime juice**

In a medium bowl, mash the avocado, and stir in the basil and juice. Cover, and chill the mixture for an hour or so to blend the flavors. Then use it instead of your usual toppings on baked potatoes, sandwiches, bagels, or crackers.

* Or substitute your favorite herb or herb combos. Coriander, cumin, garlic, and red-pepper flakes all go well with the flavor of avocado.

Yield: *About ¾ cup*

❯ Cheer Up with Chocolate

No doubt you've read about the feats dark chocolate can perform for your physical health (we'll talk more about that in Chapter 5). Well, it can also be a boon to your mental health and well-being. Specifically, it spurs your brain to release feel-good endorphins and improves your cognitive function by increasing blood flow to your brain. The secret lies in compounds called polyphenols, and 1 ounce of dark chocolate contains almost as many polyphenols as a cup of green tea, and twice as many as a glass of red wine (two widely touted sources of the compounds). Just remember that the operative word is *dark*. So look for chocolate that consists of more than 70 percent cacao. Lighter milk chocolates don't cut the mustard when it comes to polyphenol content.

⋙ RELIEVING STRESS

What's that? You say your long work hours, traffic-clogged commute, a 24-hour stream of distressing news, and a mile-long to-do list have you climbing the walls? Welcome to the 21st century! Start finding ways to ease your stress load *now* because this inescapable bugaboo of modern life has been proven to cause or complicate just about every physical and mental health problem you can name, and contributes to premature aging!

❯ Is Stress Starting to Take Its Toll?

Stress overload can reveal itself in a myriad of ways that vary greatly from one individual to another. But if you're experiencing several of these symptoms, it's a good bet you're stressed to the gills and need to mend your ways—pronto!

- Change in appetite (either heightened or lowered)
- Inability to concentrate or make decisions
- Inability to cope with even minor setbacks

NERVE-CALMING COCKTAIL

After a long, hectic day, chill out with this delicious—and healthy—cocktail.

1 part carrot juice

1 part celery juice

1 shot of Grand Marnier® (optional)

Honey to taste

Ice

Mix the ingredients in a glass. Sit back, relax, and drink up!

Yield: *1 serving*

- Frequent headaches
- Digestive problems
- Dry heaves or vomiting
- Increased susceptibility to colds and flu
- Rapid breathing
- Sleeping problems
- Tingling in your hands and feet

❯ Stress Relief to Go

Anything from a testy business meeting to a long line at the supermarket checkout counter can send your stress level soaring. For that reason, it pays to pack an aromatic weapon known for delivering instant relief. To make it, simply saturate a cotton ball with an essential oil that can calm and relax your system, and stuff it into an empty pill bottle. Then tuck it into your pocket or purse and take it wherever you go. When stress strikes, open it and take a good, long whiff. All of these fragrances are renowned for their de-stressing prowess: basil, clary sage, lavender, neroli, and vanilla.

❯ Hot Tips for Stress Reduction

When you're all hot and bothered, cayenne pepper can help reduce tension and give you a pleasant jolt of energy to boot.

Drink ⅛ teaspoon of the pepper in 8 ounces of warm water once a day. Stick with that dosage until you've gotten used to its firepower, then increase the amount of pepper to ¼ teaspoon, then ½ teaspoon. Continue this "drinking habit" until you're feeling calmer.

Keep a glass of milk, a chunk of bread, or a scoop of ice cream, yogurt, or cottage cheese close at hand to dilute any burning feeling in your mouth and to help the pepper go down a little more smoothly.

Be aware that if you're not accustomed to eating spicy foods, drinking cayenne pepper in water will burn when you swallow it *and* when it comes out the other end. Over time, your body should adjust to the heat. Or you can minimize the discomfort by taking your cayenne in capsule form. It'll perform the same stress-busting magic, just a tad more slowly.

❯ 2 Wacky Wonder Workers

Whatever is pushing your stress buttons, these unlikely sounding helpers can calm you down in a hurry. What's more, they'll also lift your spirits and boost your energy at the same time.

1. Coconut oil. Dip a fingerful out of the jar, and massage it onto your forehead and temples using circular motions. The soothing aroma of the oil combined with the gentle pressure of your fingertips will have you feeling better in no time at all.

2. Eucalyptus oil. Simply mix 15 to 20 drops of eucalyptus oil per ounce of distilled water in a spray bottle, and mist yourself anytime you're feeling anxious, down, or stressed out.

❯ Looking for Stress Relief?

It's in your sock drawer! Mix up equal parts of dried lavender, dried rosemary, and broken cinnamon sticks, all of which have aromas that are highly effective at lowering anxiety levels. Stuff a handful or so of the mixture into a clean sock until you have a lump about the size of a baseball, and tie the top closed. Then anytime you feel on edge, repeatedly squeeze the ball to release a blast of calming scent. Keep this stress buster in your sock drawer to remind yourself to start every morning off on an easygoing foot!

> **66** If you ask me what is the single most important key to longevity, I would have to say it is avoiding worry, stress, and tension. And if you didn't ask me, I'd still have to say it.
>
> —George Burns (1896–1996) **99**

MIND OVER MYTH

MYTH: Folks who run marathons, climb mountains, or hit the golf links and tennis courts on a regular basis are cleaning stress clear out of their lives.

REALITY: While it's true that exercise is a top-tier de-stresser—and absolutely essential for good health—in some cases, it can actually raise stress to dangerously high levels. That's because, for many people, engaging in competitive sports or goal-oriented recreational pursuits activates their "inner cavemen," who, by necessity, viewed life as an ongoing battle in a hostile, winner-take-all world. When these folks lose a match or fall short of the performance standards they've set for themselves, the "defeat" causes frustration, raises their blood pressure, and produces all the other ill effects of stress.

❯ Fix It or Forget It

Whenever you find yourself in a spot that's sending you into a frenzy, ask yourself these four questions:

- Is this issue really important to me?
- Would a reasonable person be upset?
- Is there anything I can do to change the matter?
- Would the fix be worth the time, energy, and possible money it would cost?

If the answer to all four questions is "yes," then leap into action, whether that means challenging your boss about a major work issue, demanding that your teenager start keeping more regular hours, or telling your philandering spouse to shape up or ship out. On the other hand, if you responded "no" one or more times, ride out the situation.

❯ Teatime

If you prefer your de-stressing drinks on the warm side, this tasty blend is just the ticket: Place 1 tablespoon of apple cider vinegar and a chamomile tea bag into 1 cup of boiling water. Reduce the heat, and let it simmer for three or four minutes. Then remove the pan from the stove, pull out the tea bag, and pour the tea into a mug. When the brew has cooled to a comfortable temperature, nestle into a cozy chair, put your feet up, and sip your cares away.

❯ Soak Your Stress Away

Sipping a soothing tea isn't the only way to fight off health-damaging stress. Relaxing in a vinegar bath will also do wonders to soothe your spirits and calm your mind. There are many excellent tub-time formulas, but this is one of the simplest: Just pour 1 quart of either apple cider or white-wine vinegar into your bathwater. Stir in a handful of mint leaves, rose petals, or chamomile (either fresh or dried). Then step into the tub, settle back, and think lovely thoughts.

❯ Sock It to Stress

Here's another way to bathe stress and tension away: First, wrap a few chamomile tea bags in a panty hose leg or a piece of gauze, and cut an orange into thin slices. Suspend the tea pouch under your bathtub spigot, and let warm water flow over it. Float the orange slices in the water, climb into the tub, and soak your troubles away. **Note:** *Be sure to cover the drain opening with gauze or panty hose, so the slices don't clog your plumbing.*

❯ Forget Synthetic Nature

Americans sure love the great outdoors—at least judging from the healthy ratings for TV nature shows and filled houses for films like *March of the Penguins*. The problem is, although folks are spending more

---

Fountain of Youth
DE-STRESSING BATH BLEND

The next time you feel your stress level rising, take it sitting down—in a bathtub filled with this calming combo.

> **4 cups of dry whole-milk powder**
>
> **2 cups of cornstarch**
>
> **4 to 5 drops of your favorite essential oil***

Mix all of the ingredients together in a blender or food processor. When it's time to unwind, add ½ cup of the mixture to hot bathwater, sink into the tub, and relax. Store the remaining mixture in an airtight container at room temperature to use later.

* Geranium, jasmine, lavender, orange, and vanilla are all good stress-busting choices.

Yield: *About 12 baths' worth*

and more hours gazing at the natural world on movie and television screens, they're venturing outdoors less. Well, don't be one of that band! Here's why:

While spending time outside is a surefire stress reliever—and a boon to your physical health to boot—numerous studies have shown that watching the natural world parade across a screen does absolutely nothing to reduce stress.

Television viewing, regardless of the subject matter, is directly linked to elevated levels of stress, anxiety, and general unhappiness (not to mention increased risk for obesity, heart disease, and other deadly physical ills).

❯ Effortless Ways to Up Your Outdoor Time

You don't have to visit a nature preserve or take a hike in the woods to lower your stress level. Study after study has shown that simply spending time outdoors—anywhere, at any time, doing anything (or nothing)—will do the trick. You say that sounds nice, but your busy

---

There Is No Substitute for Mother Nature!

In a recent study at the University of Washington, researchers had volunteers perform mildly stressful tasks for 40 minutes in two *almost* identical office settings. The only difference: One had a window overlooking a pleasant grassy area with trees and a fountain. In the other work space, the window was fitted with a 50-inch plasma-screen HDTV showing the same bucolic scene.

The researchers recorded the subjects' heart rates before, during, and after each task. They also noted when each worker looked out the window, at the screen, or at a wall. The result: The folks who had the real deal to gaze upon recovered from their stress faster—and the more time they spent looking at the view, the more quickly their heart rates dropped to normal. Meanwhile, the pretty picture on the screen had no effect on anyone's stress level. Heart rates of volunteers in the TV room fell at the same, slower pace whether they looked at the screen or at a blank wall.

Tick-Tock
TURN BACK the **CLOCK**

schedule just doesn't allow it? Poppycock! Weather permitting, lots of things you do in your house or office every day can be done just as well on a deck, porch, patio, or park bench. Here's a handful of examples:

- Exercise or practice yoga.
- Eat meals or snacks.
- Pay bills, check e-mail, or cruise the Internet on your laptop.
- Read books, the newspaper, or work materials.
- Return calls on your cell phone.

> 4 Soothing Ways to Ditch Itchy Hives

If you break out in itchy red blotches during a period of anxiety or emotional turmoil, there's a good chance that stress is the culprit. So before you try any OTC antihistamines, treat yourself to one of these nerve-calming remedies:

1. Drink a few cups of chamomile tea every day. It just may make your spots disappear right before your very eyes.

2. Add ½ cup of baking soda to a tub of warm water, and settle in for a long, soothing soak.

3. Pour 2 cups of apple cider vinegar in a tub full of warm water, and soak your itch away. (Be sure to use raw unfiltered ACV!)

4. Before breakfast, mix 1 teaspoon of cream of tartar in an 8-ounce glass of water, and drink up. In no time flat, you should be itch-free. **Note:** *This trick works best if you use it as soon as the hives first appear.*

Centenarian SECRETS 100

For centuries, savvy folks have been using chamomile tea in a gazillion and one ways to soothe their stress and enhance their health— and you can, too. But no matter how you intend to use it, the basic recipe is the same: For each serving, pour 1 cup of freshly boiled water over 1 chamomile tea bag or 1 to 2 teaspoons of dried chamomile. Cover the pot or cup to keep the herb's volatile oils from dissipating, and steep for three to five minutes. Remove the tea bag, or strain out the herbs. Add honey or lemon if you like, and drink up.

Fountain of Youth

LEEK LINIMENT

When stress (or anything else, for that matter) has your joints or muscles aching, this lovely liniment will bring quick relief.

14 leeks, chopped

Water

4 tbsp. of coconut butter

Put the leeks in a pan with enough water to cover them by 2 inches, and boil them until they're mushy. Pour off the water, reduce heat to low, and add the coconut butter. Mix until creamy. Let it cool to a comfortable temperature, then massage into any sore, painful area(s). Store, tightly covered, at room temperature.

❯ I'm Just So Tired!

If you feel constantly fatigued, the reason may be constant stress—or, rather, the lactic acid that tends to build up in your system during periods of stress. If that's the case, this trick may help: At bedtime each night, take 3 teaspoons of apple cider vinegar mixed in ⅛ cup of honey. Continue the routine until you feel like your old bouncy self. **Note:** *If your get-up-and-go hasn't returned within a few weeks, call your doctor to rule out a more serious condition.*

❯ The Eyes Have It

If your eyes are sore, tired, or puffy, stress just might be the culprit. The good news is that the dynamic duo of apple cider vinegar and blackstrap molasses can put the pep back in your peepers. It works because ACV helps improve your blood circulation, and blackstrap molasses is a potent source of vitamin B_1, which is essential for good eye health. Take this medicine either internally or externally (use twice a day for best results):

Internally. Take 2 tablespoons of apple cider vinegar mixed with 1 tablespoon of blackstrap molasses. You can slurp it straight from a spoon, or spread it on toast, bagels, or English muffins.

Externally. Mix 2 teaspoons of ACV with 1 teaspoon of blackstrap molasses, spread it onto your puffy eyelids, and leave it on for five minutes. Then gently wipe it off with a moist cotton ball.

Note: *If your puffy eyes are accompanied by blurry vision, pain, or intense discomfort, call your doctor or see an optometrist ASAP.*

10 Wacky Ways to Cure a Headache

Stress and nervous tension account for the vast majority of headaches. And over the years, folks have come up with more headache remedies than you can shake an aspirin bottle at. Here's an assortment of the weirdest—and most effective:

1. Soak for 20 to 30 minutes in a steamy hot (but not burning!) bath while holding an ice pack on your head. The combination of heat and cold will ease your pain by drawing blood away from your head and narrowing the blood vessels in your scalp.

2. Tape a fresh mint leaf on the part of your head that hurts the most, and keep it there until you feel relief.

3. Stick your tongue out about ½ inch, and bite down on it as hard as possible without hurting yourself. Hold the position for exactly 10 minutes—no less and no more.

4. Soak a large white cloth in vinegar, wring it out, and tie it tightly around your head. Keep it in place until the pain is gone.

5. Slice a fresh lime in half, and rub a cut side on the site of the ache. The pain should vanish pronto.

6. Stand up straight with your arms hanging loosely at your sides. Then swing your arms back and forth in unison (not staggered). The motion will direct blood flow away from your head to your hands, thus easing the pain.

7. Quickly drink two glasses of Gatorade® or a similar sports drink, one after the other. You'll put your electrolytes back in balance and stop the throbbing in its tracks.

8. Stuff two tennis balls into a sock. Then lie on your back and wedge the sock behind your neck with one ball on each side. They'll relax your neck muscles, thereby chasing the pain-causing tension.

9. Hold a pencil in your mouth sideways, without biting down. Your jaw muscles will relax, relieving a common cause of tension headaches: strain on the muscles that connect your jaw to your temples.

10. Guzzle a glass or two of water. Dehydration is a leading cause of headaches. If that's what triggered your pain, it should vanish in a flash.

>>> AXING ANXIETY

Everyone feels tense, nervous, and fearful from time to time—perhaps when you're facing surgery or preparing for a cross-country move after decades in your family home. But if you have a constant sense of dread, panic every time the phone rings, or feel so tense that you often break out in a cold sweat, you've moved from everyday nervous tension to the hair-raising realm of anxiety. Left untreated, it can lead to depression and chronic stress, with all the potentially lethal health consequences. Chronic anxiety can also make you look years older than you really are.

> Worry or Anxiety? The Devil Is in the Details

Not sure whether you've got a genuine anxiety disorder, or you're simply as worried as all get-out? Here's how to tell for sure:

Worry is a natural response to any distressing situation, say, when your child has a serious illness, or your company is set to downsize and your job could be on the chopping block.

Anxiety, on the other hand, generally stems from what folks used to call "borrowed trouble." Anxious people are forever fretting about disasters that may never happen and imagining worst-case scenarios in all their detail.

Note: *Spending much time watching the 24-hour news channels can easily give you a first-class ticket to anxietyland.*

> " If you can keep your head when all about you are losing theirs, it's just possible you haven't grasped the situation.
>
> —Jean Kerr (1922–2003) "

> GAD Zooks!

Generalized anxiety disorder (GAD) is by far the most common type of anxiety. Fortunately, it is also the most responsive to the kind of gentle, natural treatments presented in this chapter—in conjunction with care from a doctor or natural health provider. Here are four clues that you've got GAD:

- You're constantly worried, impatient, irritable, and restless.
- You have difficulty sleeping.
- Your nonstop fretting is giving you physical woes, such as headaches, indigestion, and muscle pain or tightness.
- Your relationships are suffering, as your family and friends get fed up with your incessant bellyaching.

▶ Let Color Calm You

If you want to create an atmosphere —indoors or out—that will *really* set your mind and spirit at ease, keep these three rules of physics in mind:

Cool tones—the colors of water, such as blue, violet, mauve, and green —make you feel calm and relaxed.

Limited color palettes—especially white with one or two pastels— impart an air of peace and restfulness.

Bright, multicolored rooms that feature furniture and decor (or flowers) in a Joseph's-coat mixture of colors can send your stress and anxiety into overdrive, no matter how visually attractive the areas may be to you.

Fountain of Youth

INCREDIBLE COMFORT CREAM

This potent but gentle cream can safely send your anxiety level plummeting.

½ cup of wheat germ oil

1 oz. of beeswax

¼ cup of plain yogurt

Contents of four 400 IU vitamin E capsules

10 drops of juniper oil

Glass jar with tight-fitting lid

Heat the wheat germ oil and beeswax in the top of a double boiler until wax is melted but cool enough to touch. Mix the yogurt and vitamin E oil in a blender on "low." With the motor running, slowly pour in the warm wax and oil, and add the juniper oil. Blend until smooth, pour into the jar, and let it cool to room temperature. Store in the fridge for up to 30 days. Several times a day, rub the cream onto your hands. The juniper's calming properties will penetrate your skin, making you feel relaxed — and giving your skin a more youthful appearance!

4 Fundamentals for Fending Off Anxiety

Coming up, you'll find an arsenal of amazing anxiety-axing remedies that carry none of the adverse side effects that anti-anxiety meds deliver. But tapping into that bag of tricks won't get you very far unless you also heed your body's need for these four essentials:

1. Fresh air and exercise
2. Good, wholesome food
3. High-quality sleep
4. Plenty of pure, clean water

By paying attention to these bottom-line basics (as Mom always told you to do), you'll relieve anxiety at its root by reducing stress hormones in your body and raising levels of soothing brain chemicals like serotonin and gamma-aminobutyric acid (GABA).

MIND OVER MYTH

MYTH: Painting your walls yellow gives you a cheery environment in which to relax and cast off your anxiety and tension.

REALITY: According to color-psychology experts, the color yellow—even in its palest shades—actually activates the anxiety center of your brain. Numerous studies show that because of this nerve-irritating effect, infants cry more in yellow nurseries, couples fight more in yellow kitchens, and divas throw more temper tantrums in yellow dressing rooms.

Lovely Lavender Tea

Lavender tea is a time-honored remedy for easing anxiety, and for good reason—it works like a charm! Just sip two or three cups throughout the day as needed to calm your nerves. The basic formula is the same as it is for any other herbal tea: 1 to 2 teaspoons of fresh or dried flowers (or more for a stronger brew) per cup of just-boiled water, with honey and lemon added to taste. But in this case, do yourself a labor-saving favor and make a batch of brew by the quart ahead of time. Then put it into the fridge, where it'll keep for three days, or freeze it in ice cube trays or plastic cups. When teatime rolls around, your potion will work the same magic, whether you warm it up, drink it cold, or eat it like an ice pop.

Don't let this or any other herbal tea sit at room temperature for any length of time. Within a few hours, it'll start to go sour.

❯ Foolproof Fixes

Anxiety relievers don't come any easier, or safer, than this terrific trio:

Pinch your fingers. Grab a handful of clip-type clothespins. Attach one to each fingertip on your left hand, so that they're pressing down on your nails, and leave them in place for seven minutes. Then repeat the process on your right hand. The pressure exerted on the nerve endings will relax your whole nervous system. Perform this routine as needed, first thing in the morning, and before, during, or immediately after a tense situation.

Serve yourself some seaweed. Kombu (available in health-food stores and Asian markets) is a type of seaweed with a remarkable ability to calm tense nerves. All you need to do is put a 3-inch strip of the stuff in a quart of water, boil it for 10 minutes, and then strain into a heat-safe container. Drink ½ cup of the tea at a time, either warmed up or at room temperature, throughout the day.

Take a stroll on a beach. If that's not possible, just turn on a sink faucet in your kitchen or bathroom. Or, install a simple fountain on your deck or in your living room. Study after study has shown that listening to the sound of waves or running water almost magically reduces anxiety and stress.

Rejuvenating Recipe

ANTI-ANXIETY NIGHTCAP

If you're battling chronic anxiety, or your stress level is soaring toward the sky, this relaxing, delicious beverage can help calm you down.

¾ cup of whole milk
¼ cup of plain almond milk
1 pinch of ground ginger
1 pinch of nutmeg

Mix the whole milk and almond milk in a saucepan, and heat until warm. Stir in the ginger and nutmeg, pour into a mug, and drink just before you go to bed. It'll help you sleep soundly and wake up ready to face the day on a more even keel.

Yield: *1 serving*

❯ Onions Tame Tension

As bizarre as it sounds, this simple topical treatment is an effective way to eliminate nervous anxiety: Grate a large raw onion, and divide the gratings between two pieces of gauze or cheesecloth about 12 inches square. Fold the sides over to form pouches. Then sit back in a chair, prop your legs up, and place a poultice on each calf. Relax for 30 minutes or so, and feel your tension drain away.

❯ Fish for Anxiety Relief

Did you know that watching fish swim around in a home aquarium is every bit as effective as biofeedback and meditation are for easing anxiety and lowering blood pressure? It's true—according to researchers at the University of Pennsylvania's Center for the Interaction of Animals & Society. So what are you waiting for? Put a few goldfish or guppies in a tank, pull up an easy chair, and feel your jitters float away!

❯ Be Prepared to Calm Down

Dreading an upcoming visit to the dentist? Or maybe your annual performance review at work? Well, getting all hot and bothered won't help you avoid the experience. But with this simple trick you'll be able to face it in a calmer mood. The morning of the big day, get up a little earlier than usual so you can mix ⅓ cup of baking soda and ⅓ cup of ground ginger in a tub of warm water and soak in it for 15 minutes or so. Your anxiety level will plummet.

Centenarian SECRETS 100

There's no doubt about it: Chronic anxiety can age you fast, in health and appearance. But if you're a regular listener to talk radio—regardless of the subject matter—you have an ultra-simple way to ease your inner turbulence. What is it? Turn off the chatter, and either put on a Mozart CD or turn the dial to a classical music station. Studies show that 30 minutes of classical music can be as calming as 10 milligrams of Valium. Of course, how often you should perform this trade-off and for how long depends on the severity of your anxiety. So experiment until you find the R_X that works for you.

▶▶ DON'T LOSE YOUR MIND

As medical science finds more and more ways to prolong our lives, for nearly all of us, one fear looms ever larger: that our minds will flicker and die long before our physical bodies give out. The good news is, there are things you can do to help ensure that your brain stays active and alert your whole life long.

▶ 4 Secrets to Sidestepping Dementia

Your daily lifestyle can go a long way toward keeping you mentally fit as you enter your senior years. These four factors hold the key to your success:

1. Mental workouts. Stimulate your brain every day by reading, playing word games, engaging in crafts or hobbies, and doing puzzles—especially crosswords. Recent studies show that working crossword puzzles at least four days a week cuts your dementia risk by 47 percent.

2. Physical exercise. Moving your body—even if it's just a stroll around the block—helps keep blood flowing to your brain and encourages the formation of new brain cells.

3. Social engagement. People who remain actively connected with friends, family, and colleagues are less likely to succumb to dementia than those who avoid social gatherings or confine their interactions to e-mail or social networking sites.

4. Weight control. Obesity in middle age doubles the odds that you'll develop dementia in later life, so lose those extra pounds as soon as possible.

> " Life loves to be taken by the lapels and told, 'I'm with you, kid. Let's go.'
> —Maya Angelou (1928–2014) "

Trip the Light Fantastic

A recent study published in *The New England Journal of Medicine* found that regular ballroom dancing—the kind requiring you to move in sync with a partner—can reduce your risk for dementia by 76 percent. Such a success rate is greater than that of any other activity studied. So haul out your dancing shoes and cut a rug!

Tick-Tock **TURN BACK** the **CLOCK**

❯ Signs That You Need to See Your Doctor

It's one thing to forget where you put your keys. But when you look at a bunch of keys and think, "What are these things?" it's time for a thorough medical checkup. Also see a doc in any of these instances:

- You have trouble performing the steps of a familiar task, such as making a pot of coffee.

- You suddenly can't remember where you are or what month it is.

- You've forgotten the names of close friends or family members.

❯ Major Misunderstandings about Alzheimer's

Misunderstanding #1: Dementia equals Alzheimer's disease.

The highly hopeful truth: Many factors can cause the severe memory loss, confusion, and chronic disorientation that are commonly identified as AD. Furthermore, it is impossible to make a definitive diagnosis of AD in a living person. Only a postmortem biopsy of the brain can detect the clumps and tangled strands of protein (amyloid and tau in medical lingo) that are the slam-dunk indicators of Alzheimer's.

Misunderstanding #2: If you do have AD, you're in for an unavoidable downhill slide.

The highly hopeful truth: Medical science has found many people who have retained their full, or nearly full, intellectual capacities well into old age—even, in some cases, close to the century mark. Only when these "escapees," as researchers term them, finally died of causes unrelated to their minds did autopsies show that their brains were in fact riddled with the unmistakable clumps and tangles of Alzheimer's.

➤ 3 Spicy Ways to Boost Your Brainpower

Numerous studies indicate that inhaling the aroma of cinnamon in any form can enhance your overall brain function and improve both your long- and short-term memory. So what are you waiting for? Try one—or all—of these terrific tricks:

1. Bake a batch of spicy cinnamon cookies (see the Brain-Boosting Cookies recipe, at right), or whip up any other recipe that has cinnamon listed as a main ingredient.

2. Toss broken cinnamon sticks into your favorite potpourri.

3. Dab a spot of cinnamon extract onto a few lightbulbs around your house. (Just make sure the bulbs are turned off and completely cool to the touch before you anoint them!)

Note: *As a bonus, the scent of cinnamon also makes you feel calmer and more relaxed.*

Rejuvenating Recipe
BRAIN-BOOSTING COOKIES

The intense cinnamon aroma of these taste-tempting treats delivers major aromatherapy that will lower your anxiety and ramp up your brainpower —besides offering up ample supplies of cinnamon's other health-giving benefits.

2 sticks of butter, softened

2¼ tsp. of ground cinnamon

½ tsp. of baking soda

½ tsp. of sea salt

1 cup of blackstrap molasses

¼ cup of brown sugar

¼ cup of dark honey

2 large eggs

½ cup of plain yogurt

4 cups of all-purpose flour

Combine the first four ingredients. Gradually add molasses, sugar, and honey. Then beat in the eggs, and stir in the yogurt and the flour. Drop rounded teaspoonfuls of dough 2 inches apart onto cookie sheets, and bake at 400°F for 12 minutes, or until lightly browned at the edges. Let cool, then enjoy!

Yield: *About 4 dozen cookies*

Losing Pounds Leads to Clearer Thinking

The mere fact of being fat fouls up the wiring in your brain that enables you to think clearly—at least according to recent research conducted at Ohio's Kent State University. To be specific, scientists found that after their obese patients underwent weight-reduction surgery, their cognitive functioning improved within just a few weeks. **Note:** *This is not to suggest that you should even consider going under the knife unless your doctor strongly advises it! There are plenty of safer, albeit slower, ways to drop your brain-fogging fat—and you'll learn about a whole lot of them coming up in Chapter 5.*

❯ Think Twice about HRT

If you're a woman heading toward menopause, you might be thinking about—or maybe already are—taking hormone-replacement therapy (HRT) as a means to keep your mind sharp. Well, I have two words of advice: Forget it! Numerous studies have found no difference in memory function between postmenopausal women who did use HRT and those who did not. **Note:** *If you're feeling mentally muddled, perhaps all those hot flashes that wake you up at night are making you too tired to think completely straight.*

❯ 2 Strategies to Corral Your Wandering Mind

As you well know if you're of a certain age, there comes a time when it's all too easy to get on a path to distraction and forgetfulness. This duo of tricks can help you stay on task (as the efficiency gurus like to say):

- Whenever you're tackling a long project, keep your mind focused by taking a five-minute break every 30 minutes.

- Never try to do several things at once. Instead, make it a point to finish one task before you start another. It works like a charm!

❯ Walking Works Wonders

A study found that people who walk regularly may be 73 percent less likely to develop dementia than people who don't. And here's even better news: You don't have to chisel a significant block of time out of your day for an extended jaunt. In fact, another study has found that taking four 10-minute walks spaced throughout the day can result in even greater control over your blood pressure than pounding a treadmill for 40 minutes—and healthy blood pressure lowers your risk of dementia.

❯ Food for Thought

Brain-derived neurotrophic factor (BDNF) is a protein that has the ability to build cells and produce new connections—especially in the areas regulating mood, memory, and cognitive skills (see "Please Pass the BDNF?!" on page 148). One key secret to fill up your mental "tank" with BDNF is to eat a diet that's low in processed foods, high in natural chow, and rich in these nutritional superstars:

Curcumin: Found in turmeric and (to a lesser extent) in curry powder

Folate: Found in asparagus, avocados, beans, broccoli, dark leafy greens (including spinach), and oranges

Omega-3 fatty acids: Found in Brussels sprouts, eggs, kale, milk, oily fish, peanut butter, pumpkin seeds, spinach, walnuts, and yogurt

Resveratrol: Found in cocoa, grape juice, peanuts, red grapes, red wine, and some berries such as blueberries, bilberries, and cranberries

Vitamin B$_{12}$: Found in beef, eggs, fish, dairy products, and poultry

---

Rejuvenating Recipe

SALMON AND TOMATOES

Ramp up your youth-enhancing supply of BDNF with this easy and tasty fix.

- 4 skinned 6-oz. salmon fillets
- 4 medium tomatoes, halved
- 2 tbsp. of extra virgin olive oil
- Sea or kosher salt and black pepper to taste
- ½ tsp. of paprika
- 8 sprigs of fresh thyme
- 4 garlic cloves, sliced

Put the salmon and tomatoes, cut side up, in a broiler-proof roasting pan or on a rimmed baking sheet. Drizzle on the oil, and season with the salt and pepper. Sprinkle the paprika on the salmon, then scatter the thyme and garlic over the fish and tomatoes. Broil until the salmon is opaque all the way through and the tomatoes are tender (8 to 10 minutes).

Yield: *4 servings*

Please Pass the BDNF?!

When you increase your BDNF level, you're primed for good moods, clear thinking, and learning new things, no matter how old you are. Here's how to produce more of this mental "Miracle-Gro®":

Move! A lifelong habit of physical activity is the very best way to boost your BDNF levels. See Chapter 7 for a variety of ways to easily get moving.

Don't get MAD. At least not often. The modern American diet (MAD), which is high in refined sugar, bad fats, and high-fructose corn syrup, greatly reduces BDNF levels. Conversely, eating a healthy diet sends those critical numbers upward (see "Food for Thought" on page 147 for a few foods that are especially helpful).

Fast on occasion. I'm not suggesting that you consider going for days— or even a whole day—without food. Rather, letting your digestive system rest periodically for as little as 12 hours triggers a tsunami of hormonal events that kick your body's repair mechanisms into high gear. It can be as simple as skipping your bedtime snack.

Use your head! As you might expect, if you want to up your supply of a substance that's brain-derived, mental stimulation is a must. And it doesn't have to be a bore to work your brain! Reading a magazine or playing a game of chess is an excellent way to give your mind a much-needed boost.

Hang out with your nearest and dearest. Spending quality time with close friends and family members is one of the best—and most pleasant— ways to boost your BDNF score.

Soak up some sun. Even just a few minutes at a time can work magic on your mind and body. (Of course, this does not mean that you should lie, baking, in the sun for hours on end!)

Reduce stress. In addition to all its other evil deeds, it cuts your BDNF production—which may be why people who are stressed out generally don't think at their peak of clarity. (See "Relieving Stress," starting on page 129, for some suggestions on how to stay calm.)

Hit the sack. And stay there for at least seven hours each night. Too-little shut-eye ranks right up there with stress as a prime robber of BDNF.

►► 'TIS THE SEASON TO BE SAD

No one is quite sure why some folks are troubled by seasonal affective disorder (SAD) while others are not, but we do know what triggers it: The absence of light during winter's gray days and long nights causes the pineal gland to turn the hormone serotonin into melatonin. And the lack of serotonin makes the chilly months miserable. And coming to dread a full quarter (or more) of every year can age you in a hurry. The good news is that if you face the problem square on, you can squelch SAD symptoms and discover— or rediscover—the joys of winter.

❯ Sinister Signals of SAD

For many folks, SAD (a.k.a. winter depression) is far more serious than a simple case of cold-weather blahs. Like any other type of depression, it can affect your whole life and well-being—and therefore decrease the likelihood that you'll live to a ripe old age. Symptoms vary greatly in their intensity from one person to another, but these are the most common signs that SAD has struck:

- Craving for sweets and starches

- Depression

- Intense desire to hibernate

- Permanent jet-lagged feeling

- Sleep disturbances

> " If the world was perfect, it wouldn't be.
> —Yogi Berra
> (1925–2015) "

Note: *If your SAD symptoms are so severe that they're hindering your ability to function through the winter, don't rely on home remedies alone. Ask your doctor to refer you to a psychiatrist or psychologist who can evaluate your condition and recommend medication if it's necessary.*

❯ Here Comes the Sun!

Even many folks who don't suffer from SAD find it hard to wake up on dark winter mornings. The simple solution: Get what's called a dawn simulator (available in catalogs and online). Essentially it's a lamp whose glow increases gradually from dim to more intense light, mimicking a natural sunrise in mid-May. All you do is program the show to begin one to three hours before wake-up time, and your body detects the increasing light through your closed eyelids. **Note:** *At any time of the year, this gentle wake-up call can be a lot more pleasant than a buzzing alarm clock.*

❯ 3 Simple SAD Solutions

A trio of the most effective ways to ease your SAD woes are also the easiest—namely these:

1. Flee your cave. Force yourself to get outdoors for part of every day, regardless of the weather. Exposure to the sun's rays, even on dim, overcast days, ups your levels of vitamin D, which in turn increases your serotonin supply. Factoid: Even during the darkest downpour, there is 30 times more light outdoors than indoors.

2. Tipple some tea. Whenever you feel a craving for carbohydrates, sip a cup of chamomile tea. It'll divert your attention from food and give you a much-needed energy boost at the same time.

3. Tipple some more tea. To curb your overall appetite—and, therefore, avoid packing on pounds—buy a bottle of fennel

Order a Blues-Beating BLT

No, not the sandwich. In this case, BLT is a remarkably simple, yet highly effective, treatment called broad-spectrum light therapy. All you do is sit in front of a desktop light box equipped with special high-intensity bulbs for a certain period of time each day. The usual Rx is 30 minutes every morning. The timing and length of exposure are highly individual though, so ask your doctor for guidance.

Tick-Tock
TURN BACK the **CLOCK**

essential oil at a health-food store or online. Then, before each meal, add 2 drops of the oil to a cup of warm water, and drink up.

❯ Feeling Blue? Think Orange!

Orange essential oil has an almost magical knack for lifting low spirits. Here's a sampling of ways you can put it to work for you:

Add a few drops of the oil to your favorite hand and body lotions.

Dab the oil onto a few lightbulbs around your house. (Make sure the bulbs are turned off and cool to the touch!)

Fill a spray bottle with water and a few drops of orange oil, and spritz the air in your home or office.

Mix a few drops of orange oil with your dishwashing liquid and household cleansers.

Note: *Whatever you do, never use any type of essential oil directly on your skin. It can be very irritating.*

❯ Follow Every Rainbow...

Right into your house. How? Simply buy as many full-spectrum lightbulbs as your budget allows, and install them in lamps and ceiling fixtures throughout your house. Because they include every color of the rainbow, these bulbs are much more like natural daylight than their ordinary counterparts are, and they'll give a big lift to your home's indoor mood.

Fountain of Youth

REKINDLE YOUR FIRE BATH

Even in its mildest forms, SAD (like any other type of depression) robs your body of essential electrolytes and makes you feel old before your time. So recharge those energizers—and soothe your spirit at the same time—with this tub-time mixer.

2 cups of Epsom salts

2 cups of sea salt

2 tbsp. of potassium

1 tbsp. of vitamin C crystals

Pour all of the ingredients into the tub while the water is running (at a temperature of your choice). Then ease yourself in and soak your troubles away for as long as you like.

MIND OVER MYTH

MYTH: SAD strikes only during the cold, gray months.

REALITY: While it is true that the vast majority of SAD attacks occur in the winter, a small number of people fall into a similar funk during the summer. Mental health pros reckon it's triggered by high heat or humidity. Unfortunately, normal air-conditioning does not generally provide relief. Summer SAD sufferers are stuck with fleeing to a cooler climate, taking antidepressants, or slogging through the heat as best they can.

In another rare variation on the theme, some folks plunge into seasonal depression in both summer and winter, while feeling just fine during the milder days of spring and fall.

> Move It and Lose It

Move your body, that is—and lose the dark clouds hanging over your head. If you're not up to joining winter sports lovers on the slopes or frozen ponds, or even taking brisk walks around your neighborhood, head for an indoor skating rink, bowling lanes, or the warmth and light of your local fitness center. Getting 30 minutes of exercise each day, in whatever form you like, will keep your system pumping out endorphins that will help you battle the blahs of a long, cold, dark winter. Just be sure to begin your exercise routine while the weather is still mild, so you have habit on your side when the gloomy-doomy season sets in.

> Plan to Fight Your Funk

When you don't have a compelling need to be out and about—showing up at work, for example—it's all too easy to hunker down under a cozy blanket and stay there all day. Well, don't do it! It'll only make the situation worse. Instead, before any chilly winds begin to blow, plan a passel of pleasant things that'll get you out of the house. If at all possible, take your annual vacation in the winter, and head straight for the sun. But don't stop at that. Make firm commitments with family and friends to attend plays or concerts, go on day or weekend trips, or throw birthday or holiday parties. In short, the more fun times you have to look forward to, the easier it will be to breeze through the blue days.

CHAPTER 5

Eat to Beat Aging

As the old adage says, you are what you eat. Well, you're also what you don't eat. Unfortunately, these days, what a whole lot of folks are eating—and failing to eat— is making them tired, sick, fat, unhappy, and old before their time. The good news is that it's never too late to clean up your act. It's a lot easier and more pleasant than you might think—and you'll grow younger with every delicious mouthful! This chapter will help you do just that.

⋙ NUTRITION IN A NUTSHELL

It's no secret that in order to stay at your peak of health and vitality at any age, you need to make sure you're getting all the nutrients your body needs. But nutritious food is especially important when you're aiming to slow down, or even reverse, the aging process. Fortunately, it doesn't take a degree in nutrition science to build yourself a better diet. All it takes is a basic understanding of what makes your system tick.

The Big 3 Nutrients

These are the key elements that power your body's engine:

Macronutrients come in three different types: protein, fats, and carbohydrates. These are the nutrients you need the most of because they provide energy; promote growth, development, and tissue repair; and regulate your bodily functions.

Micronutrients are the vitamins and minerals from A to zinc. If you don't get enough of them, you can land in *big*

> **"** Wisdom doesn't automatically come with old age. Nothing does, except wrinkles. It's true, some wines improve with age. But only if the grapes were good in the first place.
>
> —Abigail Van Buren (1918–2013) **"**

trouble because these hard workers coordinate and fine-tune the performance of *all* of your body's internal systems.

Phytonutrients (a.k.a. phytochemicals) are not vital for maintaining life itself, but they are essential for keeping you in tip-top shape (see "Fantastic Feats of Phytonutrients," below). What's more, a deficiency of these supporting players can cause significant weight gain and major difficulty shedding the extra pounds. The best known of this bunch are in fruits and vegetables (like the beta-carotene in carrots and sweet potatoes), but equally valuable are those that are found in herbs and spices, whole grains, beans, and nuts.

> Fantastic Feats of Phytonutrients

In Mother Nature's scheme of things, the mission of phytonutrients is guarding plants against diseases. And those power-packed chemicals can do the same thing for you. That's why it's important to include a variety of fruits, vegetables, and herbs in your diet. Here's a fistful of deeds this fix-it team can perform:

- Boost your body's ability to repair damaged cells and expel waste products and toxic compounds

- Enhance your immune system, thereby shoring up your defenses against illnesses of all kinds

- Fight off free radicals and reduce the oxidation that causes Alzheimer's and other degenerative diseases

- Help prevent damage from such cancer-causing agents as UV rays, secondhand smoke, and environmental pollutants

- Reduce inflammation throughout your body

❯ 4 Reasons to Get Enough Vitamins

A serious lack of certain vitamins can result in some gruesome diseases, the most infamous being beriberi (vitamin B_1, a.k.a. thiamine), pellagra (vitamin B_3, a.k.a niacin), rickets (vitamin D), and scurvy (vitamin C). Fortunately, those horrors are all but extinct in the United States and other developed countries, but less severe underdoses of vitamins can—and routinely do—cause trouble for hordes of Americans who could easily mend their ways. Just consider these four sobering examples:

1. A low intake of vitamin A can lead to intestinal and lung infections.

2. Too little vitamin B_2 (a.k.a. riboflavin) can cause a multitude of woes, ranging from digestive problems to slowed mental processes, dizzy spells, insomnia, cataracts, skin rashes, and hair loss.

3. A diet that's low in vitamin C has been found to increase your likelihood of developing high blood pressure, diabetes, heart disease, and certain forms of cancer, as well as memory loss, urinary tract infections, and muscle soreness after exercise—and that's just for starters. Yikes!

4. A shortage of vitamin D can contribute directly to bone diseases, hypertension, and certain forms of cancer.

Tap Into the Magic of Magnesium

Magnesium is essential for maintaining such crucial bodily functions as muscle control, tissue healing, the elimination of harmful toxins, and the processes that control your heart and circulatory system. Most of us don't get enough magnesium in our daily diets, and supplements could give you a toxic overdose. What to do? Three times a week, pour 2 cups of Epsom salts into a tub of warm water, and soak for 20 minutes. If you like, add ½ cup of your favorite bath oil. But don't use soap of any kind—it'll interfere with the action of the salts. Besides improving your blood circulation, lowering your stress level, and relieving general aches and pains, this powerful soak can help alleviate major and minor health conditions, including arthritis, bruises, gout, hives, kidney stones, and sciatica.

MYTH: Going on a fat-free diet is a fast, healthy way to slim down.

REALITY: Fast—maybe. Healthy—not by a long shot. In fact, eating a fat-free diet for any length of time will actually kill you. That's because you'd deprive yourself of the four vitamins necessary for life. Although vitamin C and the entire B group are soluble in water, your system cannot absorb and use vitamins A, D, E, and K without the presence of dietary fat. And if those micronutrients can't do their jobs, your days are numbered. If that statement sounds extreme, consider these biological facts: Both your immune system and eyesight depend upon a steady supply of vitamin A. Vitamin D works with calcium and other minerals to build and maintain bones. Vitamin K makes blood clot as it should (thereby preventing you from hemorrhaging to death), and vitamin E is a key player in limiting the formation of free radicals that wreak havoc on every cell in your body.

❯ Mighty Minerals Demystified

Medical science has identified 28 minerals that perform specific, essential functions in your body and 12 others that are just as crucial to our health but whose roles are not yet fully understood. As you might expect, there are hundreds of mineral supplements for sale, and like most folks, you are probably confused about what, if any, are necessary for your diet. So let's set the record straight.

Misconception #1: Minerals are solo performers.

Fact: While it is true that, for instance, calcium builds strong bones and iron gives you strong blood, neither one does its job alone. In reality, minerals team up with vitamins, enzymes, and other minerals to perform these and other highly complex processes.

Misconception #2: If you show signs of a deficiency, all you need to do is pump more of the lacking mineral into your body.

Fact: A short supply of any mineral is rarely the only cause of any condition exhibited by your body. In fact, very often, you may have plenty of the needed mineral, but your system can't use it effectively because one of its essential teammates is AWOL.

Misconception #3: You should always take the standard recommended daily allowance (RDA) of every mineral.

Fact: Individual mineral requirements vary tremendously, depending on scads of factors, including your age, sex, size, metabolism, health condition, activity level, and (yes) even your personality, the type of work you do, and the climate you live in.

Misconception #4: To correct a mineral deficiency, you need to take one or more supplements.

Fact: Sometimes, yes, depending on the nature and severity of the problem, you may need a supplemental boost, at least temporarily. But in many, if not most, cases, eating more of the right foods will do the trick just fine.

› Beware of Overdosing!

Getting too much of just about any vitamin or mineral is likely to cause bothersome side effects such as stomach pain, nausea, skin rashes, vomiting, and diarrhea. But in some cases, taking too big a dose for a prolonged period of time can have even worse consequences. Here are five worst-case scenarios a supplemental megadose can cause:

- An excess of vitamin A raises the risk for osteoporosis and hip fracture in postmenopausal women, and it may increase your chances of death from all serious health conditions.

- Massive amounts of magnesium can lead to extremely low blood pressure and ultimately to cardiac arrest and death.

Centenarian SECRETS 100

If you've had a stroke or know someone who has, this news will be music to your ears: The journal *Nutritional Neuroscience* reported the results of a study involving 26 volunteers who had recently suffered a stroke. Half of the folks were given 20 milligrams of zinc each day for a month, while the rest took no supplements. At the end of 30 days, the zinc-takers had a 30 percent greater recovery in brain function than those who had not taken the mineral. And here's even better news: You don't have to take zinc supplements to get your brain-boosting quota. You can easily get 20 milligrams or more simply by eating plenty of zinc-rich foods, such as plain yogurt, lean meat, oysters, crab, lentils, and the dark meat of turkey and chicken.

- Overdoing it with vitamin E may trigger hemorrhaging and hemorrhagic stroke.
- Iron overload (a.k.a. hemochromatosis) can cause fatal damage to your liver, pancreas, and heart.
- Taking too much potassium can result in potentially deadly cardiac arrhythmia.

▶ The Multivitamin Debate

It's probably safe to say that most of us have been taking a daily multivitamin or mineral pill for years. But do you really need it? The answer depends on whom you talk to. Natural health pros and conventional MDs are unanimous in the conviction that it's best to get all of your nutrients from a wholesome, well-balanced diet. But most experts also realize that for the majority of us, that is highly impractical. For that reason, in addition to eating the healthiest diet you can, doctors generally recommend one of two options:

Take individual supplements to fill in nutritional gaps—extra vitamin C if you tend to shortchange yourself of C-rich fruits and vegetables, or iron if you eat little or no red meat.

Down a daily multivitamin or mineral blend to make sure all your bases are covered.

Note: *If you're on medications or suffer from a chronic condition, check with your doctor before you start taking any supplement— even basic multivitamin or mineral pills.*

Rejuvenating Recipe

MULTINUTRIENT SMOOTHIE

With this simple formula there's no excuse for depriving yourself of essential nutrients. This tasty beverage delivers almost all the vitamins and minerals needed each day for tip-top health.

- **1 banana, peeled**
- **1 cup of green grapes**
- **1 cup of vanilla yogurt (preferably full-fat)**
- **½ apple, chopped (but not peeled)**
- **1½ cups of fresh spinach**
- **1 tbsp. of flaxseeds**
- **1 cup of ice cubes**

Add all the ingredients to a blender in the order listed, and blend for 45 seconds, or until thoroughly liquefied and freely circulating. Then drink up!

Yield: *1 serving*

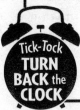

Liberate Your Minerals

Dark leafy greens pack potent loads of iron and calcium. Unfortunately, the leaves also contain compounds that restrict the absorption of those essential minerals. The secret to freeing up the flow: Douse the greens with vinegar (any kind is fine). It'll liberate those health-giving minerals so that none of their power goes to waste.

Tick-Tock
**TURN
BACK** the
CLOCK

❯ You Probably Don't Need Calcium Supplements

For years, the medical community has promoted the use of calcium supplements to alleviate, prevent, or slow the onset of osteoporosis. But now, bone-health experts are questioning that conventional wisdom for three reasons:

- Most parts of the world have lower rates of osteoporosis than we have in the United States, *and* folks in those areas consume less calcium than we do.

- Studies show that taking calcium supplements only cuts your risk of osteoporosis by a mere 1 to 2 percent.

- It seems highly likely that vitamin D and other nutrients play larger bone-building roles than calcium does.

The new R$_x$ for strong bones: Up your vitamin D intake by spending more quality time in the sun, and shape up your lifestyle to eliminate two factors that deplete calcium from your system: lack of physical activity and a diet that's too high in protein, salt, sugar, and fat. **Note:** *If you've already been prescribed calcium supplements, check with your doctor before you quit them cold turkey.*

❯ 3 Keys to Success with Multis

To ensure that your daily vitamin or mineral dose packs the biggest possible punch and keeps you fit as a fiddle, keep these three pointers in mind:

1. Choose your product wisely. It's best to select one with 100 percent of the daily values for most of the essential vitamins and minerals.

2. Take it at mealtime. Which meal is your call, but make sure the menu includes a little fat so that your body can readily absorb the fat-soluble vitamins A, D, E, and K. It doesn't take very much. For example, a small handful of nuts, a tablespoon of olive oil in your salad dressing, or full-fat milk on your cereal will do the trick nicely.

3. Chase it with a drink. A glass of orange or tomato juice at breakfast, for instance, will help the pill dissolve quickly.

❯ Secrets to Safe Supplement Shopping

With literally tens of thousands of nutritional supplements crowding store shelves and streaming across the Internet, how do you tell the real deal from expensive snake oil? Whether you're looking for daily multivitamins, mineral pills, or a super-sophisticated health enhancer, follow these simple guidelines:

Check the label for a gold stamp saying "USP Verified," which indicates the product has been tested and approved by the U.S. Pharmacopeial Convention. Bear in mind, though, that the absence of the stamp does not necessarily mean the stuff didn't pass muster. The manufacturer may simply have chosen not to pay for the verification process.

Look for a scientific advisory board listed on the company's website. If you don't see one, skip that brand.

Pick up the phone and call the manufacturer if you have any concerns. If you can't reach a human being who can answer your questions—or, worse yet, if there is no contact information on the package—don't even think of putting the stuff in your mouth!

When You're Beyond Thirsty

If a big thirst or a change in urine color is your only sign of dehydration, upping your fluid intake should solve the problem quickly. But if you have more severe symptoms, like dizziness; a bad headache; burning stomach; or dry skin, eyes, lips, and mouth—especially after exercising in a hot climate or following a bout of vomiting or diarrhea—get to the ER fast. You may need an IV drip to head off major trouble.

❯ Words to the Wise about Water

We all know that to maintain your good health (and youthful good looks), you should drink eight glasses of water a day, right? Wrong! While it is true that a steady supply of H_2O is essential for your well-being, no scientific research supports the magic number eight. According to a study in the *American Journal of Physiology*, here's the truth of the matter:

- There's no need to count. Your body will tell you when it's time to drink up. Clue: You'll feel thirsty (surprise!).

- Look at your urine output. Brown or dark yellow urine indicates that you're dehydrated, and you need to chug more liquid. On the other hand, if that bodily fluid is clear or close to it, you're doing just fine.

- You don't have to guzzle water. To keep your body healthily hydrated, beverages of all kinds, including juice, milk, tea, and (yes, nutritionists now tell us) coffee, deliver the elixir of life. So do fruits, vegetables, and plenty of other foods.

❯❯ SMART SHOPPING

Contrary to what a lot of folks think, eating a healthier, youth-enhancing diet does not have to mean dropping a lot more dough on food. In fact, a few simple strategies to up the quality of your edibles can actually help reduce your grocery budget—not to mention save you buckets of bucks on health-care costs.

❯ 2 Bonus Benefits of Organic Food

Avoiding pesticides, herbicides, and other dangerous substances is a mighty powerful reason to opt for organic foods whenever you possibly can. But crud-free chow has a couple of other feathers in its cap that you should know about:

1. It tastes better. According to consumer studies, organic foods have richer flavor than those of the same variety that are grown with synthetic fertilizers and sprayed with chemical pesticides.

2. It's better for you. Synthetic fertilizers kill off beneficial microorganisms in the soil that supply fruits and vegetables with their life-giving nutrients. In fact, in a recent survey that examined more than 40 years' worth of scientific studies, organic produce was found to have much higher levels of vitamin C, iron, magnesium, and phosphorous than conventionally grown versions.

❯ The Truth about Organic Food Prices

True or false? Organic food is a gigantic rip-off.

Sometimes true, but more often false. While some supermarkets and specialty stores do jack up prices to target dedicated organic-food shoppers, in most cases there is a valid reason behind those bigger numbers. Growing organic produce or raising organic-grade livestock on a commercial scale involves a whole lot more than just saying "No!" to synthetic chemicals, genetically modified organisms (GMOs), and antibiotics. It demands systematic, long-term planning, detailed record keeping to meet government certification standards, and a major investment in equipment and supplies— which all add up to the higher prices.

> " I am prepared to meet my Maker. Whether my Maker is prepared for the great ordeal of meeting me is another matter.
>
> —Winston Churchill (1874–1965) "

Exceptions to the rule: Organic foods don't always cost more than their conventional counterparts. In my supermarket, the price of a box of cherry tomatoes is the same for both varieties. The same is true for pasta in all shapes and sizes. Just like everything else, organic foods go on sale frequently, and the cost often drops below the prices of conventional brands. So keep your eyes open—a healthy diet could cost less than you think!

❯ Head Down to the Farm

One of the best ways to cut the high cost of organic food—and have a lot of fun at the same time—is to buy your fruits, vegetables, eggs, meats, and dairy products directly from the source. Chances are, a short drive from home will take you to organic farms with roadside stands or, better yet, pick-your-own fields, where you'll find excellent edibles at a fraction of the cost your local supermarket probably charges. If there's no room in your schedule for a country jaunt, visit a nearby farmers' market that includes organic growers. Besides fresh-picked produce, you're also likely to find cut flowers, homemade jams and jellies, yummy baked goods, and sometimes even free entertainment. For a listing of organic farms and markets in your area, check out www.localharvest.org.

❯ The Dirty Dozen and the Clean 15

Each year, the Environmental Working Group (EWG) releases two lists that make it a whole lot easier to eat healthier without the time and expense it can take to go fully organic. The Dirty Dozen list presents the 12 conventionally grown fruits and vegetables that EWG's scientists have analyzed and found to retain the largest amounts of pesticide residue. The most recent twelve are (in order of likely pesticide content) strawberries, apples, nectarines, peaches, celery, grapes, cherries, spinach, tomatoes, sweet bell peppers, cherry tomatoes, and

MIND OVER MYTH

MYTH: When you see the word *natural* on a food label, it means that what's inside is wholesome and always healthy.

REALITY: Not necessarily. A "natural" label is just a designation the food companies apply to any product that has received relatively little processing and has no chemical preservatives. It may or may not be any different from the regular, unmarked version of the same product, even if it sports a higher price tag. Furthermore, it could easily contain GMOs and a lot of other stuff you'd rather not put into your body. So don't be hoodwinked by a buzzword: Before you pop any packaged food item into your grocery cart, read the ingredients list carefully.

cucumbers. The Clean 15 identifies the least pesticide-laden types of produce that you're likely to find in your local supermarket. The most recent list (starting with the cleanest) includes avocados, sweet corn, pineapples, cabbage, sweet peas (frozen), onions, asparagus, mangoes, papayas, kiwi, eggplant, honeydew melon, grapefruit, cantaloupe, and cauliflower. **Note:** *To download the most up-to-date lists, visit the EWG website at https://www.ewg.org/foodnews/.*

❯ Eat Better for Less

Even if your local supermarket doesn't offer a big supply of organic foods, or you just need to keep an eagle eye on your food budget, you can still reduce your chemical intake considerably. Here are two simple ways to enjoy a healthier diet without going completely organic:

Consider what you consume. Remember that when pesticides are sprayed onto produce such as leafy greens, tomatoes, broccoli, berries, or grapes, the chemicals go directly onto (and often into) the edible plant parts. For that reason, these foods belong at the top of your buy-organic list. On the other hand, root vegetables like carrots, beets, and onions, as well as thick-skinned fruits like melons, have more natural protection, so less of the sprayed substance will reach the parts you eat. That means you can rest a little easier with buying the conventionally grown versions of these foods.

Consider your eating habits. Most likely, there are certain foods that you and your family consume in quantity nearly every day—maybe milk, bananas, or tomatoes, or processed foods like cereals

Make Your Meats Organic

Studies show that meat, milk, and other dairy products retain more pesticide residue than vegetables and fruits do—in addition to harboring antibiotics and other toxic crap that is routinely pumped into conventionally raised livestock. So do yourself a favor and buy organic versions of any animal-derived foods, even if it means trimming your overall intake of those menu items or pinching pennies elsewhere in your budget.

Tick-Tock
TURN BACK the CLOCK

and ketchup—and others that you eat less often. Simply by seeking out organic versions of your steady favorites, you'll cut your potential chemical intake dramatically, even if everything else in your shopping cart comes from a traditional agri-business.

❯ 2 Labels to Look For

Unless you've been living in a cave for the past decade or so, you know that genetically modified organisms are running rampant in just about every kind of processed food on the supermarket shelves. The jury is still out on the degree of danger these ingredients pose for human health, but extensive animal testing has shown that foods containing GMOs cause health problems ranging from gastrointestinal upsets and infertility to organ damage, immune system impairment, and—yes—accelerated aging. You can make shopping a lot easier and avoid unhealthy food by looking for one or both of these labels on the packaging:

1. Certified Organic. By law, any food that sports this label must be produced without genetic engineering, most synthetic pesticides and fertilizers (including sewer sludge), growth hormones, irradiation, and antibiotics. It also must be certified as meeting those standards by the United States Department of Agriculture (USDA) and various other state

---

Fountain of Youth
PERFECT PRODUCE CLEANER

If you buy fruits or vegetables that are not organically grown—even if they're not on the Dirty Dozen list (see page 163)—it's all but guaranteed they contain some chemical residue. Even commercially grown organic produce is sprayed with a botanical pesticide like rotenone or pyrethrum, or with something you'd rather not eat, like garlic oil. This powerful potion will get rid of all types of unwanted surface additives:

1 cup of white vinegar
1 tbsp. of baking soda
Juice of ½ lemon
1 cup of water

Combine the ingredients in a spray bottle, and shake. Before eating fresh produce, or using in a recipe, spritz and let sit for five minutes. Rinse well, and you're good to go.

governments. Just about any edible product—whether it's fresh, dried, frozen, or canned—is eligible for the organic designation. That includes fruits and vegetables, grains, meat, dairy products, eggs, coffee and tea, and even processed foods like ketchup and salad dressings.

2. Non-GMO Project Verified. This designation by the Non-GMO Project takes organic certification one step further. Not only does it tell you that the food in question contains no GMOs, but it also tests foods to ensure they have not been contaminated with pollen from nonorganic farms. It only certifies products that have less than 0.9 percent GMO contamination.

❯ Food Expiration Dates Demystified

If you're confused by all of the expiration dates on food packages, you are not alone. Some believe it's a deliberate move by food companies to make you toss out perfectly good edibles before their time, but here's the lowdown on what that label lingo really means:

"Sell by" denotes that the store should move the product off its shelves by that date, but you still have ample time at home to consume it before the quality and nutrient content go downhill. Take milk, for example. If the date says, "Sell by July 25," you have a good week or so to consume it before it will actually be unsafe (or at least highly unpalatable) to drink.

"Best if used by" is a form of quality assurance. It's provided by the manufacturer to suggest how long the product will be at its peak of flavor and freshness. Usually, a package label will say something like "Best if used by July 25." Again, this is only a guideline. It doesn't mean, for instance, that your bag of walnuts will suddenly become inedible at midnight of that day. They will simply begin to slowly decline in flavor, texture, and (in most cases) nutrients.

"Use by" or "Expires on" is a whole other thing. In this case, if you don't use it by the date listed, you are likely to see a marked deterioration in product quality, safety, or both.

❯ Liven Up Limp Vegetables

Just because the vegetables in your produce drawer are looking droopy doesn't mean they're over the hill. While the vitamin content will have diminished, it won't have vanished, and it's a snap to restore the crispness and flavor. Depending on the type of veggies, use one of these two methods:

- Salad greens—add 1 teaspoon of white or apple cider vinegar to a pan of water, and let the greens soak in it for 15 minutes.

- Other veggies—dunk them briefly in hot tap water, then immediately drop them into a bowl of ice water with 1 tablespoon of either white or apple cider vinegar mixed into it. In a few minutes, they'll perk right up!

❯ Is Fresh Produce Really Better for You?

A lot of so-called dietary experts are constantly telling us that fresh fruits and vegetables are far superior to frozen and canned versions.

Eye-Opening Facts about Tomatoes

Before you reach for tomatoes at your supermarket, bear in mind that those red orbs were probably picked when they weren't nearly so rosy—and that could make them much less valuable dietary allies than you might think. Studies have proven that vine-ripened tomatoes contain nearly twice as much vitamin C and beta-carotene as their green counterparts. And don't be hoodwinked by signs saying "Vine-Ripened." Unless it's high tomato season and they were grown locally (which in a big chain store is unlikely), they won't be up to snuff. Although tomatoes can be ripened on the vine in greenhouses, they aren't nearly as nutritious as the ones raised in the fresh air and hot summer sun.

And that is true when you pick fully ripe, organic fruits and veggies fresh from your own garden or buy them, fresh picked, from a local organic farmer and eat them the same day. But the picture-perfect stuff you see in supermarkets has serious nutritional shortcomings—even if it was grown organically. There are two major reasons:

The vast majority of produce sold in big stores has traveled a long way to get there. In the process, it's been exposed to extreme temperatures and other conditions that deplete both flavor and nutrients. (Vitamins A and C are especially prone to going AWOL during long road trips.)

Fruits and vegetables pack their full nutritional punch only when they've ripened completely. But, by necessity, most produce that will be shipped a considerable distance is harvested before the vitamins and other nutrients have had a chance to fully develop.

➤ Frozen Is Fine—but Shop with Care!

While it is a fact that frozen produce is often healthier than its fresh counterparts—especially when you have a choice between, let's say, a bag of frozen organic blueberries and a box of fresh ones that have been treated with pesticides and herbicides—there is one caveat: When frozen food is allowed to thaw and refreeze, it loses boatloads of vitamins. So before you toss those packages into your shopping

---

More Is Better—Period!

If you're like most folks, you don't eat nearly as many health-giving fruits and vegetables as you should. So take a tip from top nutritionists: Quit fretting about which form of produce is best. Instead, focus on simply adding more of it to your diet. Calling on a combination of fresh, frozen, and canned fruits and vegetables will help ensure that you meet the ideal intake of five servings each day—or at least come a lot closer to your target.

Tick-Tock **TURN BACK** the **CLOCK**

cart, put 'em to the test. Here's what to check for:

- Fruits and veggies that come in individual pieces, like peas, corn, or berries, should move around loosely or break apart easily in the bag. If you pick up what feels like a solid chunk of ice, put it right back where you got it!

- When you lift a box of pureed squash, spinach, or other greens, the weight should be evenly distributed. If it's all lumped on one side of the package, give it a pass.

Once you've made your way through the checkout line, hightail it home and stash your bounty in the freezer. Everything should keep all its flavor and goodness for up to six months.

❯ The Bewildering Bashing of Canned Produce

Canned fruits and vegetables have gotten a bum rap in recent years. Do they deserve it? In a word, no. Granted, they're rarely photogenic enough to grace the pages of a fancy food magazine. But that's no reason to banish canned foods from your diet. Let's consider the pros and cons of these traditional pantry staples.

Rejuvenating Recipe
KALE-MUSTARD TOPPER

Kale and apple cider vinegar are full of nutrients that help hold back the hands of time. And mustard powder packs an army of phytonutrients, omega-3 fatty acids, and antioxidants. Put this trio together, and you've got a simple, versatile, and delicious way to supercharge your diet.

> 2 cups of kale, rinsed and torn into pieces
> ¼ cup of unfiltered apple cider vinegar
> ¼ cup of water
> 2 tbsp. of dry mustard powder (such as Colman's®)

Whirl all of the ingredients together in a blender or food processor. Use the blend as a topping for chicken, fish, baked potatoes, or pasta, or as a tasty dip for crackers, corn chips, or raw vegetables.

Yield: *About 1½ cups*

First, the highly exaggerated cons:

- During the canning process, vegetables and fruits can lose some of their vitamin C content, but when they're processed quickly—in your kitchen or at the processing plant—the majority of nutrients are locked in and retained, just as they are in frozen foods.

- Canned vegetables are high in sodium and may contain other undesirable ingredients. The simple solution to these potential drawbacks: Read labels carefully to avoid harmful additives, and whenever possible, choose organic brands and low- or no-sodium versions. **Note:** *Rinse canned vegetables to remove a lot of the salt.*

Second, the highly practical pros:

- Canned foods have a shelf life of two to four years or more, compared with six months for frozen types and a week or so max for most fresh fruits and vegetables. Better yet, unlike their fridge- and freezer-bound counterparts, canned goods sail through even the longest power outages in fine fettle.

- Depending on the season and where you live, canned vegetables and fruits may cost considerably less than fresh versions.

- Because foods must be heated before canning, they're less prone to contamination than fresh vittles can be.

- Foods intended for canning (or freezing) are generally picked at their peak of ripeness and processed close to the source, before valuable vitamins have a chance to fly the coop.

❯ 3 Sneaky Ways to Up Your Produce Intake

Are you and your family eating all the fruits and vegetables you need each day to maintain good health—much less reverse the aging process? If you're like the vast majority of Americans, the answer is no. It's not always easy to eat a well-balanced diet when you're on the go almost nonstop—and who isn't these days? But this roundup of simple tricks can help you come a lot closer to your daily quota:

1. Invite temptation. Fill eye-catching bowls with grapes, cherries, or grape tomatoes, and set them out in well-trafficked spots around your house. It's all but guaranteed that you—and everyone else who passes by—will grab a healthy handful.

2. Put 'em by the door. Pile bananas, apples, oranges, and other fruits in a basket by the door. On your way out, you're bound to snatch one to snack on later.

3. Top it off. Get in the habit of making fortified vinegars. These are thickened blends of fruits or vegetables mixed with herbs and spices. Whip them up in a blender to use as dips, salad dressings, or toppings. The Kale-Mustard Topper recipe (page 169) is one superpowered example; for other clever combo ideas, see "Top Off Your Nutrient 'Tank'" (below).

TOP OFF YOUR NUTRIENT "TANK"

Fortified vinegars provide one of the easiest and tastiest ways to pack more fruits and vegetables into your diet (see "3 Sneaky Ways to Up Your Produce Intake," at left). The roster of possibilities is virtually limitless, but here's a handful of my favorite age-defying champs. The simple recipe: Puree the ingredients in a blender or food processor.

Fortified Vinegar	Ingredients
Carrot	1 cup of sliced carrots, ½ cup of apple cider vinegar, ½ cup of water, 3–4 tbsp. of raw honey (optional)
Cucumber, celery & onion	1 cucumber, 2 cups of chopped celery, 1 chopped onion, 1 cup of champagne vinegar, 1 cup of water
Melon	2 cups of chopped cantaloupe or honeydew melon, ¼ cup of champagne vinegar, ¼ cup of water
Raspberry	1 cup of raspberries (either fresh or frozen), 3 tbsp. of red-wine vinegar
Strawberry	2 cups of fresh strawberries, 1 cup of sugar, ½ cup of champagne vinegar

>>> FOOD Rx

Hippocrates, the Father of Medicine, routinely advised his patients to "Let food be thy medicine and medicine be thy food." Well, he wasn't just blowing them off so he could flee his office and spend the day on the golf course! He knew then what we're beginning to learn now: that the answer to curing everyday ills and fending off or alleviating even the most serious diseases—as well as restoring your youthful vitality—may be as close as your local supermarket.

> Terrific Tricks for Tossing Cancer Sticks

Trying to quit smoking? Congratulations! Nothing can make that process pleasant, but this trio of tricks can help ease your constant desire for hand-to-mouth gratification. Whenever you crave a smoke, try one of these healthy alternatives:

Grab a raw carrot, and chomp away. It'll give you a big antioxidant boost and satisfy your craving at the same time.

> "Old age is like everything else. To make a success of it, you've got to start young.
> —Fred Astaire (1899–1987)"

Reach for a cinnamon stick, and suck on it, or brew a cup of cinnamon tea and sip it slowly until the feeling passes.

Suck on a lime. Besides curbing your desire for tobacco, it will replace some of the vitamins, phosphates, and calcium that frequent smoking may have drained from your system.

Note: *For more ways to become a successful quitter, see "Kicking the Nastiest Habit of All" on page 34.*

> The Astounding Deeds of Sunflower Seeds

Looking at a sunflower seed, you'd never take it for a grow-younger superstar. But it is! Believe it or not, eating just a handful of the unsalted seeds every day can help reduce your cravings for alcohol and tobacco, lower your LDL (bad) cholesterol levels, prevent tooth decay, relieve constipation, improve your memory—and much more.

❯ Spicy Help for Body and Mind

Curcumin, the active ingredient in turmeric, is one of the most powerful, naturally occurring anti-inflammatory substances ever identified—and, therefore, one of your most potent weapons in the fight against chronic diseases and premature aging. What's more, turmeric has also been shown to have strong anti-cancer properties and to reduce the buildup of plaque in your brain that causes Alzheimer's and cognitive decline. Your Rx for good health: Simply add turmeric to your favorite soups, stews, and other foods as often as you can—the more, the merrier!

❯ Bring on the Berries!

The same compounds that give berries their beautiful colors—namely anthocyanins—also make them a boon for your body and your brain. To be specific, here's a sampling of the wonders these jewel-toned powerhouses can work for you:

Lessen your risk of chronic diseases by protecting your body's cells from damage

MIND OVER MYTH

MYTH: You can be healthier and live longer by packing your diet with certain anti-aging "superfoods."

REALITY: Despite all the hoopla you hear about "superfoods," reputable nutritionists and dieticians tell us there is no such thing. Rather, the term is merely a marketing ploy. That being said, there are a great many foods, like the ones singled out in this chapter, that contain large concentrations of powerful nutrients. But no single type of edible can do anything on its own. Rather, the key to regaining and retaining a younger-feeling you for as long as possible is to eat a varied, well-balanced diet that provides all the essential nutrients you need for good health—and, of course, to couple wholesome eating habits with plenty of sleep and regular exercise.

Improve your eyesight, reduce inflammation, relieve pain, and help ward off cancer and coronary heart disease

Enhance your overall brain function, improve your memory, and possibly reduce your risk of developing Parkinson's disease

But that's not all! Researchers have even found that eating two or more servings of blueberries and strawberries a week may also delay cognitive aging by as much as two and a half years.

❯ Become Eagle-Eyed

Fresh bilberries are hard to come by in supermarkets, but they are widely available via the Internet in both dried and frozen forms—and they're well worth seeking out if you have eye problems of any kind. These blueberry relatives are especially renowned for their power to sharpen your vision and help your eyes adjust quickly from light to darkness. In fact, they're so effective that during World War II the British Royal Air Force included generous supplies of bilberry jam in their pilots' ration kits.

❯ 7 Dirt-Cheap, Age-Defying Foods

These days, a couple of exotic berries by the names goji and acai are getting a whole lot of airplay for their potent supplies of anti-aging

Nothin' Beats Home Cookin'!

If you've heard that old adage once, you've heard it a zillion times. But it turns out that those fresh-from-your-kitchen vittles don't just taste better than restaurant fare. A recent study published in the journal *Public Health Nutrition* found that people who cooked their meals at home at least five times a week lived longer than those who didn't. The likely reasons: When you whip up your own grub, you know exactly what ingredients are going into it—and you control the portion sizes to boot. So what are you waiting for? Clear off the counters, haul out the gear, and start holding back the hands of time!

Tick-Tock
TURN BACK the **CLOCK**

antioxidants. Well, guess what? You can stroll into your local supermarket and pick up a passel of foods that are as effective in the fight against free radicals as those fancy little fruits are—for a lot less money. Just include heaping helpings of these winners in your diet, and you'll be fortifying your system against everything from arthritis to Alzheimer's and cancer to cardiovascular disease.

- Apples
- Black rice
- Coffee
- Cranberries
- Dried beans
- Sweet potatoes
- Tea

> Freaky Food Fixes

It's a fact that what you put on your skin goes into your body—and that's the secret behind these amazing antidotes to cure a half-dozen hindering health problems:

Banish skin troubles. Stuff a cotton drawstring bag or panty hose leg with a cup or two of uncooked oatmeal. Toss it into your tub as you run cool to lukewarm water, then settle in and relax for 15 to 20 minutes. If possible, let yourself air-dry when you're finished, and bid bye-bye to the pain, itch, and inflammation of wind- and sunburn, insect bites, poison-plant rashes, contact allergies, or eczema.

Clear up conjunctivitis. Grate a large, peeled apple, and spread the gratings in the center of a piece of damp cheesecloth that's about 12 inches square. Fold it to form a pouch, lie down, and place it over your eyes for 30 minutes. Within a day or two, all should be well again.

Fountain of Youth

SORE SKIN SOLUTION

Here's a straight-from-the-kitchen emollient for treating psoriasis or other painful and itchy skin irritations, ranging from chapped hands to cold sores, shingles, and (attention, grandparents!) diaper rash.

4 tbsp. of sweet almond oil

Juice of 1 lemon or lime

Mix the oil and juice, and apply the mixture generously to the afflicted skin. Repeat as needed until you feel relief. Then store any leftover salve in a tightly closed jar at room temperature, to use later.

Build Stronger Bones

Attention, ladies of a certain age! If you're taking calcium supplements to help fend off osteoporosis, here's something you should know: Those high doses of calcium can impair your body's ability to absorb manganese, which is a crucial bone-building compound. But that doesn't mean you should give up on doctor-prescribed calcium! Instead, simply include a tablespoon or so of parsley in your daily diet. It enhances manganese absorption, especially when you eat it with foods that are high in copper and zinc, such as shellfish, poultry, and whole grains.

Eradicate athlete's foot. Simply rub plain yogurt directly onto the affected skin. For good measure, eat a cup or two of yogurt each day until the fungus has flown the coop.

Heal cuts. Blend or chop ¼ cup or so of cranberries (either fresh or frozen), apply the mash to the cut, and cover it with a bandage. Change the dressing every few hours until the wound has healed.

Treat hemorrhoids. Chop a cabbage, lay the pieces on a towel, and sit on them for 30 minutes or so. And don't forget to take your pants off first!

Quell a cold. At bedtime, put a slice of raw onion on the sole of each foot, and hold the slices in place with thick, wool socks. Overnight, the curative compounds in the onion will draw out the infection and lower your fever. (Be forewarned: They'll also leave you with onion breath in the morning!)

❯ 2 Super Reasons to Say "Yes!" to Spuds

The average American eats more than 130 pounds of potatoes each year. Unfortunately, about half of that load comes in the form of potato chips, French fries, and other junk-food treats. For that reason, nutritionists have largely overlooked the nutritional gold mine lurking inside the humble spud. But an article published in the *Journal of Nutrition* has food gurus changing their tune. Specifically, they're now singing the praises of colorful—and far more flavorful—types of taters because of these two valuable nutrients:

1. Anthocyanins—found in pink, red, blue, and purple potatoes—

are the same phytonutrients that give many berries their potent antioxidant kick. Reap the benefits with choices like All Red, All Blue, and Mountain Rose.

2. Carotenoids—hidden in yellow-fleshed potatoes (like the popular Yukon Gold)—help boost essential vitamin A action. Some lesser-known varieties rapidly gaining in popularity are Yellow Finn, Carola, and Charlotte.

These colorful characters are turning up in more and more local supermarkets and farmers' markets—so toss 'em into your cart!

➤ Shrink Your Prostate

Medical statisticians estimate that one out of every three men over the age of 60 has some kind of prostate problem. And, according to natural health practitioners, one of the most effective ways to help relieve an enlarged prostate is to eat ½ cup of shelled, unsalted pumpkin seeds every day. One reason may be that the prostate contains 10 times more zinc than most other organs in your body, and pumpkin seeds are packed with that mineral. **Note:** *Check with your doctor before you use this remedy.*

➤ A Big Hand for Hen Fruit!

Back when fat phobia was sweeping the country, eggs were about as desirable as lumps of coal in a Christmas stocking. How times change! Now these barnyard gems rank high on every nutritionist's list of healthiest foods—especially for aging adults. The reason: As we get older, our appetites tend to shrink, so it's important to make sure that everything that goes into our bodies benefits the bottom line in some way. And each egg is neatly "wrapped" with five essential assets in one tasty, versatile, and easily digestible package. Here's the breakdown:

> " Part of the secret of success in life is to eat what you like and let the food fight it out inside.
>
> —Mark Twain (1835–1910) "

Choline. One egg provides 20 percent of the recommended daily allowance of choline, which not only enhances memory and cognition but also helps reduce chronic inflammation, which has been linked to the development of Alzheimer's disease.

Iron. Older adults often have a mild iron deficiency, which can lower their energy level. That, in turn, can also lead to less physical activity. Egg yolks provide iron in a more absorbable form than supplements can.

Protein. A single large egg offers up to 6 grams of protein. The older we get, the more important this is because the ability of tissue to renew and repair itself slows down with age, meaning that wounds take longer to heal and become more susceptible to infection.

Tryptophan. Eggs are full of this important amino acid, which your body converts to mood-lifting serotonin.

Vitamin D. A single egg yolk has about 40 IUs of vitamin D, which joins with calcium to promote bone health and decrease the risk for fractures and osteoporosis. (For one tasty way to put this duo to work, see the Anti-Aging Egg Salad recipe at left).

❯ Medicinal Marvels of Chocolate

By now you've probably heard that chocolate is good for your health.

Rejuvenating Recipe

ANTI-AGING EGG SALAD

If the thought of egg salad makes you turn up your nose, this version will put it back in place pronto!

> 2 large, hard-boiled eggs, chopped
>
> 1 tbsp. of plain yogurt
>
> 1 tsp. of lemon juice
>
> 1 rib of celery, washed and chopped
>
> ½ bunch of chives, chopped
>
> Freshly ground pepper and salt (optional)

Mix the first three ingredients in a bowl until they're blended but the texture is still chunky. If necessary, add more yogurt for moisture. Stir in the celery and chives, and season to taste with the pepper and salt. Sandwich the mixture between two slices of whole-grain bread, eat it all by itself, or use it as a topping for a green salad or baked potato.

Yield: *1 serving*

Well, that's true! Compounds in dark chocolate can perform these fabulous feats:

- Decrease inflammation in cardio-vascular tissues, thereby reducing your risk of stroke

- Make blood platelets less likely to stick together and form harmful clots, while at the same time promoting normal clotting and improving your circulation

- Improve cognitive function by increasing blood flow to your brain

- Lower your risk for tooth decay by hardening your tooth enamel (Of course, you do still need to practice good dental hygiene!)

- Boost your mood by spurring your brain to release feel-good endorphins

❯ 3 Reasons to Take a Break!

Earlier, I told you that intermittent fasting (as medical pros call it) can increase your levels of brain-derived neurotrophic factor (BDNF), a protein that dramatically enhances your brain's health and performance. Better-functioning gray matter isn't the only reward you'll reap by letting your digestive system rest periodically for as little as 12 hours. More and more research is showing that simply by skipping your after-dinner snack once in a while, you trigger a tsunami of hormones that can perform heroic feats in your body, including these:

1. Make weight loss easier. If you reduce your calorie intake every day, your metabolism slows down, so it's hard to continue losing weight. But when you fast intermittently and eat normally

Centenarian SECRETS 100

Adopting a 12-hour fasting habit can do more than help you conquer conditions ranging from obesity to heart disease. It can also help you live a longer, healthier life. Most likely, the docs figure, this is because going without any food from dinner until breakfast puts your body into the natural sleep-wake-eat rhythm that nature intended—and the one that just happens to be business as usual in the parts of the world where people live, and stay youthful, the longest.

the rest of the time, your metabolism stays high, so the pounds keep flowing off.

2. Prevent leaky gut syndrome. This is *big* because more and more research is showing the connection of leaky gut and impaired gut flora to all manner of diseases.

3. Prevent or reverse dreaded conditions including diabetes, heart disease, and cancer.

❯ Common Food Cures

Believe it or not, the solution to a whole lot of nagging health problems may be right in your kitchen—or as close as your local supermarket. Here's a quartet of ultra-common foods that can work wonders for you:

Ease your achin' joints with apples. The next time your knees, elbows, or other joints start hurting—or better yet, before the pain starts—eat a few apples. Their potent load of boron can relieve joint pain and stiffness and actually seems to protect against arthritis.

Lower your blood pressure with avocados. Their mega-supply of potassium prevents the thickening of your artery walls and also helps regulate your body's fluid levels, which are crucial to regulating your blood pressure.

Rout out gout with cherries. They help clear toxins from your body and clean your kidneys, which puts them at the top of the gout-relief list. The easy R_X: Eat 1 to 12 fresh or frozen cherries a day, or a handful of dried cherries. Drinking 100 percent cherry juice will also ease gout pain.

Stave off PMS with pork 'n' beans. This classic combo is rich in thiamine and riboflavin, both of which have been proven to keep these monthly miseries at bay. Eating a 3-ounce serving of pork and a cup of cooked beans on a regular basis will do the trick just fine.

Anti-Aging Dietary Duos

We all know it takes teamwork to win a baseball game. Well, guess what? That same strategy can also help you slow down—or even reverse—the aging process. Each one of these foods all by itself is an anti-aging all-star. But when you team them up, stand back and watch 'em light up your scoreboard!

Almonds + red wine. Vitamin E in the almonds works with resveratrol in the wine to thin your blood and help to boost the health of your blood vessel linings. *The result: a happier, healthier heart!*

Bananas + yogurt. A fiber called inulin in the bananas revs up the growth of yogurt's healthy bacteria. *The result: improved digestion and a ramped-up immune system.*

Blueberries + walnuts. Antioxidants, called anthocyanins, in the berries guard your brain cells against damage from free radicals, and the omega-3 fatty acids in walnuts boost your brainpower. *The result: improved memory, enhanced mental function, and possibly a lowered risk for Parkinson's disease.*

Chicken + carrots. The zinc in chicken enables your body to convert the carrots' beta-carotene into vitamin A. *The result: a rugged immune system, stronger eyes, and healthier skin.*

Dark chocolate + raspberries. The catechin in chocolate and quercetin found in raspberries intensify each other's disease-fighting prowess. *The result: thinner blood and a healthier heart.*

Eggs + cheese. The vitamin D in the egg yolks makes the calcium in the cheese more readily available to your body. *The result: stronger bones, clearer thinking, and a healthier heart—plus reduced PMS symptoms and easier weight-loss labors.*

Onions + garlic. Working together increases the potency of their artery-clearing compounds. *The result: cleaner blood vessels and reduced risk for arteriosclerosis.*

Peanut butter + whole-grain bread. The classic peanut butter sandwich packs all nine of the amino acids that your body needs to build muscles, bones, and hormones. *The result: a stronger, healthier you.*

Tomatoes + olive oil. The oil makes your body better able to use the tomatoes' disease-fighting lycopene. *The result: improved ability to prevent cancer and heart disease.*

>>> DRINK TO YOUR HEALTH!

Solid food isn't the only dietary dynamo in your grow-younger arsenal. Plenty of liquid refreshments are also chock-full of nutrients to help fend off or alleviate health problems that can make you old—in body and mind—long before your time.

> The Truth about Tea

Study after study has shown that tea, whether black, green, white, or oolong (all of which are made from the leaves of the *Camellia sinensis* shrub), can fight inflammation, boost your immune system, preserve your brainpower, and help prevent diabetes, osteoporosis, and many types of cancer—and that's just for starters. Unfortunately, a few misconceptions have arisen about this bracing beverage, so let's set the record straight right now.

Tall tale #1: Adding milk to tea destroys its health benefits.
The truth: Although some studies a while back suggested that was the case, recent research, including a study published in the *Journal of Agricultural and Food Chemistry*, has found that tea offers up about the same potent load of antioxidants whether it's laced with milk or not.

Tall tale #2: To get the biggest health boost from tea, you should drink it plain.
The truth: There are a couple of additives that actually increase the health-giving properties of tea. When you're brewing it ahead, say for iced tea, squeezing some lemon, lime, or orange juice into the pitcher helps preserve the flavonoids that deliver many of tea's health benefits. Furthermore, drinking tea with honey stirred into it seems to enhance your ability to

> " They say some of my stars drink whiskey, but I have found that the ones who drink milk shakes don't win any ball games.
>
> —Casey Stengel (1890–1975 "

work more productively—apparently by activating the areas of your brain that control concentration.

Tall tale #3: Tea never goes bad. **The truth:** While tea does not spoil in the way that meat or produce does, after about six months, its antioxidant supply starts to diminish. To maintain full potency as long as possible, always store tea (whether it's loose or in bags) in a sealed container in a cool, dark place.

❯ 2 Tips to Treat Cataracts

No nutrient can cure cataracts, but studies show that quercetin, a strong antioxidant, may help delay their formation or slow their development. And dried tea leaves (both green and black) contain more quercetin than any other food. There's one catch: Brewed tea contains almost no quercetin. But you can still enjoy its benefits in two easy ways:

1. Brew your tea using loose leaves, and don't strain it before sipping. Just drink it down, leaves and all.

2. Add a teaspoon or two of tea leaves to a delicious smoothie recipe, or stir them into your favorite yogurt.

There is no specific recommended dosage for cataract avoidance—so make tea leaves part of your regular diet, along with a few other quercetin-rich foods, like apples, cranberries, onions, and peppers.

❯ The Hidden Healing Power of Lemonade

For generations of Americans, nothing has shouted "Summertime!"

> # Centenarian SECRETS 100
>
> Here's great news, ladies! Studies show that drinking as little as one cup of black or green tea a day may preserve your bone density well into your senior years. The reason is that as your natural estrogen levels decline during menopause (thereby hindering your bones' ability to absorb calcium), the natural phytoestrogens in tea can take over to boost your absorption of this essential mineral. Of course, it's best to start your cup-a-day routine in the year or so leading up to menopause, when your body starts to produce less and less estrogen.

Rejuvenating Recipe
CLASSIC LEMONADE

This is the ultimate, old-time recipe. Feel free to increase the ingredients if you're serving a crowd, but stick to the same proportions for best results.

- **1 cup of sugar (or less to taste)**
- **1 cup of water (for simple syrup)**
- **1 cup of freshly squeezed lemon juice (4–6 lemons)**
- **3–4 cups of cold water**

Make a simple syrup by heating 1 cup of water in a pan, and then stirring in the sugar until it's dissolved. Mix the syrup and lemon juice in a pitcher, and add enough cold water to reach the desired strength. Refrigerate, covered, for 30 to 40 minutes. If the lemonade is too sweet for your liking, add more straight lemon juice, and use less sugar. Serve it up in ice-filled glasses, garnished with lemon slices.

Yield: *6 servings*

like a tall, cold glass of lemonade. Well, guess what? Medical experts now tell us that this sweet and tangy treat can help resolve or prevent a passel of serious health problems. That's because lemons are rich in phytonutrients that are associated with the prevention and treatment of at least four of the leading causes of death in Western countries: cancer, cardiovascular disease, diabetes, and hypertension. What's more, though lemons are acidic, they increase the alkalinity of our bodily fluids—and an alkaline system is key to maintaining good health. Here's a sampling of the fabulous feats that a daily glass of real lemonade (not the powdered stuff) can perform for you:

- Boost your immune system
- Cleanse your system of toxins and impurities
- Conquer cravings for cigarettes, alcohol, and junk food
- Improve your mood
- Increase your energy level
- Prevent kidney stones
- Protect against adult asthma and other respiratory ailments
- Reduce acid reflux
- Speed weight loss

Note: *For best results, make your own lemonade from scratch using freshly squeezed lemon juice and sugar (see the Classic Lemonade recipe above).*

❯ 7 Surprising Secrets of Carrot Juice

In many parts of the world, folks consider carrot juice to be the "king of juices," and for good reason: Drinking an 8-ounce glass of this golden treasure several times a week can work wonders for your health and well-being. Like these, for instance:

1. Help fend off asthma attacks and other respiratory ailments

2. Guard against the effects of secondhand smoke

3. Fortify your blood and help prevent anemia

4. Balance your blood sugar levels

5. Cleanse your liver

6. Prevent water retention

7. Strengthen your immune system

Note: *You can get all of these benefits from pure, bottled carrot juice, but the kind you make in your own home juicer or buy fresh from the machine at your local juice bar is far more potent.*

❯ Cabbage Juice Cures Ulcers

For centuries, folk-medicine gurus have sworn by cabbage and cabbage juice as top-notch ulcer remedies. Well, it turns out they're right. Recently, numerous medical studies (including one at the Stanford University School of Medicine) have found that drinking 8 ounces of pure cabbage juice four times a day can heal both gastric and duodenal ulcers in anywhere from 2 to 10 days. Eating raw cabbage can perform the same miraculous feat. So if you'd rather not drink a quart of cabbage juice every

The Unsavory Scoop on Non-Dairy Creamers

Attention, coffee drinkers! Thanks to its brimming boatload of antioxidants, your beloved beverage can be a powerful part of your health-care arsenal. That is, unless you add non-dairy creamer to your cup. A study published in the *Journal of Nutrition* found that these dairy stand-ins may block the absorption of the phenolic acids that give java its disease-fighting firepower. On the other hand, neither half-and-half nor milk disrupts your body's antioxidant uptake. So do yourself a favor: Drink your coffee either black or with the real deal mixed in.

day, you can substitute a wedge of raw cabbage or about 1 cup of sliced or shredded cabbage for each 8-ounce cup of juice.

❯ Say No to "Diet" Drinks and Sweeteners

Two of the most consumed "diet" products in America are diet soda and artificial sweeteners. Yet the population continues to grow in girth. What gives? The truth of the matter is that far from stemming our obesity epidemic, diet sodas and sugar substitutes may actually be fueling it.

"Diet" is deceptive. Diet soda drinkers are actually 65 percent more likely to be overweight than non-soda drinkers. What's more, they are more likely to be overweight than folks who drink regular soda.

Type 2 diabetes. Numerous studies have found that diet soda drinkers are at increased risk of developing type 2 diabetes. The jury is out on the exact cause. It may be hormonal reactions triggered by the chemicals in the sweeteners, or it could be that people eat unhealthy foods that undo any calorie-saving effects.

Slow metabolism. Regular consumption of artificial sweeteners, particularly in beverages, slows down your metabolism, which makes it easier to pack on pounds and harder to lose them.

The zero-calorie con. In nature, there is no such thing as sweetness without calories. When you consume zero-calorie sugar substitutes that are anywhere from 200 to 7,000 times sweeter than the real deal, it triggers hormonal processes that ramp up your brain's craving for real food. Research

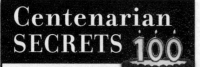

Centenarian SECRETS 100

An old Russian folk remedy calls on pumpkin seed "tea" to relieve inflammation of the bladder and prostate. To make it, simmer ½ cup of whole (unshelled) pumpkin seeds in a quart of boiling water for 20 minutes. Let it cool to room temperature, and pour it into a wide-mouthed jar with a tight cover. Do not strain out the seeds; just let them settle to the bottom of the jar. Stir thoroughly before using the potion. Drink 6 to 8 ounces three times a day, or as needed to relieve pain. **Note:** *This is not a substitute for professional medical care. If you suspect that you have either bladder or prostate problems, see your doctor.*

suggests that artificial sweeteners actually prevent your body from producing GLP-1, a hormone that controls your blood sugar levels and feelings of fullness. As a result, you can easily wind up eating a whole lot more than you would if you allowed yourself to enjoy moderate amounts of sugar.

Cardiovascular complications. A recent study at the University of Iowa Hospitals and Clinics found that women who drink two or more diet beverages a day are 30 percent more likely than non-diet pop drinkers to have a heart attack or similar cardiovascular "event" and 50 percent more likely to die from the experience.

❯ Swig Some Blueberry Sore-Throat Relief

Like any other kind of pain, a sore throat can make you feel like the years are ganging up on you. Plenty of beverages can ease that blasted discomfort, but one of the most effective comfort givers is good old blueberry juice. If you can't find pure juice at your local supermarket or health-food store, liquefy a handful of the berries in a juicer, blender, or food processor, and drink up. (Add a little water to taste if the flavor is too intense for you.)

Fountain of Youth
SWEET & SPICY THROAT CURE

This two-timing gargle makes a sore throat scurry in a hurry!

⅛ tsp. of cayenne pepper
⅛ tsp. of ground ginger
8 oz. of hot water
Ice-cold pineapple juice

Mix the spices in the water. Pour the juice into a glass, and set it aside. First, gargle with a swig of the spicy mix. Then follow up by gargling with the pineapple juice. Keep alternating between the hot and cold liquids until both glasses are empty. Repeat routine several times a day. The combination of hot and cold liquids will ease the burning sensation. The dual action of the spices and bromelain (an enzyme in pineapple) will also loosen that irritating mucus stuck in your throat.

❯ 3 Blackberry Beverages to Cure the Big Ds

Since biblical times, folks have been using blackberries in one form of liquid or another to cure diarrhea and dysentery. How you take your tasty medicine is up to you, but you should drink one of these lovely libations every four hours:

- 1½ ounces of blackberry brandy
- 2 ounces of blackberry wine
- 6 ounces of pure blackberry juice

Note: *If the sufferer is an infant or young child, lose the liquor and instead give the tot 2 or 3 tablespoons of pure blackberry juice four times a day.*

❯ Make Peace with Moo Juice

Lactose intolerance is caused by a deficiency of an enzyme that breaks down the sugar in milk. It's not a dangerous health condition, but it can be highly annoying if you love things like milk, ice cream, and cheese. Plus, avoiding dairy makes it harder to have enough calcium in your diet. In many supermarkets, you can buy lactose-free dairy products marketed under the Lactaid® label. Simpler yet, pick up some Lactaid drops or tablets (available over the counter at drugstores), and take a dose before downing your favorite dairy treats.

❯ Rev Up Your Circulation

Are your hands and feet always cold, no matter what season it is? Well, don't let that stop you from getting your share of outdoor exercise!

Soothe a Sour Stomach

Does it seem as though the roster of foods that trouble your tummy gets longer by the year? If so, here's a remarkable remedy you ought to know: Whenever you've overindulged, grate a raw potato, and squeeze it through cheesecloth into a bowl. Mix 1 tablespoon of the juice with ½ cup of warm water. Drink the potion slowly, and before you know it, you'll be feeling right as rain!

Tick-Tock
**TURN
BACK** the
CLOCK

Onion "tea" can send your blood flowing to those extremities and get you back in the swing of things: Boil four to six chopped, medium-size onions in a quart of water for 10 to 15 minutes. Strain out the cooked onions, and stir in 2 tablespoons of honey. Store the brew in the refrigerator, and drink one or two warmed-up cups each day. But if your circulation doesn't start improving within a couple of weeks, consult with your doctor. **Note:** *This bracing brew can help soothe the burning sensation of a urinary tract infection.*

Belly Up to the Juice Bar...

And head off or relieve a whole lot of health problems—major and minor. Here's a sampling of super powered juices and the fabulous, age-defying feats they can perform for you:

Cranberry juice. It's been shown to clear up urinary tract infections (UTIs), even in people with antibiotic-resistant strains of the bacteria. The recommended R_X: At the first sign of burning, start drinking 2 cups of unsweetened cranberry juice every hour.

Grape juice. Both the purple and red varieties contain many of the same heart-healthy chemicals found in red wine.

Orange juice. In addition to combating cold and flu viruses, good old O.J. delivers a potent load of the B vitamins that are necessary to keep both your heart and your brain in good working order.

Papaya juice. It's just the ticket for reducing heartburn, soothing indigestion, and clearing up gassiness and cramping. Just add 1 teaspoon of sugar and two pinches of cardamom to 1 cup of papaya juice, and drink it down.

Alleviate Arthritis Aches

Here's an ultra-simple way to ease the pain in your joints: Twice a day, mix 1/8 teaspoon of cayenne pepper in a glass of water or fruit juice, and drink up. The capsaicin in the pepper will block the debilitating pain. If you can't take the pepper's heat, get out of the kitchen, and head for the closest health-food store. Buy cayenne pepper capsules, and take two a day as recommended, washed down with either water or fruit juice.

CHOCOLATE-VINEGAR COOLER

For years, medical science has been singing the praises of dark chocolate for its ability to perform health-giving feats of all kinds. And balsamic vinegar is loaded with compounds that fight cancer, strengthen your immune system, and destroy the free radicals that can cause premature aging and hardening of the arteries. Put 'em together, and you've got one delicious powerhouse of a beverage!

¼ cup of balsamic vinegar

1 cup of dark-chocolate chips

Sparkling water

1–2 oz of vodka (optional)

Mix the vinegar and chocolate chips in a small saucepan, and warm the mix over medium heat until chocolate is melted. Then whisk the mixture until it's smooth. Put 2–3 tablespoons of the blend into each tall glass, mix it with sparkling water, and add ice. Add vodka to taste, if desired.

Yield: *4–6 servings*

Pomegranate juice. It helps keep your arteries clear by interfering with the process that makes cholesterol stick to the artery walls. Just one word of warning: Don't be taken in by any health claims on pomegranate soda pop labels. These beverages contain too little juice to do much of anything.

❯ Drink Green for Good Health

Like many other herbs, parsley makes a tea that's just right for performing a passel of youth-enhancing health-care feats. To make it, steep 1 teaspoon of dried or (preferably) 2 tablespoons of fresh parsley in 8 ounces of freshly boiled water for 10 minutes. When the tea is ready to drink, it'll be a vibrant green color. Strain it, and store it, covered, in the refrigerator. Then drink 3 or 4 cups of the tea each day, either cold or warmed up, to work any of these wonders:

- Detoxify your kidneys, liver, and bladder

- Eliminate kidney stones

- Reduce prostate swelling

- Relieve urinary tract infections

Note: *Consult with your doctor before you use parsley tea (or any homemade healer) to treat any of these conditions.*

CHAPTER 6

Look Your Best

Let's face it: No matter how hard you try to retain the dewy-fresh appearance you had in your youth, it isn't gonna happen. But armed with the helpful hints, timely tricks, and savvy solutions in this chapter, you can keep your face and entire body looking their best your whole life long. The secret lies in a combination of the healthy diet and lifestyle strategies we've been talking about throughout this book, along with some mighty maneuvers targeted specifically for your excellent exterior.

>>> PUT YOUR BEST FACE FORWARD

There's no getting around it: Day after day, your face is on full display for all the world (or at least all of your neighborhood) to see. So it only stands to reason that when you're fixin' to grow younger, this is the place to start!

> The Lowdown on Botox®

Since this wrinkle remover first appeared on the cosmetic scene in 1989, tens of millions of people have shelled out anywhere from a few hundred to a thousand dollars a pop for injections that temporarily erase facial lines without the dangers of plastic surgery. But are Botox and copycat products truly safe alternatives? Not by a long shot! In technical terms, Botox is a neurotoxin—a killer of nerve cells. It's made from the botulinum toxin, the same bacterium that causes botulism. Although it's lethal in large doses or when administered improperly, botulinum won't kill you in smaller

> "I'm tired of all this nonsense about beauty being only skin-deep. That's deep enough. What do you want—an adorable pancreas?"
>
> —Jean Kerr (1922–2003)

quantities, injected by an expert (preferably a cosmetic surgeon). It merely paralyzes the nerve endings in your face, immobilizing the muscles that make you frown, squint, or smile. Your face stays essentially frozen, so it's unable to create lines and crow's-feet. The results last for three to six months. Then you'll need another treatment to keep life's souvenirs at bay.

But the expense and pain are far from the only reasons to give Botox a pass. The fact is that regular users don't wind up looking younger at all. Instead, they often bear a striking resemblance to zombies in old-time horror movies.

Note: *The FDA has approved two other products, Dysport® and Xeomin®, that work the same way Botox does. But, like Kleenex® and Vaseline®, the Big B brand has become so familiar that it's almost universally used as a generic term.*

❯ Who Needs It?!

You say you'd just as soon not go through all that discomfort and potential danger for the sake of ditching a few signs of experience? I don't blame you! Fortunately, there are plenty of safer, cheaper, and longer-lasting ways to make your skin smoother and younger-looking—beginning with these simple ploys:

Use a cream or lotion that contains alpha-hydroxy acids (AHAs). These natural substances, which come from fruit, milk, and sugarcane, work their magic in two ways: They remove dead cells from the surface of your skin, and they boost the growth of collagen, which fills in wrinkles. **Note:** *Although AHAs are harmless, they can irritate your skin, so test the product on a small area. If it hasn't turned red by the next day, you're good to go.*

Hit high C. Pack your diet with fruits and vegetables that deliver megadoses of vitamin C and other antioxidants, and for good measure, use a face cream that contains at least 5 percent vitamin C. It boosts collagen production and, according to recent research, can help minimize signs of aging after just six months of use. (Coming up, you'll find scads of specific foods, a.k.a. nutraceuticals, that help nourish and rejuvenate your skin—from the outside *and* inside.)

Drink plenty of water. In addition to being essential for good health, a steady supply of H_2O flushes toxins from your skin cells and helps keep them plump and youthful.

Exercise for 20 to 30 minutes every day, or as close to it as you can (a brisk walk is perfect). It'll quickly send nourishing, beautifying blood and oxygen flowing to the capillaries in your face and throughout your body.

Quit smoking! It damages the capillaries in your skin, breaking down the collagen and elastin that are vital to its structure. This is why smokers get wrinkles years before nonsmokers do.

Go easy on the booze. It's true that moderate drinking can boost your health, but overdoing it can age you fast. (See Chapter 1 for tips on tossing tobacco and trimming your alcohol consumption.)

Seek a Super Serum

Anti-wrinkle serums are the latest "miracle" products on the grow-younger scene. They're meant to be used in conjunction with moisturizing creams or lotions. As you might expect, brands vary widely in price and effectiveness, but here's the shocker: You don't always get what you pay for. Several websites rate serums according to the safety of their ingredients, as well as their ability to improve skin firmness and texture, reduce wrinkles, and stimulate collagen production—and some of the most expensive brands rank low on the lists. Conversely, some moderately priced formulas earn top marks in every category. Your best bet: In addition to checking product ratings online, get firsthand recommendations from friends and dermatologists.

Tick-Tock
TURN BACK the CLOCK

▶ 3 Secrets to Conquering Crow's-Feet

Everyone gets these eye wrinkles eventually. You can delay their onset and keep their visibility to a minimum. Here's your three-part plan:

1. Don't squint. Like any other repetitive facial movement, squinting overworks the relevant muscles and makes grooves below your skin's surface. Eventually those unseen grooves become full-fledged wrinkles. So if you have to squint to see the words on the page or the smartphone screen in front of you, get reading glasses—*now!*

2. Don't rub your eyes. Consistently rubbing that thin, tender skin will also make it crinkle years before its time. It's human instinct to rub your eyes when you feel tired, or when your peepers are dry, itchy, or irritated. But do your best to resist the impulse. You'll find plenty of skin-friendlier ways to baby your sore orbs coming up.

3. Never tug or rub at your skin when you apply or remove eye cosmetics. The pressure will cause the collagen to break down, leading to puffiness, broken blood vessels, and wrinkles. Instead, always tap eye cream gently onto your skin with your ring finger (don't rub it in!), and make sure to use an eyeliner that glides on smoothly (with no tugging required). The best way to take off stubborn makeup is to apply a bit of remover with a cotton swab, give it a few seconds to dissolve, and then wipe it off.

❯ Soothe Your Achin' Eyes

Eyes that are tired, strained, itchy, or sore all but cry out to be rubbed. Well, don't do it! If you do, you're begging for wrinkles (see "3 Secrets to Conquering Crow's-Feet," at left). Instead, reach for one of these gentler remedies:

- Put a few drops of sterile saline solution in each eye.
- Lay a cold, wet tea bag over each closed orb, lie down, and relax for half an hour or so. (Green, black, and chamomile versions all work like magic.)
- Soak two small cotton pads in witch hazel, and put one over each closed eye. Lie back and relax for about 10 minutes.

Whichever fix-it method you choose, it should leave you bright-eyed and ready for action.

❯ Bag the Bags

When aging trouble strikes in the form of dark circles and sagging skin, don't just stand there. Tighten your skin with one of these kitchen-counter cures:

Cut two thick slices from a peeled avocado, lie down, and lay a wedge under each eye. Leave the fruit in place for about 20 minutes, then rinse off the residue.

Grind three or four shelled pistachios in a food processor or coffee grinder, and mix the powder with 1 teaspoon of whole milk. Gently dab the mixture onto the skin around your eyes. Leave it on for 30 minutes and wash it off with lukewarm water.

Lighten Up!

Has your under-eye area gotten so dark that you refuse to leave the house without wearing concealer? Well, here's a remedy that may set you free from makeup prison: Blend a small handful of fresh parsley and 2 tablespoons of plain yogurt in a blender or food processor until you have a creamy paste. Apply it generously (and gently) to the skin under your eyes. Lie back and relax for 20 minutes or so, and then rinse the mixture off with lukewarm water. Treat yourself to this restful routine twice a week. After four or five treatments, you should start to see your skin getting lighter and brighter.

Dab unsweetened 100 percent pineapple juice onto your under-eye area. Wait for 20 minutes, and rinse with lukewarm water.

Repeat your remedy of choice once a day until your droopy skin has gone to the lost-baggage area. Be sure not to get any of these treatments in your eyes. **Note:** *These don't work overnight, so don't give up too soon!*

MIND OVER MYTH

MYTH: If your mother has (or had) lots of wrinkles and age spots, you'll get them, too. Or vice versa: If her skin was smooth and clear her whole life, you can rest easy.

REALITY: Your genes play a small role in how your skin ages, but for the most part, you call the shots. The way you care for your skin and your body in general—such as your diet, exercise, and basic lifestyle habits—is what really determines how long and to what degree your skin retains its youthful appearance. For example, if you've spent countless hours baking in the summer sun, you can bet your bikini bottom that you'll pay the price in the form of alligator skin. If your mother smoked and you've never acquired the nasty habit, it's highly likely that your body's outer covering will stay younger-looking than hers did.

❯ Thicken Lashes and Brows

As you age, your eyelashes naturally become thinner. To make them thicker and fuller again, just rub a little castor oil over the base of your lashes before bed. It'll prevent thinning and promote rapid growth of the hair. To thicken your eyebrows—whether they've become naturally sparse over time, or you've plucked them more thoroughly than you'd intended to—wipe a little castor oil over your brow line each night.

❯ Screen Out Wrinkles

We hear it often, but it bears repeating: Always apply sunscreen to exposed skin before you go outdoors. But when you do, keep these three guidelines in mind:

- For optimal protection, choose a product with a sun protection factor (SPF) that's between 30 and 50.

- Always buy sunscreen labeled "full-spectrum," which means it's been proven to protect against both UVB rays, which burn your skin and increase your risk for skin cancer, and UVA rays, which damage collagen and accelerate the aging process.

• Bypass chemical-based sunscreens whenever possible. Avoid any that contain oxybenzone, retinyl palmitate, or parabens (these generally appear on ingredient lists last; look for methylparaben, propylparaben, and/or butylparaben). The jury is still out on how dangerous these substances are, but why take any chances?

▶ 5 Reasons to Give Stress the Boot...

And put the bloom back in your cheeks. Stress ranks right up there with smoking and obesity as a major cause of health problems. It can also destroy your youthful good looks. Consider this handful of ways that stress can make a royal mess of your complexion:

1. It can bring on blemishes. Overproduction of the stress hormone cortisol causes acne and similar skin flare-ups (yes, at any age) by hindering your body's ability to regulate inflammation.

2. It causes wrinkles. Cortisol makes your blood sugar levels spike, and those excess sugar molecules can bond to the proteins in your skin's collagen fibers, causing them to harden and crack. The result: loose skin and deep (or deeper) wrinkles.

3. It cuts collagen production. Increased levels of the stress hormone epinephrine constrict your blood vessels. This in turn reduces the flow of oxygen and nutrients that your skin needs to stay smooth and supple.

> ### *Rejuvenating Recipe*
> ### TUNA SALAD SANDWICHES
>
> Tuna, whole-grain breads, and avocados all rank high on lists of stress-relieving foods. Try this quick and easy twist on a classic lunchtime treat.
>
> 1 can (12 oz.) of tuna, drained and flaked*
> 1 avocado, mashed
> 4 tbsp. of mayonnaise
> 1 hard-boiled egg, mashed
> Freshly ground pepper to taste
> 4 slices of whole-grain bread
> Cheese slices (optional)
>
> Mix the first five ingredients together. Cover bread slices with your choice of cheese, if desired, and top each one with half of the tuna mixture and enjoy!
> *Tuna packed in olive oil is best.*
> **Yield:** *2 servings*

4. It dries out your skin. Stress disrupts your skin's ability to retain moisture—it's as simple as that.

5. It encourages poor skin care. After a long, hectic day "riding" on the 21st Century Unlimited, it's all too easy to fall into bed without even removing your makeup, much less taking the time to tone and moisturize your skin.

So don't just sit there watching the years pile up! Read and heed the stress-busting tips and tricks in Chapter 4.

❯ Wash with Care

Few things feel more invigorating than a freshly washed face. But unfortunately, tap water and many commercial soaps can strip your skin of moisture and the natural oils that guard against wrinkles. So, unless your "mug" has gotten dirty, don't wash it more than twice a day. And whenever you do the job, always use a mild soap or cleanser that contains natural moisturizers (goat's milk and olive oil are two big winners). Or opt for one of the dandy DIY cleansing formulas coming up.

❯ Power Up Your Cleanser

If you prefer to use a commercial cleansing cream, give it some real—but gentle—razzmatazz with one of these amazing add-ins:

Laugh and Look Younger

Science has proven beyond a shadow of a doubt that laughing on a regular basis delivers benefits galore for your physical and mental health (see "Laughter Really *Is* the Best Medicine" on page 122). Well, it can also shave years from your appearance. It works in two ways. A hearty laugh increases your intake of oxygen-rich air, which triggers your brain to release more stress-busting endorphins—and chronic stress can add years to your appearance (see "5 Reasons to Give Stress the Boot..." on page 197). The same ramped-up blood flow that relaxes tense muscles also makes your skin more radiant and younger-looking.

Tick-Tock
TURN BACK the **CLOCK**

Oatmeal + cornmeal. Blend ½ cup of uncooked oatmeal and 1 tablespoon of cornmeal in a food processor until you get a fine powder, and store it in an airtight container. Two or three times a week, add ½ teaspoon of the combo to your favorite cleanser. It'll help even out your skin tone, diminish fine lines, and make your complexion gleam like the sun!

Avocado pit powder. Slice open three or four fresh avocados, remove their pits, and place the pits in a heavy-duty plastic bag. Smash them with a hammer until the pieces are about the size of green peas. Spread the little chunks out on a baking sheet to dry for one or two days. Then grind them with a food processor into a powder that's about the consistency of ground coffee. Again, spread them out to dry. After a few days, store them in an airtight container (a clamp-top canning jar is perfect). When you wash your face, add a teaspoon of the ground pits to your favorite liquid soap for a fantastic finish.

Baking soda + water. Keep a jar of baking soda by your bathroom sink. Then, after you wash your face, mix 3 parts soda to 1 part water, and gently massage the mixture into your damp skin. Rinse with cool water, and pat dry. It'll lift out the traces of oil, dirt, and makeup that even the best cleansers can leave behind.

Fountain of Youth
NOURISHING FACIAL SCRUB

To deep-cleanse, soften, and liven up dry, mature skin, use this gentle formula once a week.

- **6 oz. of plain whole-milk yogurt**
- **¼ cup of ground uncooked oatmeal***
- **2 tsp. of raw honey**
- **1 tsp. of lemon or orange juice**

Mix all of the ingredients together in a bowl. Massage the mixture onto your freshly washed face and neck using small circular motions. Let it dry, and rinse it off with warm water. Pat dry, and follow up with your usual moisturizer.

* *Use a coffee grinder, blender, or food processor.*

▶ A Trio of Triple-Threat Cleansers

There are some excellent all-natural facial cleansers on the market. But these DIY versions will clean, nourish, and rejuvenate your skin as well as any of their commercial counterparts—at a fraction of the cost.

1. Mash two or three blackberries in a bowl, and mix in 2 tablespoons of plain yogurt and 1 teaspoon of distilled rose water. Massage the mixture into your skin for about 30 seconds. Rinse with cool water, and moisturize.

2. Mix the freshly squeezed juice of half an orange with enough cornmeal to make a paste (about ¼ cup should do the trick). Massage it onto your face and neck for three minutes and rinse it off with warm water. Follow up with your usual moisturizer.

3. Bring ½ cup of water to a rolling boil, pour it into a heat-proof bowl, and add two green-tea bags. Let them steep until the water is cool to the touch. Then stir in 3 tablespoons of sugar. Saturate a clean washcloth with the solution, and massage your skin using small circular motions. Rinse thoroughly with lukewarm water, and apply a moisturizer. Do this once a week to keep your skin clear, glowing, and younger-looking.

▶ Tone, Don't Dry

Toners are invaluable for removing excess cold cream or cleansers from

---

Hate Turns You into a Hag

Just as laughter and a sunny disposition can make you look years younger than you really are, the opposite is also true: Harboring negative emotions such as hate, vindictiveness, and jealousy takes a major toll on your looks as well as your health. Don't get me wrong! If someone treats you badly or a relationship breaks up in a nasty, or even violent, way, you don't have to pretend that everything's fine. But for the sake of your looks, as well as your physical and mental health, it's vital that you learn to let go of the anger raging inside, stop playing the blame game, and focus on the positive facets of your life. So do what it takes, whether it's joining a support group, getting professional help, seeking spiritual counseling, or all of the above. In the meantime, see Chapter 4 for guaranteed ways to lift your spirits and ease the stress your bad experience has caused.

your face. Unfortunately, many commercial toners, which are generally alcohol-based, can be extremely drying to your skin—and everyone's skin grows drier as it ages. Enter these much gentler, all-natural alternatives:

Honey-mint. Mix 1 tablespoon of honey in ¼ cup of hot water, and stir in ¼ cup of apple cider vinegar. Then add ½ cup of peppermint infusion to the container, and mix thoroughly. Pour the blend into a bottle with a tight-fitting cap. Store it at room temperature, and use it as you would any other toner, shaking occasionally between uses. **Note:** *To make peppermint infusion, cover 2 heaping tablespoons of peppermint leaves (fresh or dried) with 1 cup of freshly boiled water, cover the container, and steep for 15 minutes. Strain the liquid, and use ½ cup of it for the toner.*

Watermelon. Mix 1 tablespoon of vodka and 2 tablespoons each of fresh watermelon juice, witch hazel, and distilled water in a bowl, and pour the potion into a clean, capped glass bottle. **Note:** *To make fresh watermelon juice, liquefy ¼ cup of melon chunks in a blender and strain out the solids.*

Witch hazel and company. Mix ½ cup each of witch hazel and water, and 4 tablespoons each of aloe vera gel, rose water, and glycerin, in a bottle with a tight-fitting cap. Store it at room temperature, shaking it occasionally and before each use.

In each case, after washing with your usual cleanser, apply the toner to your face and neck with a clean cotton pad. Follow up with your favorite moisturizer. That's all there is to it!

Centenarian SECRETS 100

This ultra-simple DIY cream can perform almost miraculous results on mature, extra-dry skin. To make it, mix together the contents of a 13-ounce jar of petroleum jelly, a 15-ounce bottle of baby lotion (not oil), and a 16-ounce jar of vitamin E cream in a large bowl. (If you like, nuke the jelly in the microwave for a few seconds to soften it up.) The texture of the finished product should be somewhere between that of whipped topping and whipped butter. Store it at room temperature in a widemouthed, lidded container, and use it as you would any other cream. You should start seeing softer, more radiant skin almost immediately.

❯ Cleanse, Tone, *and* Moisturize!

When it comes to time- and money-saving beauty treatments, this triple-threat, anti-aging mask is the berries. Mash four medium-size ripe strawberries, and puree them in a blender or food processor with 1 tablespoon each of heavy cream and organic honey. (You'll want to sneak a lick, but hold off! You can always make another batch for eating later.) Spread the mixture on your face and neck, keeping it away from your eyes. Wait 10 minutes, rinse with lukewarm water, and pat dry.

❯ Smooth Wrinkles

You don't need an expensive wrinkle-fighting cream to "iron out" your signs of experience. This trio of anti-aging treatments works just as well as any of them—if not better. The formulas range from simple to simplest:

- Simple: Mix 1 cup of milk, 2 tablespoons of lemon juice, and 1 tablespoon of brandy in a medium-size pan. Bring the combo to a boil, then remove the pan from the heat. When the mixture has cooled down to room temperature, gently apply the solution to your crinkly lines. Let it dry thoroughly, then rinse your face with lukewarm water.

- Simpler: Combine 2 tablespoons of heavy cream, 1 tablespoon of honey, and the contents of one vitamin E capsule until the mixture has a smooth, creamy consistency. Spread it onto your face and neck, and leave it in place for 15 to 20 minutes. Then rinse it off with lukewarm water.

- Simplest: Smooth a dollop of honey over your whole face, and leave it on for 20 minutes (or longer if you'd like). Then rinse the mask off with warm water, and pat dry.

You can either choose the routine you like the best and stick with it, or alternate treatments, based on the amount of available time you have or the mood you're in. In any case, repeat the process every week or so to keep your skin youthful and vibrant.

Mind Your Makeup

Believe it or not, your makeup routine may be making you look older, not younger. That's because, no matter how much TLC you give your skin, it gets drier and thinner with age. So the same products that gave you a healthy glow a few years ago could—and probably do—make you look quite matronly today. According to skin-care gurus, if you're old enough to have laugh lines, this is your best plan of action:

Prime before you "paint." Apply your moisturizer, then top it with a high-quality primer to fill in small wrinkles. Follow up with a light liquid foundation for additional skin-plumping moisture. For best results, tap it on gently with a sponge rather than rubbing it on.

Direct eyes to your eyes. As you age, your eyelids tend to droop. There's nothing you can do about that, but you can divert attention away from your lids toward your eyes. Apply eyeliner in a thin streak along the line where your lashes begin—top and bottom. This will enhance the shape of your eyes and make your lashes appear thicker. For good measure, use eye shadow that's a natural shade, and apply it with a light touch.

Enhance your eyebrows. They're important because they frame your face, but with each passing year, they tend to grow thinner and grayer. The easy solution: Draw them back on using eyebrow pencil that complements your hair color, then dab on powder to help the pencil stay put. Whatever you do, don't have your brows permanently tattooed—both *Consumer Reports* and the Food and Drug Administration (FDA) have raised serious safety concerns about this invasive (and painful) procedure.

Give 'em lip service. Lipstick (like any other cream) makes a beeline for low spaces—in this case, the lines around your lips. To keep the color in place, first coat your lips with moisturizer, followed by foundation. Next, line your lips with pencil and fill them in. Finally, brush on a lip-plumping lipstick in a color that's attractive but not over-the-top bright.

Don't clown around. Applying flattering makeup demands precision. If you don't see as well as you used to, do yourself a favor and invest in a top-notch magnifying mirror. Otherwise, you could wind up looking like Clarabel the Clown.

>>> KEEP YOUR BODY BEAUTIFUL

Just like your face, the rest of your body can look years younger than it really is. All it takes is a few simple strategies—along with some dynamic DIY formulas—that are specially geared to slowing down the sands of time.

> Scrub-a-Dub-Dub

Store cosmetic counters are filled with youth-enhancing body scrubs that cost an arm and a leg—and contain chemicals that you can't even pronounce, much less recall from high school chemistry class. So give 'em a pass, and make your own. Here are two of the best:

- Put a peeled and seeded mango into a blender with ½ cup of sugar, 2 tablespoons of whole milk, and 1 tablespoon of honey. Blend thoroughly, pour the mixture into a shatterproof bowl, step into the shower, and rub the scrub vigorously all over your body. Rinse with warm water, followed by cold water.

- Melt ½ cup of coconut oil over very low heat, then pour it over 1 cup of brown sugar or coarse salt (whichever you have on hand), and mix thoroughly. If you like, stir in 5 drops of pure vanilla extract or your favorite essential oil. To use, massage the mixture into your skin from neck to toes, then rinse it off with warm water.

> **Middle age is when your classmates are so gray and wrinkled and bald they don't recognize you.**
> —Bennett Cerf
> (1898–1971)

Whichever scrub you use, after rinsing, pat dry and follow up with your favorite body lotion.

> An A-Peeling Body Scrub

There's no doubt about it: Sugar- and salt-based body scrubs are effective, but when you don't have time to put one together—or you just don't feel inclined to slather on a grainy, potentially messy concoction—grab an orange. Peel it, and wrap the rind in a large piece of gauze or cheesecloth. Then hop into the shower, and rub the scrubber all over your body. The acid and vitamin C in the peel will firm your skin, help even out its tone, and refresh you from head to toe.

❯ Post-Sun Softener

Even if you don't burn, a day (or even a few hours) in the sun can leave your skin dry and parched— thereby hastening the aging process. This powerful but oh-so-gentle spray will solve that problem in a hurry. To make it, follow this ultra-easy three-step process:

Gather the goods. You'll need a 4-ounce spray bottle plus these ingredients: 3 tablespoons of rose water, 2 tablespoons of aloe vera gel (preferably organic), ½ tablespoon of apple cider vinegar, 1 teaspoon of glycerin, 5 drops of peppermint oil, and distilled water. (Feel free to double the recipe—in which case, of course, you'll need two 4-ounce spray bottles or a single 8-ounce version.)

Mix the first five ingredients in the bottle(s), and shake hard until the aloe is thoroughly blended

---

Fountain of Youth
BEAUTIFYING BODY CLEANSER

Ever since the days of ancient Egypt, milk has played a key role in skin care. This vinegar-powered dairy delight will leave your skin luxuriously soft, clean, and younger-looking (and feeling).

- ½ cucumber, scrubbed but not peeled, and diced
- ½ lemon, peeled and seeded, and diced
- ¼ russet potato, scrubbed but not peeled, and diced
- ¼ cup of baking soda
- 2 tbsp. of chopped strawberries
- 2 tbsp. of whole milk
- 2 tsp. of apple cider vinegar

Mix ingredients in a blender on medium-high speed for 60 seconds, or until smooth. Moisten your skin with warm water, and massage the mixture all over your body— but not your face. Rinse with warm, then cool, water. Cover any leftover cleanser, and pop it into the refrigerator, where it'll keep for two days.

in (this may take several minutes). Fill the balance of the bottle(s) with distilled water.

Store the potion in the refrigerator. This is essential because the all-natural formula contains no preservatives. Plus, the chilled fluid will feel cool and refreshing on your hot, scratchy skin.

Immediately following your time in the sun, spray the mixture on all exposed areas, and let it air-dry before covering your skin. **Note:** *In a pinch, you can substitute distilled water for the rose water, but try not to because rose water is much more effective at soothing irritated skin.*

❯ Lovely Lavender Bath Vinegar

For centuries, herbalists have touted the relaxing, skin-toning, youth-enhancing effects of aromatic, floral bath vinegars. This is one of the best: Mix 1 cup of distilled water, 1 cup of white vinegar, and ¾ cup of fresh lavender flowers in a glass jar with a tight-fitting lid. Shake the jar, and store it in a cool, dark place for 30 days, shaking it every week or so. When the time's up, give the jar a final shake, strain out the flowers, and pour the floral vinegar into a decorative glass bottle. Use ½ cup or so for each tub of water (the temperature is your call). Store the remaining blend, with the lid tightly closed, at room temperature; it will keep for two to six months.

Soak Your Cares Away...

And make your skin look years younger at the same time. How? Just pour 4 cups of red wine and 1 cup of raw honey into your bathtub as you fill it with very warm (but not burning hot!) water. Settle in and relax for 20 to 30 minutes. The warm, steamy air will open your pores so they can absorb the wine's beautifying antioxidants and complex amino acids. The honey, a powerful humectant, will help your skin retain moisture. When you're done soaking, rinse off with clear water, and pat dry. **Note:** *Don't waste good wine on this venture! Instead, buy the cheapest red vino you can find, or collect leftovers until you have enough for a bath.*

Tick-Tock **TURN BACK** the **CLOCK**

❯ Land of Milk and Honey

Ever since Cleopatra's day, women have been tapping into the beautifying powers of milk and honey. Here are two ways you can put them to work here in the 21st century:

- Pour 1 to 2 cups of whole milk and ½ cup of raw honey under warm water as it flows from the spigot into your bathtub. Swish the water around with your hand to mix the ingredients, and settle in. Close your eyes, relax, and think lovely thoughts for about 20 minutes. Then step out, pat dry, and apply your usual moisturizer. **Note:** *To get the maximum softening and exfoliating effects, lightly brush your skin in circular motions with a dry brush before you get into the tub.*

- Mix equal parts of honey and whole milk; starting at your feet, massage the lotion into your thirsty skin. Then step into the shower and rinse yourself off.

Note: *Don't use reduced-fat milk for these or any other skin-softening routines. This job demands the heavy-hitting power of full-strength moo juice.*

❯ 5-Step DIY Body Butter

Rejuvenate and soften your skin from your neck to your toes with the magic-making combo of coconut oil and honey. It's a treat worthy of

---

MIND OVER MYTH

MYTH: Cellulite is simply an annoying cosmetic issue.

REALITY: Those unattractive pockets of fat could indicate that your lymphatic system is not functioning at its peak—and that lackadaisical performance will hinder your body's ability to eliminate toxins and other waste products. It can also throw your immune system out of whack, leaving you wide open to infectious diseases. So take those ugly patches as a wake-up call, and get your act together. Start by revamping your diet and getting regular, moderate exercise. You'll reenergize your lymphatic system—and also bid "Good riddance!" to that nasty-looking skin. And to speed up the exit process, use one or all of the simple strategies in "So Long, Cellulite!" (see page 208). **Note:** *Whatever you do, steer clear of trendy and potentially dangerous detox diets!*

a fancy spa—for a fraction of the cost. Here's the simple five-step routine:

1. Round up 2 tablespoons of extra virgin coconut oil, 1 tablespoon of raw honey, 2 drops of pure vanilla extract or peppermint oil (optional), a small bowl, and enough soft cotton bath towels to cover your body.

2. Mix all of the ingredients together in the bowl. (If necessary, heat the coconut oil on the stove or in the microwave until it's soft enough to blend with the honey.)

3. Spread the towels out in your bathtub, and dampen them with water that's as hot as your comfort range will allow.

4. Rub the butter all over your body, settle into the tub, and wrap yourself in the hot towels. Then lie back and relax until the towels have cooled to room temperature.

5. Rinse yourself off, pat dry, and smooth coconut oil (by itself) onto your skin to seal in the moisture.

❯ So Long, Cellulite!

In addition to healthy eating habits and regular exercise, external treatments can be highly effective at removing cellulite. You could fork out big bucks for an anti-cellulite wrap at a fancy spa. Or you could whip up one of these highly effective alternatives for a tiny fraction of the cost:

Scrub it away. Mix 2 teaspoons of freshly grated, peeled ginger with ½ cup of sugar, ¼ cup of olive oil, and the zest of one lemon in a shatterproof bowl. In the shower or bath, gather up handfuls of the mixture, and scrub your body lightly. Rinse well, and pat dry.

Massage it off. In a blender or food processor, blend 1 cup of strawberries with 1 tablespoon of ground coffee to make a paste. Massage the mixture vigorously into your skin using circular motions, then immediately rinse it off.

Wrap it up. Mix ½ cup of grapefruit juice and 2 teaspoons of dried thyme with 1 cup of corn oil. Massage the mixture into your thighs, hips, and buttocks. Cover the area with plastic wrap, and hold a heating pad over each body part for five minutes.

Flush it out. Mix 2 tablespoons of fresh, minced ginger with 1 cup of Epsom salts and 4 tablespoons of mustard powder. Pour 2 tablespoons of the combo into a tub of hot water. Swirl the mixture around until it dissolves, then settle in and soak for 15 to 30 minutes. Follow up with a tall, cool glass of water to help flush out the toxins from your body. Store the remaining mixture in a tightly closed glass jar. **Note:** *Don't rush as you get out of the tub—your body expends a lot of energy in the detoxifying process.*

Repeat your chosen strategy once a week. After several treatments, you should start to see an improvement.

❯ Put on Your Lime and Go to Sleep

Lime and milk team up in an overnight whole-body moisturizer that can't be beat. Just before you go to bed at night, bring 1 cup of milk to a boil, and mix in 1 teaspoon of glycerin and the freshly squeezed juice of one lime. Let the mixture cool to room temperature, then massage it into your face, hands, and feet, and hop under the covers. Store any extra moisturizer, tightly covered, in the refrigerator, and use it within a week or so.

Dress for Lifetime Success

Once you've passed your 40th birthday, the key to retaining a youthful appearance is to edit out the practices that make you look like a 20-something wannabe. In particular, *don't*:

- Put on too much makeup or lipstick
- Overprocess or overstyle your hair
- Grow your nails too long
- Overload yourself with jewelry and other accessories
- Adopt overly young-looking trends

Accentuate the Positive

The secret to looking classy and elegant at any age is to play up your best assets and downplay the parts of your body that are less attractive. For example, if your upper arms are slender and toned, by all means say yes to sleeveless or cap-sleeved dresses and blouses. On the other hand, if your arms are jiggly or on the heavy side, stick with long or three-quarter sleeves.

Likewise, if you have a slender waist and hips, highlight your figure with eye-catching belts or dresses that are nipped in at the waist. To help camouflage excess weight, choose clothes with a trim but easy fit. Garments that are either baggy or snug will exaggerate your plumpness. In particular, steer clear of the currently trendy skintight stretch pants, as well as anything in a big, bold print.

Put Yourself in the Driver's Seat

Forget websites that try to tell you what clothes and accessories you should buy and how celebrities your age are dressing this year. Wear what makes you happy, is both comfortable and attractive, and fits your lifestyle. After all, a woman who works in an upscale clothing boutique needs an entirely different kind of wardrobe than, let's say, a first-grade teacher, a corporate executive, or the proprietor of a home-based Internet business. But you can't go wrong if you follow these guidelines:

- Know your likes and dislikes, and shop accordingly.
- Never buy—or wear—anything that doesn't fit well.
- Before you walk out of a clothing store with any purchase, check yourself out in a three-way mirror.

⟩⟩ TERRIFIC TREATS FOR HANDS & FEET

It's often said that a woman's hands reveal her age even more than her face does. The same goes for your feet when you take your shoes off. Fortunately, the age you reveal doesn't have to match up with the numbers on your birth certificate. A little timely TLC can help your appendages "lie" like crazy!

⟩ 4 Fine Solutions to Fade Dark Spots

Many middle-aged people, especially those with fair skin, develop large, flat brown marks (a.k.a. age or liver spots) on their hands and faces. These may be caused by the sun or by a nutritional deficiency. In most cases, the spots are perfectly harmless. But who needs the unsightly things? Here's a quartet of ways to make 'em vamoose:

1. Mix 1 tablespoon of fresh onion juice with 2 teaspoons of apple cider vinegar. Massage the mixture into the discolored areas twice a day until you no longer see spots before your eyes.

2. Finely grate a 4-inch piece of fresh horseradish, and mix the pieces with ¼ cup of apple cider vinegar in a clean, lidded jar. Let the mixture sit for two weeks, but shake the jar daily. Strain the liquid into a second jar, and store it in the refrigerator. Then, three times a day, rub the potion into your problem areas with a cotton ball or swab.

3. Dissolve a pinch of sugar in 2 tablespoons of lemon juice, and rub the mixture onto each blotch with a cotton ball or swab. Repeat the procedure every day or two until the spots have lightened up.

4. Once a day, mix 1 teaspoon of honey with 1 teaspoon of plain yogurt. Apply the mixture to the problem areas, and let it dry. Wait another 30 minutes, and

> " As a graduate of the Zsa Zsa Gabor School of Creative Mathematics, I honestly do not know how old I am.
> —Erma Bombeck (1927–1996) "

wash it off. Besides bleaching the marks, it will also soften your skin.

Note: *In any case, it may be a few months before you start to see results, but be patient: It took years for the pigment to build up, so you can't expect it to vanish overnight!*

❯ Hand It to Buttermilk

The next time your hands need some TLC, try this nourishing routine: Mix ¼ cup of buttermilk and ½ cup of dry milk to form a smooth paste. Using a soft paint-brush or pastry brush, spread an even layer of the mixture onto each hand. Leave it on for 20 minutes, or until it's dried. Rinse with cool water, and pat dry. Your skin should be soft and smooth, with a healthy, youthful glow.

❯ Smooth Moves for Rough Skin

It doesn't take much for hardworking (or hard-playing) hands and feet to become overly rough, dry, and old-looking. Either of these two fabulous formulas can bring the youthful glow back to your skin—fast.

Formula #1. Mix the juice of half a lemon, ½ cup of brown or raw sugar, and 2 tablespoons of almond oil in a bowl. If you like, add a few drops of essential oil (lavender, mint, and rosemary are good choices).

Formula #2. Pulverize ¼ cup of freshly grated ginger in a blender or food processor. Then mix it with ½ cup of lukewarm olive oil, ½ cup of salt, and the juice of two limes to make a soft, gritty paste.

To use either formula, massage the mixture into your skin with gentle circular motions. Then rinse it off with warm water, and follow up by slathering on your favorite body lotion to seal in the moisture.

Centenarian SECRETS 100

This old-time secret for soothing raw, chapped hands works just as well today as it did in the days of yore: Just mix some ultra-rich hand cream with an equal amount of vinegar (any kind will do), and smooth it on your paws every time after washing them. Within days, your skin will be smooth and young-looking again.

› Intensive Care Treatments

You say your hands or feet are not just chapped—they're raw and sore as the dickens? Not to worry! Here are two treatments that can solve the problem in a flash:

- Mix 3 tablespoons of finely ground oatmeal, 2 tablespoons of rose water, and 2 teaspoons of almond oil in bowl, and nuke the mixture until it's warm (not hot). Spread the paste on your hands or feet, and cover them with plastic wrap. Leave the mask on until its cooled, then take off the wrap and rinse with warm water. Perform this routine as needed until your skin is no longer sore.

- Combine equal parts of petroleum jelly and sugar, and stir in a few drops of your favorite essential oil. Wipe the mixture generously onto your freshly washed hands or feet, and put on cotton gloves or socks. Wait 30 minutes, and then scrub the combo off with a pumice stone. Repeat the process every day until your skin is silky and pain-free.

› Give Your Rough Heels Some Skin

After you've made the Avocado Hand Treatment (at right), don't throw the peel away. Instead, scrape it clean of any remaining fruit, and sprinkle a few drops of lemon juice on the surface. Then rub it across each of your heels. It'll feel a little strange at first, but your dry skin will love it—guaranteed! (This trick works to soften up your knees and elbows too.)

Fountain of Youth

AVOCADO HAND TREATMENT

When work or play leaves you with chapped, old-looking, or sore hands, treat them to this super-soothing routine.

- ¼ avocado, peeled and pitted
- 1 egg white
- 2 tbsp. of uncooked oatmeal
- 1 tsp. of freshly squeezed lemon or lime juice

Mash the avocado in a bowl, add the remaining ingredients, and mix thoroughly. Rub the mixture into your skin, leave it on for 20 minutes, then rinse with warm water.

❯ Fill in the Cracks

Dry, cracked feet are no fun, and that's putting it mildly. Not only are they unsightly, but they can also be painful to walk on. Try this intensive overnight treatment for a simple solution:

Just before bedtime, whisk ¼ cup of extra virgin olive oil and ¼ cup of mild, unscented body lotion in a bowl, and heat it in the microwave for 15 to 20 seconds. (You want it to be pleasantly warm, but not hot.)

While the oil-lotion combo is heating, tear off two long sections of plastic wrap, and set them aside.

Apply a generous layer of the mixture to both feet, and cover them with plastic wrap to lock in the warmth and moisture.

Put on thick socks, and head off to dreamland. Come morning, remove the socks and plastic wrap.

❯ Preventive Maintenance

Once your feet are soft and crack-free, keep them that way by using a lotion made from 2 drops of essential oil (either lavender or lemon) per 1 tablespoon of extra virgin olive oil. Combine the oils in a sterilized bottle with a tight-fitting cap, and shake it until well combined. Store at room temperature, and shake the bottle before each use. Massage the lotion into your feet a few times a week, or as often as needed to maintain picture-perfect appendages.

❯ 3 Steps to Sandal Season

Keeping your feet young-looking and rarin' to be bare all through the warm-weather months is as easy as 1, 2, 3!

1. Mix 1 cup of sea salt, ¼ cup of coconut oil, ¼ cup of vitamin E oil, and 3 or 4 drops of essential oil (lavender, orange blossom, and rose are all excellent choices).

2. Massage a tablespoon or so of the mixture into each foot, then rinse with cool water.

3. Store the blend at room temperature in a jar with a tight-fitting lid, and use it as needed.

❯ Wintertime Foot Freshener

Your feet can develop unpleasant aromas at any time of the year, but they're at especially high risk when you wear boots all day, as many women do in the winter. That's when it pays to know this four-step trick:

- Mix 1 cup of coarse sea salt, ½ cup of minced fresh mint, 5 tablespoons of olive or coconut oil, and 1 tablespoon of cocoa powder.

- Soak your feet in a basin of warm water for 10 to 15 minutes.

- Starting at your toes, massage the mixture into your skin with your fingertips, making small circular motions. Pay special attention to your soles and any rough areas.

- Rinse thoroughly, and apply your favorite moisturizer.

Off with the Old...

Skin, that is. When your feet are showing signs of wear and tear, fill a pan or foot basin with 10 cups of hot water, and mix in the juice of two freshly squeezed lemons, 1 cup of apple cider vinegar, and ½ cup of sea salt. Soak your dogs for 15 minutes, pat dry, and use a pumice stone to slough off any dead or flaky skin. Then hop into the shower to rinse off the salad dressing aroma, and follow up with your favorite skin cream.

Tick-Tock TURN BACK the CLOCK

Olive Oil: A Solo Act

For centuries, women in the Mediterranean region have relied on extra virgin olive oil as the key—and often only—product in their beauty-care routines. It'll work just as well for you. Here's a sampling of possibilities:

Condition your hair. After shampooing, section your damp hair, and apply a light coat of oil from the roots to the ends. Then style your hair as usual. (This is an especially effective way to moisturize coarse gray hair and make it more manageable.)

Fade scars. Rub a thin film of oil onto the marks every day. With time they should vanish, or at least greatly diminish in appearance.

Gloss your lips. Put a dab of oil on your fingertip, and rub it across your lips to lock in the moisture and make them gleam.

Minimize wrinkles. Each night at bedtime, massage oil into the lined areas of your face and neck. In the morning, wash the oil off with lukewarm water, then splash your skin with cold water.

Moisturize daily. Use it as you would any other moisturizer. To avoid greasiness, smooth it on when your skin is damp, and blot the oil dry before you apply any makeup.

Remove eye makeup. Simply moisten a cotton pad or ball with oil, and gently rub it across your eyelids and lashes.

Shave clean, shave close. Wipe oil onto your legs and underarms, and have at it. For you guys, olive oil works just as well on your face, and it's healthier than shaving creams that contain alcohol and chemicals.

Shine your nails. Rub oil onto your nails and cuticles each night to keep your nails glossy and your cuticles healthy and pliable.

Soften your skin. Add a tablespoon or so of oil to your bathwater. It's the simplest all-over moisturizer you can find.

Banish acne. After washing your face with mild soap and hot water, apply a thin layer of olive oil, and let your skin absorb it—don't wash it off. Repeat the procedure three times a day, and within a week your skin should be smooth and clear. After that, use the treatment once a day to prevent further outbreaks.

▶▶ HAVE A GOOD-HAIR DAY—EVERY DAY!

Your crowning glory got its moniker for a reason. The hair on your head is probably your most noticeable feature—and the one that can announce your age more than any other part of your body. Armed with the tips in this section, you can make sure that "shout-out" is the lowest number possible.

▶ To Color or Not to Color?

That is the question every mature woman (and, it seems, quite a few men) must answer at some point. If you choose to celebrate your silver strands, go for it! But if you do decide to cover the gray, beauty experts caution that to look your best—and youngest—you should avoid making a drastic change. Instead, follow these three guidelines:

If you want to emulate someone else's hair color, make sure your role model is within 10 years of your age.

Don't make an abrupt switch from, let's say, brunette to blonde or vice versa. Rather, stay within two or three shades lighter or darker than the natural color you had in your younger days.

Include highlights to make the color look natural. An old-fashioned monotone will cover the gray all right, but it will make you look older—not younger. You can do this whether you choose to color your hair at home or have a pro do the job. **Note:** *Highlights can also add shine and sparkle to hair that's lost its youthful zip but hasn't yet gone gray.*

> " There is still no cure for the common birthday.
> —John Glenn (1921–2016) "

▶ The Long and Short of It

Contrary to what many women assume, the most flattering hair length depends on your height and the proportions of your face and body—not your age. If you're tall, you'll look fine with hair that's past your shoulders. If you're shorter, you're better off with a style that's no longer than shoulder length.

❯ Let's Face It

Just as your height helps determine your most flattering hair length, your best style depends on the shape and muscle tone of your face. My advice: Find a hairstylist who is especially skilled at working with women in your age group. But don't simply rely on an Internet search. When you see someone around your age who has a great hairstyle—even if you've never met her—be brazen: Ask who did her "do." Other good intel sources for expert hairstylists (and makeup artists) are the folks who work at high-end stores, such as Lord & Taylor, Nordstrom, and Saks Fifth Avenue.

MIND OVER MYTH

MYTH: Coloring your hair dries it out and damages the strands.

REALITY: Once upon a time that was the case, but most newer dye formulas actually deposit moisture and protein in your hair, making it both stronger and healthier than before. Since these ingredients work their magic only at the roots, you need to keep coloring the regrowth as it comes in. So if you opt to conceal the gray, don't procrastinate between cover-up sessions!

❯ About Layers and Bangs

These features can be effective when you want to modify the style of your hair without dramatically changing it or hacking a lot off. But if you're not careful, these seemingly minor tweaks can wind up adding years to your appearance—not subtracting them. Again, a top-notch hairstylist can help you make winning decisions, but here are a couple of pointers:

- Bangs. They're a surefire way to hide forehead wrinkles, but if you have a round face, forget bangs that hang straight down; instead they should be longer and swept to one side to counteract the roundness. If your face is long, give short bangs a shot.

- Layers. It is true that layering your hair can help soften your face, but only if the layers are brushed slightly back and up. If you keep your hair close to your face in an attempt to hide wrinkles, it will visually draw all your facial features down-ward—making you look older in the process.

> All-Natural Shampoos

Many commercial shampoos sport the word *natural* in big letters on the label, but when you read the fine print on the back, you usually see a bunch of ingredients that you can't even pronounce. These DIY versions come straight from Mother Nature herself, and are cheap too:

All-purpose shampoo.

Thoroughly mix 2 tablespoons of extra virgin olive oil, 1 table-spoon of lemon juice, 1 teaspoon of unfiltered apple cider vinegar, and 1 egg in a blender. Pour the mixture into a plastic bottle, and use it as you would any shampoo. **Note:** *This recipe must be made up just before you're ready to use it.*

Color-keeper shampoo. Mix 6 ounces of liquid castile soap, 1 teaspoon of melted coconut oil, and ½ teaspoon of avocado oil in a

---

Fountain of Youth
HAIR-GROWTH TONIC

It happens to most women at least once: You impulsively opt for a new short, perky hairstyle, only to find that it doesn't suit you at all. Well, don't fret. Your hair will grow back to a more flattering length, and this formula can help speed up the process.

- **1 ½ tbsp. of organic raw honey**
- **1 ½ tbsp. of plain yogurt**
- **1 tbsp. of coconut oil**
- **1 tsp. of extra virgin olive oil**

Mix all of the ingredients together in a small bowl. Gently brush your hair, then use your fingers to apply the mixture to your scalp, and work it through to your ends. Put on a shower cap, or cover your head with a plastic bag, and keep it on for at least 60 minutes. Then wash and condition your hair as usual. Repeat once a week or so until you're happy—or at least happier—with the length of your locks.

When your hair is so dry it feels like it's about to split all the way up the shafts, this sweet and pungent potion will replace the moisture in a flash. To make it, mix 2 tablespoons of garlic oil and 1 teaspoon of honey in a bowl, then beat in one egg yolk. Rub the mixture into your hair a small section at a time. Cover your head with a shower cap or a plastic bag, and wait 30 minutes. Rinse thoroughly, and shampoo. Bingo—lively, lovely looking locks.

plastic bottle with a flip spout (a pre-used shampoo or conditioner bottle is perfect).

Extra-gentle chamomile shampoo. Steep four chamomile tea bags in 1 ½ cups of just-boiled (not boiling!) water for 10 minutes. Remove the tea bags, add 4 tablespoons of pure soap flakes, and let the mixture stand until the soap softens, stirring occasionally. Add 1 ½ tablespoons of glycerin, stir to blend thoroughly, and pour it into a plastic bottle.

❯ 3 Ways to Get the Gunk Out

Over time, hair sprays, gels, and other styling products can build up in your hair, making it downright dull, drab, and old-looking. Here's a trio of tricks to rout that residue:

1. Mix equal parts vinegar and water in a spray bottle. After shampooing, spritz the mixture onto your hair, and massage it into your scalp. Let it sit for about three three minutes or so, and then rinse with clear water. You'll soon have soft, shiny, silky smooth hair that's easy to manage.

2. Massage ½ cup of plain yogurt into your damp hair, and leave it on for 20 minutes. Rinse it off with warm water, then with cool water. Follow up with your usual shampoo and conditioner.

3. Grate a medium-size carrot and massage the gratings through your hair. Wait 15 minutes, and rinse the carrot slaw out. (Either perform this maneuver over your kitchen garbage disposal, or cover your sink drain with a piece of screen or old panty hose so that the carrot pieces don't clog your plumbing.)

❯ The Perfect Pair for Your Hair

Forget about those commercial two-in-one products that shampoo and condition your hair in one step! Instead, do it yourself: Puree a peeled, diced cucumber and a peeled, sliced lemon in a blender or food processor. Strain out the seeds, wash your hair as usual with the dynamic duo, and rinse it out. The lemon cleans your tresses like nobody's business, while the cuke acts as a terrific conditioning agent.

❯ Beautiful Balancing Conditioner

The acids in tomatoes help balance the pH levels in your hair, thereby making your locks shinier and more manageable. To perform this balancing act, just mix 1 teaspoon of cornstarch into 1 cup of tomato juice, and comb the solution through your clean, wet hair. Leave it on for 10 minutes, and rinse well.

❯ Help for Harried Swimmers

When it comes to "hair pollution," styling products cannot hold a candle to the high doses of chlorine and other chemicals used in public swimming pools. That crud calls for more intensive treatment—like one of these two tough but gentle routines:

- If you're a blonde: Thoroughly mix ¼ cup of freshly squeezed lemon juice, 2 tablespoons of baking soda, and 1 teaspoon of mild

---

Keep the Bright Lights Shining

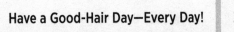

When you hair starts looking dingy, any of the tricks at left will bring back the youthful shine (see "3 Ways to Get the Gunk Out"). But why wait for the lights to dim? At least once a week, pour about 1 teaspoon of baking soda into the palm of your hand, and mix it with your regular shampoo. Then wash your hair as usual, and rinse thoroughly. Your tresses will keep their gleaming good looks no matter what styling products you use to arrange your "do." (This trick is ideal for color-treated hair.)

Tick-Tock TURN BACK the CLOCK

shampoo. Then wet your hair with water, and work the mixture thoroughly into your scalp and hair, clear down to the tips. Cover your locks with a shower cap or plastic bag, and go about your business for about half an hour. Rinse well, and shampoo as usual.

- If you're a brunette: Blend 1 egg, 2 tablespoons of extra virgin olive oil, and one-quarter of a peeled, chopped cucumber in a blender or food processor until you've got a rich, creamy consistency. Spread the mixture evenly through your hair, and leave it on for 15 minutes or so. Then rinse thoroughly and follow up with your usual shampoo.

Repeat as needed for ongoing damage control. The frequency will depend on how often you swim and how thoroughly you rinse your hair after each dip.

❯ Prevent Hair Loss...

Or at least slow it down. Even on the best-endowed heads, hair falls out and regrows constantly. But if you seem to be shedding more and growing less—which comes naturally as we age—try this easy remedy: Combine equal parts of olive oil and rosemary oil in a bottle, and shake to mix thoroughly. At bedtime, massage the mixture into your scalp, and cover it with a shower cap. In the morning, wash your hair with a gentle shampoo, and rinse with 1 tablespoon of apple cider vinegar mixed into 1 quart of warm water. Repeat this procedure each night for a few weeks. By that time, your hair income should exceed the outgo. **Note:** *Some people claim this routine will even work to stop male pattern baldness, but it's not guaranteed.*

A Rummy Good Keeper

Once you've got your full head of hair back, help keep those locks in place with this simple routine: Chop a medium-size onion and soak it overnight, peels and all, in an 8-ounce glass of dark rum (don't refrigerate it). Strain out the solids, and massage the liquid into your scalp. Then shampoo, condition, and style your hair as usual. Repeat the procedure every week or so, and your hair should stay well rooted.

▶ 5 Reasons for Excessive Hair Loss

While sparser hair growth is part and parcel of the aging process, if you're losing more than seems natural, the reason could be any of these:

1. Stress. Both chronic stress and specific stressful events, such as childbirth, surgery, or a death in the family, can trigger the loss of hair—sometimes as much as 70 percent of your crop. In nearly all cases, your mane will grow back once you've recovered from the experience. (See Chapter 4 for hints to help reduce stress.)

2. Hormonal disruptions. If your thyroid is either overactive or underactive, you could experience hair loss as a side effect. Also, an imbalance of male and female hormones (a.k.a. androgens and estrogens) can cause hair loss. In either case, once the problem is corrected, the shedding should stop.

3. Medications. Chemotherapy is notorious for making hair vanish, but it's not the only culprit. Some blood thinners, antidepressants, and drugs prescribed to combat arthritis, gout, high blood pressure, and high cholesterol can also trigger a major crop drop. So can high doses of vitamin A supplements. In this case, you need to consult your doctor to learn whether a change in meds might stop the shedding. (See Chapter 3 for safer, natural ways to combat chronic conditions of all kinds.)

4. Dietary deficiencies. Eating disorders, as well as too little iron, protein, and zinc, can take a major toll on your hair's health and staying power. Your simple mission: Follow the general Eat to Beat Aging guidelines in Chapter 5.

MIND OVER MYTH

MYTH: Stress and worry make your hair turn gray.

REALITY: While stress can make your hair fall out (see "5 Reasons for Excessive Hair Loss," at left), it can't be blamed for putting you on the fast-graying express. Pigment-producing cells called melanocytes are genetically programmed to stop manufacturing hair pigment when you reach a certain age, and there's not a blasted thing that your emotions have to do with it.

5. Diseases. Type 2 diabetes, as well as lupus and various other autoimmune disorders, can cause your strands to abandon ship. So if you experience excessive hair loss that you can't explain—and you haven't been diagnosed with any of those problems—see your doctor pronto.

❯ Brunettes, Take Note!

To put glistening highlights in your brown locks, boil a large unpeeled potato in a quart of water, then dip a pastry brush into the liquid, and saturate your hair. (Be careful not to get the spud water in your eyes!) Wait 30 minutes, then rinse with cool water. Repeat every two to three weeks to retain your "spud-tacular" new highlights.

❯ A Great Gray Cover-Up

No matter what your natural hair color is, this all-natural treatment can help conceal the encroaching silver strands in your hair without the time and expense of beauty shop visits. To make the potion, bring 2 cups of water to a boil, and add in a handful each of dried sage and rosemary. Reduce the heat, and let the mixture simmer for 30 minutes. Remove it from the stove, pour it into a container, and let it steep for several hours or (better yet) overnight. Strain out the herbs, massage the liquid into your hair, and let it air-dry. Then shampoo, condition, and style as usual. Repeat the procedure every three to five days.

Centenarian SECRETS 100

In recent years, beef has gotten a bum rap in certain circles—and, yes, in large quantities, it's far from the healthiest stuff you could put on your plate. But the fact is (as any nutritionist will tell you), beef is the most potent source of three nutrients that are essential for the health and appearance of your hair and nails—namely iron, protein, and zinc. So unless you're a dedicated vegetarian, don't hesitate to help yourself to a steak, chop, or burger every now and then. For a quick, easy hair (and nail) helper, see the Simple Sirloin Steaks recipe at right.

> Rev Up the Color

You say your hair hasn't turned gray yet, but the color is starting to turn dull and drab? No worries! There is a passel of simple, natural (and inexpensive) ways to make your tresses' tones richer and more radiant. Your best choice depends on your natural hair color.

Blonde or light brown. To put glistening highlights in your locks, steep 4 tablespoons of dried chamomile in 2 cups of just-boiled water for two hours, then strain out the solids. Shampoo and rinse as usual, then massage the tea through your hair.

Dark brown or black. Steep two black-tea bags in 2 cups of boiling water for 10 minutes. Let the tea cool to room temperature, and pour it over your wet, freshly washed hair, rubbing it through as you would with shampoo. Leave the rinse on for 10 minutes, then shampoo again, and apply your usual conditioner.

Medium brown. Mix ½ cup of plain yogurt, ½ cup of cocoa powder, 1 teaspoon of honey, and 1 teaspoon of apple cider vinegar to form a smooth paste. Apply the mixture to your freshly shampooed hair. Rinse after two or three minutes.

Reddish-brown. Steep a pinch of leek seeds (available in garden centers and online) in a cup of just-boiled water for 10 minutes. Strain out the seeds, and let the tea cool to room temperature. Shampoo, then pour the rinse through your hair.

Rejuvenating Recipe
SIMPLE SIRLOIN STEAKS

Fresh off the grill, this is one of the simplest and most delicious hair-pleasing treats you can eat.

½ cup of unsalted butter

2 tsp. of garlic powder

4 garlic cloves, minced

4 lbs. of top sirloin steaks

Salt and pepper to taste

Melt the butter in a small pan over medium-low heat, and stir in the garlic powder and garlic cloves. Sprinkle both sides of each steak with salt and pepper. Then grill them to your (and your dinner guests') desired degree of doneness. Brush the tops with the garlic butter, and serve.

Yield: *8 servings*

Red. In a blender or food processor, mix 3 tablespoons of plain yogurt, 2 tablespoons of honey, and three medium-size chopped carrots to get a coarse paste. After shampooing, work the mixture through your hair. Leave it on for one to two minutes, and then rinse it out. Follow up with your usual styling routine. **Note:** *If you want copper undertones, substitute ½ cup of cranberries for the carrots.*

⟩⟩⟩ YOUNGER-LOOKING NAILS—NOW

It's a fact: Ill-kempt fingernails can make even the most coddled hands look old and tired. The same goes for neglected toenails— you sure don't want to show 'em off when sandal season rolls around! In this section, you'll find plenty of pointers for keeping your nails as shipshape as your hands and feet.

⟩ 4 Formulas to Fortify Your Fingernails

All kinds of things, ranging from household cleaners to cold air, can draw moisture out of your fingernails, leaving them brittle and weak. Fortunately, any of these fabulous feats can put the moisture and strength back into them:

1. Add a finely minced garlic clove to a bottle of nail polish (either clear or your favorite shade), and let it sit for a few days. Then paint it onto your nails in the usual way. Afterward, remove any garlic odor by washing your hands with freshly squeezed lemon juice.

2. Mix 3 tablespoons of olive oil and 1 tablespoon of freshly squeezed lemon juice in a bowl, and heat it until it's lukewarm. At bedtime, use a cotton swab to brush the mixture onto each nail, including the undersides and the surrounding cuticles. Put on a pair of soft, clean cotton gloves, and hit the sack. Repeat the process every night, until your "claws" are in fighting form again.

3. Mix 2 teaspoons of castor oil with 2 teaspoons of salt and 1 teaspoon of wheat germ, and pour the mixture into a bottle with a tight-fitting cap. Give the bottle a good shake, and rub the treatment onto your nails with a cotton ball or swab.

4. At bedtime, massage vegetable oil or vegetable shortening into your hands and nails, and put on a pair of rubber gloves, which will force the oil to penetrate your skin. Leave the gloves on overnight, and by morning, you should see signs of improvement. Repeat the treatment each night until your nails are in good shape.

No matter which procedure you choose, repeat it once every few weeks, or as needed, to maintain the strength and youthful appearance of your nails. **Note:** *If you don't start to see improvement within a couple of weeks, call your doctor. Fingernail problems can sometimes indicate an underlying health condition.*

❯ Ginger Nails It

To make your fingernails lighter and brighter, soak them for 10 minutes twice a week in a small bowl of ginger ale. The soluble salts, like sodium benzoate and potassium sorbate, found in most commercial ginger ales act as natural bleaching agents. They'll quickly clean up dingy nails and keep them a whiter shade of pale.

> " How old would you be if you didn't know how old you were?
>
> —Satchel Paige (1906–1982) "

❯ Soften Your Cuticles

Dry, damaged cuticles don't merely make your hands look old. They're also as painful as all get-out! Any of these cuticle conditioners will have them feeling better—and looking younger—in a jiffy:

Avocado oil. Mix 1 tablespoon of avocado oil and 5 drops of tea tree oil in a small bottle. Once or twice a day, dampen the skin on your affected fingers and/or toes. Then apply a drop of the mixture to each cuticle, and massage the oil in thoroughly. Use a cuticle stick to gently push the cuticle back off the nail. You should start seeing rather dramatic results within a few days.

Olive oil. Combine 1 teaspoon of olive oil with 1 teaspoon of vitamin E oil, and massage the mixture into your cuticles. Repeat as needed to keep them strong and supple.

Cocoa butter. Warm 4 tablespoons of cocoa butter over low heat until it liquefies. Stir in 4 tablespoons of castor oil, and pour the mixture into a deep bowl. Let the potion cool to a comfortable temperature, then soak your fingertips and nails for 15 minutes. Rinse your fingers in warm water, and gently push back your cuticles. Store any leftover conditioner in a lidded jar for up to three months at room temperature.

Baking soda. Dip a moistened nail brush in baking soda, and scrub. You'll clean your nails and soften your cuticles simultaneously.

❯ Make Your Polish Linger Longer

Whether you paint your nails in a classic shade of red or pink, or a trendy, multicolored design, it's frustrating when your handiwork starts chipping off almost before the polish is dry. Well, don't get all hot and bothered about it. Instead, just adopt this simple prep routine: Soak your nails in vinegar (any kind will do) for about 60 seconds. Wait until they've dried thoroughly, and then paint the surfaces as usual. The vinegar will remove the natural oils from the surface of your nails, so instead of sliding off, your polish will hang on tight!

Fight Yellow with Yellow

Prolonged exposure to sunlight, wearing nail polish for too long, and smoking can all turn your fingernails yellow and downright old-looking. Fortunately, there's a simple solution. Just fill a shallow bowl with enough lemon juice to cover your nails, and soak them for five or six minutes. Then wash and rinse your hands, and apply your favorite moisturizer. Repeat the treatment once a day (or as close to it as you can). You should start seeing results in five to seven days. **Note:** *Fresh, frozen, and bottled lemon juice all work fine. But before you proceed, make sure your fingers are free of cuts and scrapes, or you'll get a stinging surprise!*

Tick-Tock **TURN BACK** the **CLOCK**

❯ Foil Foul Fungi

There are few skin afflictions more annoying—or more unsightly—than a finger- or toenail fungus. This can be treated with powerful prescription medications that can easily cure the foul fungi from the inside—and quickly. There's just one problem. These meds can deliver side effects, including kidney damage, that are a lot worse than the pain, itch, and ugly appearance of your infected digit. So why take chances? Use one of these simple and safe alternatives instead:

- Paint your nails with tea tree oil three times a day.

- Twice a day, coat the afflicted nail(s) and surrounding skin with mentholated rub.

- Soak your affected hand or foot for 15 to 20 minutes every day in a solution made from 1 part vinegar to 2 parts warm water.

- Cover the infected nail with a thick layer of plain yogurt, wrap it with a bandage or piece of gauze. Soak it overnight, then rinse off the residue. Repeat the procedure each night until your fungus has flown the coop.

Keep your nails short and unpolished, and if the "victims" are your toes, go barefoot or wear open sandals as often as you can. This way, you'll maximize your nails' exposure to air, which encourages faster healing. Before you know it, the fungus won't be among us anymore!

Note: *If the infection hasn't cleared up after a week or two, call your doctor.*

Fountain of Youth
HARD AS NAILS TONIC

Just like every other part of your body, your finger- and toenails reflect what you eat. If your nails are soft, chances are that you're not getting enough protein in your diet. This tasty supplement should solve your problem fast.

1 cup of milk

1 tsp. of blackstrap molasses

1 tsp. of unflavored gelatin

¼ tsp. of peanut oil

Heat (but don't boil) the milk, pour it into a mug, and stir in the other ingredients.* Drink the potion three times a day, and you should start seeing results within a few weeks.

If the gelatin doesn't dissolve, pop the mug into the microwave for 30 seconds.

Dodge Nail Salon Nightmares

A professional manicure or pedicure can make your hands and feet look years younger in a flash. But if the salon you choose isn't spotlessly clean and hygienic—and many are not—your rejuvenating treat could deliver potentially deadly viruses. So always take these simple precautions:

- Make sure that the salon is fully licensed and the aestheticians' licenses are posted.

- Look for a UV sterilizer tool that disinfects all instruments.

- Ask the manager or a technician to describe the shop's general hygiene practices. Between uses, workstations and soaking vessels should be thoroughly sterilized with disinfectants labeled "germicidal."

- Go the extra mile, and bring your own tools, soaking bowl, and/or foot basin (or plastic liner) to the shop.

- Before the procedure begins, ask the technician whether she's washed her hands after working on her previous client. If the answer is no, politely request that she do so.

BAR THE DOOR ON GERMS

Bacteria, fungi, and viruses can weasel their way into your body through even the teeniest-tiniest entryways. For that reason, even if your chosen salon meets the highest hygienic standards, don't take chances. Lock the doors using these no-fail defenses:

- If you have any open cuts, cracks, scratches, bug bites, or rashes—no matter how small—on your hands or feet, postpone your appointment until after they've healed.

- Wait at least 24 hours after shaving, waxing, or using a hair-removal cream on your legs before getting a pedicure.

- Nix fake nails. They can lift up from the base of your natural nails, providing a dandy entry point for dangerous germs.

- Never let anyone cut into your skin, using either a cuticle clipper or a credo blade (which many salons use to remove calluses, even though it's illegal in most states).

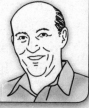

Live HAPPIER

In a sense, the final part of the book takes up where Chapter 4 left off. There, we focused on the most important factor in growing younger: maintaining a positive, upbeat outlook on life. Now, we'll delve deeper into three specific elements that are crucial to remaining happy and young at heart. You'll find practical pointers and surprising secrets for nurturing joy- and health-giving relationships with the people (and pets) in your life. You'll also discover savvy strategies for remaining productive and creative well into your senior years. And first off, we'll get moving with a treasure trove of tips, tricks, and techniques that'll keep you fit as a fiddle and rarin' to relish all the years ahead.

CHAPTER 7

Get a Move On

It's no coincidence that the longest-lived people on the planet are those who have been physically active in one form or another for their entire lives. The fact is that the less you use your body, the sooner it goes downhill. Conversely, keeping your body in motion, as Mother Nature intended, is a guaranteed way to grow—and stay—younger. Best of all, that's true whether you choose to adopt a formal exercise program, take up a sport (or several), or simply work more movement into your daily routine.

>>> GET OFF THE COUCH!

We all know that in order to lose weight, you need to burn more calories than you take in. But here's a shocker: Scientists have proven that even slender folks can build up dangerous amounts of internal fat if they don't move around enough—and, let's face it, in this day and age, most of us don't. Now for the good news: There are scads of ways you can incorporate health-giving, youth-enhancing movement into your day without taking up running, hiring a personal trainer, or spending hours a week at the gym.

> Moving Makes You Younger

Just take a gander at the benefits you'll gain simply by keeping your body in motion, whether you plunge into a formal exercise program, engage in sports, or simply tackle your household chores with gusto.

Keep your heart healthy. Regular physical activity lowers your blood pressure, boosts HDL (good) cholesterol, and decreases both

LDL (bad) cholesterol and unhealthy triglycerides. This one-two punch keeps your blood flowing smoothly, which decreases your risk for cardiovascular disease.

Fend off or manage other dastardly diseases. Exercise also helps prevent or mitigate the effects of stroke, metabolic syndrome, type 2 diabetes, and numerous types of cancer.

Keep your joints jumpin'. Moving your body around increases flexibility in your joints and helps avoid or relieve osteoarthritis.

Prevent osteoporosis. Weight-bearing exercises (such as walking, dancing, and skating) are especially helpful for increasing bone density.

Boost your stamina. Regular exercise strengthens your muscles and increases your lung capacity. The result: greater endurance and energy, whether you're performing your daily chores, romping with your grandchildren, or taking off on a whirlwind world tour.

Elevate your mood. Physical activity of any kind triggers an outpouring of various brain chemicals that leave you feeling happier and more relaxed.

Help you sleep better. Shifting into action mode on a routine basis can help you fall asleep faster and snooze deeper. Just one "but": Avoid vigorous exercise within a couple hours of bedtime, or you may find yourself too wired to summon the sandman!

Liven up your sex life. In addition to upping your energy level and improving your physical appearance—both of which can lead to more bedroom activity—regular exercise has been shown to enhance arousal in women and help resolve erectile dysfunction in men.

> "If you rest, you rust.
> —Helen Hayes (1900–1993)"

Expand your social circle. Games, sports, and other physical activities give you an ideal chance to spend happy times with family and friends and to make new pals. (See Chapter 8 for more on the ways that social interaction can help you grow younger.)

❯ Don't Commit Suicide by Sitting!

If you think that headline is an exaggeration, consider this factoid: On average, Americans spend 56 hours or more per week planted on their butts—either at work, in their cars, or slouched in front of their televisions. The health consequences of that immobility are so severe that a whole new field of medicine, called inactivity physiology, has sprung up to explore the deadly new epidemic that researchers have dubbed "sitting disease" (see "What's the Big Deal?" at left). The good news is that to save yourself from sitting disease, you don't have to give up your day job, or even embark on a formal exercise plan. All you need to do is move your body every chance you get or, as physiologists put it, ramp up your daily non-exercise activity thermogenesis (NEAT). That's a fancy term for the calories you burn doing everything *but* exercising—such as folding laundry, feeding the dog, or strolling to the water cooler.

What's the Big Deal?

Why all the fuss about sitting? Here's why: The human body was designed to move, and until recently, daily survival demanded almost constant movement in one form or another. Now, thanks to modern technology, you can make a living, pay bills, deposit checks, keep up with friends, and shop for everything from bedsheets to baby clothes without even getting out of your chair. Add that to longer workdays, long-haul commutes, and traffic-clogged highways, and you've got a population that moves about as much as a picket fence. If you're one of those couch, car-seat, or office-chair potatoes, you're begging for cardiovascular disease, diabetes, chronic back pain, depression, severe stress, and breast and colon cancer—not to mention simply growing old before your time.

❯ 6 Tricks to NEATen Up Your Day

By now, I hope you're thinking about how you can squeeze more movement into your daily routine. Here are six positively painless pointers for getting off your duff more often:

At Work:

1. Stand up at least every 30 minutes, and grab every chance you get to walk around your cubicle—for instance, while you're reading, talking on the phone, or chatting with a visitor.

2. Rather than phoning or e-mailing a coworker, step down the hall for a personal conversation.

3. Instead of holding sit-down meetings, gather your colleagues for a walking conference in the corridors or (better yet) outdoors.

On Your Own Time:

1. Whenever you have the option of standing up or sitting down to do a chore—whether it's opening the mail, peeling potatoes, or writing checks—opt for the upright position for at least part of the time.

2. When you arrive for an appointment and find that you'll need to wait, don't sit in a chair. Instead, stroll around the block, down the hall, or however far time permits.

3. Practice intentional inefficiency. For example, anytime you need to carry a couple of boxes from your car to the house or from one room to another, make separate trips, even if you could easily manage both packages at the same time.

❯ Mobility Can Be Habit-Forming

Here are four other simple ways to work more movement into your daily life, whether you're at home, at work, or on the go:

- Shun the elevator—at least for most trips. Unless you're on an upper floor in a high-rise building, or carrying a lot of baggage,

MIND OVER MYTH

MYTH: Regular exercise makes you immune to sitting disease.

REALITY: Even working out for 30 minutes every day cannot counteract the detrimental effects of sitting. If your muscles—especially the ones in your legs—are immobile for extended periods of time, your metabolic processes begin to shut down. One sobering example: If you sit for a full, eight-hour day, your fat-burning enzymes drop by 50 percent. The bottom line: The more time you spend sitting each day, the more likely you are to die early. Conversely, the more you move, the younger you'll grow (well, up to a point, of course).

make it a habit to walk down the stairs. Likewise, if you're only going up a few flights, take the steps.

- Step right along. Whenever you're on an escalator or a moving walkway, like the ones at airports, don't just stand there—keep walking. As a plus, you'll reach your destination faster.

- Opt out of auto-pay. Instead, write checks and walk them to a mailbox. In addition to getting some exercise, you're likely to pay more attention to the bills—thereby catching any overcharges or other mistakes quickly. (You can always switch back to auto-pay temporarily if you're going away for an extended period of time.)

- Cook at home more often. You'll be forced to move around as you prep the food, set the table, and clean up afterward—as opposed to sitting like a bump on a log in a restaurant while you wait for your meal to be delivered to your table. As a bonus, the money you save could pay for sports equipment or lessons, a swim or health club membership, or an action-oriented vacation.

⫸ BEYOND BASIC MOVEMENT

While it is true that any kind of physical activity improves the health of your body and your mind, the more you move around, the more you'll benefit. Don't get me wrong! If you'd like to start on a formal exercise routine, by all means go for it. But it's not necessary. In fact, most of the longest-lived folks on the planet stay in tip-top shape simply by incorporating plenty of movement into their daily lives—and you can, too.

❯ The Core Four

One key to growing younger, physically and mentally, is to create a repertoire of activities that includes each of the four basic types of movement. How you choose to work them into your daily routine depends on personal preference, as well as your current condition.

Coming up, we'll cover each category in more depth, but in the meantime, here's the roster:

Aerobic activities increase your breathing and heart rate. Any form of continued, brisk movement belongs in this group. Walking, dancing, swimming, biking, and mowing your lawn can all give you a first-class aerobic workout.

Strength exercises do what the name implies: They make your muscles stronger. Lifting weights or using a resistance band is the formal way to accomplish this goal. But plenty of sports, including golf, tennis, bowling, and squash, also increase your muscle power. So do scads of everyday chores, ranging from digging garden beds to washing your car.

Stretching, a.k.a. flexibility exercises, helps your body stay limber and able to function at its youthful peak. Many fitness experts recommend doing stretching exercises in conjunction with sports and other strenuous activities to help prevent injuries.

Balance-enhancing activities play a crucial role as we grow older because they help prevent falls. Dancing, horseback riding, and skating are excellent ways to keep your balance on the beam.

Note: *Get your doctor's okay before you begin any formal exercise program or dramatically up your daily activity level.*

Focus on Function

One of the hottest trends in exercise circles for seniors is functional fitness. This program focuses on your ability to perform everyday activities, such as carrying groceries, lifting a toddler out of his car seat, or turning your neck far enough to see a car that's coming up behind you. Do you need it? It all depends on your physical condition. If you're doing just fine, thank you, then give it a pass. But if you're struggling to get through your daily routine, functional fitness exercises can help improve your balance, agility, and muscle strength; reduce the risk of falls; and generally improve your quality of life. To find a helpful gym near you, simply do an online search for (you guessed it!) functional fitness.

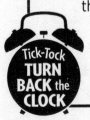

> The Very Best Exercise of All...

Is whatever you enjoy enough to do it regularly. Granted, there may be times—when you're recovering from surgery or an injury—that you have to endure some therapist-prescribed rehab exercises, no matter how much you may hate them. But don't force yourself to (let's say) jog on a treadmill, swim laps, or bounce through a Pilates routine when your mind is saying, "I know this is good for me, but I can't wait to get it over with." You'll defeat your purpose by bringing on stress and robbing yourself of the happiness you could—and should—be getting from your physical endeavors. That is, if you don't quit first. Focus on a variety of activities that include each of the four basic types of movement and that you enjoy, or that produce tangible results that give you satisfaction, such as planting a garden, painting the living room, or de-cluttering your home.

> Walk to a Younger You

Across the board, medical pros will tell you that simply walking for 30 minutes a day can not only help you lose weight and tone your leg muscles, but also lower your stress level, reduce your risk for lethal

---

MIND OVER MYTH

MYTH: You will need to exercise long and hard to see any beneficial results from physical activity.

REALITY: At one time, that was the commonly accepted belief. But now, medical pros tell us that all you really need for good health (and a younger you) is 30 minutes a day of moderate physical activity such as the kind you get from taking a brisk walk or from doing any manner of jobs around the house (see "Shape Up with the Power of Household Chores" on page 242). And here's more good news: You don't have to get your whole 30 minutes in one fell swoop. Two 15-minute or even three 10-minute sessions will do the trick just fine.

diseases, and even make you happier and more youthful. One of the simplest ways to reach that target—and combat sitting disease at the same time—is to get out of your car for 30 minutes a day, and spend that time walking instead of driving.

Of course, you don't have to limit your daily walks to half an hour. Nor do you need to rack up the time in one fell swoop, or hit the full 30-minute mark each and every day. The bottom line is that the more minutes you devote to this transportation trade-off throughout the day, the more rewards you'll reap! Consider these six no-fuss ways you can replace horsepower with foot power:

- Walk to and from work, church, errands, and social gatherings whenever you can. When that's not possible, drive to within 15 minutes of your destination, park, and hoof it the rest of the way.

- If you routinely drive to and from lunch, walk instead. The return portion of the jaunt is especially effective for weight loss (or weight maintenance) because walking within 30 minutes after eating increases calorie burning by as much as 30 percent. So when you only have time for a one-way trek, get a ride to the restaurant and take the shoe-leather express back to the office.

- When you drive downtown or out to the mall, don't circle the block or the parking lot until you find the vacant spot that's closest to the door. Do the opposite: Ease into a space that's a healthy distance away from the building entrance.

- Nix drive-up windows at places like banks, coffee shops, and the post office. Instead, park the car and amble inside.

- When you take public transportation, get off a stop or two early, and walk to your destination.

- At work, use restrooms, copy machines, and so on that are farther away than your nearest ones.

> " I believe every human has an infinite number of heartbeats. I don't intend to waste any of mine running around doing exercises.
> —Neil Armstrong (1930–2012) "

> 3 Terrific Tips for Happy Hoofing

Unlike most athletic pursuits and exercise routines, walking requires absolutely no special clothing or equipment. But to maximize your comfort level (and, therefore, the likelihood that you'll stick with the program), keep these pointers in mind:

1. Baby your feet. Wear the most comfortable shoes you can find. For longer distances (say, when you're doing 15 minutes or more at a single stretch), shoes that are specially made for running or power walking are your best bet. For short strolls or occasions that call for something a little dressier than sneakers, simply wear whatever footgear feels best to you and goes well with your outfit. Whatever you do, though, steer clear of high, spiky heels because with every step you take, they subject the balls of your feet to as much as (are you ready for this?) 2,000 pounds of pressure! And that takes an enormous toll on your knee and hip joints.

2. Accessorize your outfit. Consider purchasing an inexpensive pedometer that you can clip to your belt, waistband, or coat. You'll find that counting the steps you take each day is a lot like watching your savings account: The more the numbers increase, the more motivated you are to nudge them upward even further.

3. Lose the luggage. Granted, there may be times (when you're on your way to work, for instance) when you have to tote a purse, a briefcase, or both. But whenever possible, leave those carrying cases at home. Instead, wear clothes that have enough pockets to hold any essential take-alongs, such as your cell phone, wallet, reading glasses, and/or shopping list. It's a fact: The less stuff you have to lug along, the more enjoyable your trek will be.

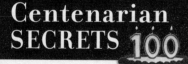

Centenarian SECRETS

Studies show that the average American takes between 3,000 and 5,000 steps a day. Medical experts say that in order to stay healthy, fend off chronic diseases, and live to a ripe old age, a person should take at least 10,000 steps a day, which comes out to roughly five miles. So start steppin'!

Walk More, Spend Less

While your health earns big bucks each time you leave your car behind and walk to your destination, your body isn't the only beneficiary of this deal. It's also a boon to your bank account. For starters, the less you drive, the less you'll have to shell out for gasoline and all the other liquids that your gas guzzler consumes, including motor oil, antifreeze, and brake or transmission fluid. What's more, you'll reduce wear and tear on your car, which will translate into lower maintenance costs and, ultimately, a longer life for old Betsy. Most likely, you'll also save money on parking fees. Depending on how often you leave your vehicle behind, you could even qualify for a discount on your auto insurance policy. That's because insurance underwriters know that the less time you spend behind the wheel, the less likely you are to be involved in an accident. (Chalk up yet another health benefit of walking rather than driving!)

The Power of the Pedal

If you'd rather cycle than stroll, I have even better news for you: Replacing a 30-minute drive with a half-hour bike ride will help you

---

Rejuvenating Recipe
EASY ENERGY BARS

Whether you're walking on city sidewalks, cycling through the suburbs, or trotting across a parking lot, you can suddenly find yourself craving an energy boost. Keep a few of these tasty and nutritious treats handy, and reach for one whenever you need a power fix.

1 egg

½ cup of brown sugar

1 tsp. of vanilla extract

1 cup of granola

½ cup of chopped, dried fruit

½ cup of chopped nuts

3 tbsp. of dark chocolate chips (preferably organic)

Grease an 8-by-8-inch baking pan with butter. Combine the egg, brown sugar, and vanilla extract in a bowl. Stir in the granola, dried fruit, nuts, and chocolate chips until combined. Scrape the mixture into the pan, pressing firmly, to make sure the surface is covered evenly. Bake for 25 minutes at 350°F. Cool, cut into bars, and wrap in wax paper or aluminum foil.

shed even more weight and give a bigger boost to your heart rate than walking for the same amount of time. That's because you'll be moving your legs faster and traveling a lot farther. To be specific, walking for 30 minutes at the rate of 3 miles per hour will burn a little over 128 calories. Riding a bicycle for the same length of time at 12.4 miles per hour will burn roughly 274 calories. The exact numbers will vary depending on your age and weight, but the bottom line is a win-win trade-off!

❯ Shape Up with the Power of Household Chores

Lots of folks love the camaraderie of working out at a gym, where they're surrounded and encouraged by their fellow grow-younger warriors. But if you're not that social by nature, you don't care for formal workout routines—or you simply don't have the time or money to squander on a health club membership—don't fret: By performing routine chores around the old homestead, you'll roast calories galore, ramp up your blood flow, and tone your muscles. Here's just a handful of examples:

- Digging in your yard burns about 630 calories per hour, in addition to toning the muscles in your calves, thighs, arms,

---

Push for Fitness

If you'd like to give a down-home boost to your shape-up labors—and you have a small, fairly flat lawn—here's a "reel" sweet idea: Exchange your powered lawn mower for a manual reel mower. Using it to mow your lawn will burn about 400 calories an hour, compared with 250 for a powered push mower and 175 for the riding version. Plus, it'll tone your muscles and rev up your heart rate far beyond what you'd achieve with any powered machine. (If the only reel mower you've ever known was the one you muscled around your parents' lawn on Saturday mornings, don't worry: That old dinosaur has been reborn, with a much lighter body and smoother-working parts.) So do your body a favor, and take one for a test drive, er, test push.

Tick-Tock
TURN BACK the **CLOCK**

and shoulders. Plus, if you go at it vigorously for 20 minutes or more, you'll increase your heart rate and strengthen your whole cardiovascular system.

- Raking leaves for an hour burns 450 calories, and the resistance offered by the leaves helps tone all your major muscle groups.

- Scrubbing your bathroom burns 400 calories an hour, while toning your arm and shoulder muscles.

- Sweeping and mopping the floor burn about 240 calories an hour and give you a great upper- and lower-body workout.

- Washing your car burns 286 calories an hour and helps tone your arms and abdominal muscles.

Note: *The calorie counts above are estimates. The exact number burned during any activity varies greatly, depending on your gender, age, and weight, as well as your individual metabolism. An Internet search for "calorie burn calculator" will bring up scads of sites where you can type in your vital stats and learn how many calories you'll expend on common chores, ranging from loading your dishwasher to washing your dog, in addition to more athletic endeavors such as swimming, dancing, and lifting weights.*

❯ The Superstar of Domestic Exercise

The next time you look out your window and see your driveway covered with a thick white blanket, consider this fact: Shoveling snow or pushing a heavy snow blower is more strenuous than running on a treadmill set at full throttle. For that reason, clearing away several inches of snow is a dandy way to get a first-class workout—but only if you're healthy and fit. Otherwise, you could find yourself being rushed to the ER with a heart attack or severe back injury, as tens of

When to Shun the Shovel

If you're out of shape or have a history of back injuries or heart disease, don't even think about shoveling snow! Likewise, farm the job out to someone who's strong and fit if you're obese, diabetic, or have high blood pressure— all of which put you at ultra-high risk for a heart attack or stroke.

thousands of folks are each winter. Even if you are (or think you are) in pretty good shape, following these half-dozen guidelines can literally spell the difference between life and death:

Warm up. Do some light exercises and stretches inside the house before you head outdoors.

Dress for success. Wear warm, slip-resistant boots, and dress in layers, so you can peel one off while you're working, then put it back on during breaks.

Work smart. Whenever possible, push the snow out of the way instead of lifting it. When hoisting is necessary, shovel many light loads instead of fewer heavy ones. And never throw the snow over your shoulder or to the side because the twisting motion can wrench your back. Instead, turn slowly and gently, so you can toss the load forward. And always be sure to bend your knees, and lift with your legs—not with your back!

Pace yourself. Take frequent breaks, drink plenty of water, and don't try to do the whole job in one stint. Especially if you're not used to exercising or you've had even minor back problems, shovel (or snow-blow) for 5 to 10 minutes, then go back inside for 10 to 20 minutes.

Forget perfection. Do not try to remove every speck of white from your snow-covered surfaces. Instead, tackle the areas that could pose problems for cars or pedestrians, and let Mother Nature take care of the rest in her own good time.

Know when to quit. Stop immediately if you feel light-headed or short of breath, your heart begins to race, your chest starts hurting, or you feel any other alarming physical sensation. If you even suspect that you're having a heart attack, call 911.

❯ May I Have This Dance?

Good old-fashioned ballroom dancing is one of the very best forms of exercise that you'll ever hope to find. Whether you are waltzing in elegant Viennese style or cuttin' a rug to a swing, tango, or polka tune, moving rhythmically in sync with a partner has an almost magical way of peeling off the years. In addition to roasting the same number of calories as swimming and cycling (between 200 and 400 per hour), dancing also performs these youth-enhancing feats:

- Lowers your cholesterol and blood pressure
- Conditions your entire cardiovascular system
- Increases your lung capacity and general stamina
- Helps maintain bone density
- Improves balance
- Tones and strengthens muscles in your calves, thighs, and buttocks

As a plus, guys, if the choreography involves dipping or lifting your partner, you can get a darn good upper-body workout as well. **Note:** *Orthopedic surgeons tell us that because of its low-impact nature, ballroom dancing is an especially effective way to rehabilitate your knees after surgery.*

❯ More Reasons to Shake a Leg

Aside from its purely physical advantages, dancing on a regular basis— or taking lessons—gives you a dandy opportunity to grow younger by socializing with old pals and making new ones. Plus, research galore has shown that the kind of melodic music you hear on a ballroom dance floor has prodigious power to reignite memories, enhance your ability to learn new things, generally stimulate your brain, and even help manage pain without drugs. All this is on top of a landmark study showing that ballroom dancing can greatly reduce your risk for dementia (see "Trip the Light Fantastic" on page 144).

>>> AEROBIC EXERCISES

Throughout this chapter and the rest of the book, I've been preaching the gospel of vigorous physical activity as a major player in any grow-younger effort. In fact, because of its ability to do everything from maintaining your ideal weight to strengthening your heart, boosting your mood, and helping you sleep soundly, you could say that aerobic exercise is the two-word secret to living a longer, healthier, happier life. In this section, you'll discover some simple ways to make this magic bullet even more effective at hitting its target.

> Variety Is the Spice of Life

It's also crucial to the success of your aerobic endeavors. That's true for a trio of reasons:

It heads off aches and pains. When you confine exercise to any single sport or activity, you put undue stress on a specific set of muscles. That puts them at high risk for injuries caused by repetitive use and makes your other muscles vulnerable to weakness-related strains. By regularly engaging in several kinds of exercise, you will condition your whole body.

It broadens your options. Let's say you arrive at the pool for your morning swim, only to find that it's closed for repairs. No problem! You can head to the skating rink or go for a bike ride instead. Conversely, if a twisted ankle nixes your usual squash game, you can jump in the pool and swim laps, do aquatic exercises, or even run (see "5 Fine Reasons to Run Deep," at right).

It reduces boredom. Chances are that if you perform the same type of exercise day after day for months, it'll get pretty darn old. (After all, people were bred to be physically active in a variety of ways in their daily lives—not to simply jog 3 miles every morning.) Fortunately, as we've seen earlier in this chapter, when it comes to healthy aerobic exercise, the sky's the limit.

➤ 5 Fine Reasons to Run Deep

There's no denying that running can give you one of the best aerobic workouts on the planet. There's just one problem: Over time, it's murder on your knees. If you've already learned that the hard way, consider plunging into deep-water running. A flotation device keeps your head comfortably out of the water, so you can breathe normally and run—or perform other exercises—in much the same way as you would on dry land, with none of the pounding. But wait! The benefits of deep-water running don't stop there.

1. In the water, your musculoskeletal system bears virtually no weight at all, so you can get a full cardiovascular workout even if you're recovering from injuries or strains you suffered on dry land.

2. Water creates resistance to movement in all directions. By simply changing the speed of any action, you automatically increase or decrease its intensity. Exercising in water is like having an adjustable weight machine surrounding your body.

3. With every move you make, the water massages your muscles—thereby revving up your circulation, promoting physical and mental relaxation, and helping stress and tension float away.

4. Simply being up to your neck in water produces physiological changes that enhance the removal of metabolic waste, improve heart function, lower blood pressure, and support tissue healing.

5. Finally, deep-water running or any other aquatic exercise is ideal for people who like being in the water but find swimming laps boring.

Centenarian SECRETS 100

Remember all the games you loved as a child? Well, there is no law that says you can't keep right on playing them, and it's a no-fail way to add variety to your aerobic exercise routine. Even if the old gang isn't here to join in, you can still jump rope, skip around the block, build snowmen, or play tag with your grandchildren or the neighborhood kids. You'll have a ball and get a top-notch workout at the same time. Well, don't just stand there—you're It!

› Walking in Water

When you step into a body of water—whether it's a pool, lake, or the open ocean—a simple stroll becomes a genuine power walk. To ensure best results, wear water shoes to help you maintain traction and hand webs to provide resistance, thereby strengthening your arms as they move through the water (as shown in illustration A). Start off at whatever speed and distance feel comfortable to you, and work up from there at your own pace. Here's the basic procedure:

1. Stand straight up in waist-deep water, keeping your stomach and buttock muscles firm and your shoulders back.

2. Step forward just as you do on land, putting your heel down first and rolling onto the ball of your foot. Don't go onto your tiptoes! As you move, keep your back erect and your stomach muscles taut.

3. Keep your arms straight and your palms turned out. When reaching out with your leg, bring your opposite arm ahead, and vice versa.

4. If you want to tone different muscle groups, walk forward eight steps, then back four steps.

5. Once you're comfortable walking in waist-deep water, gradually increase the depth—thereby upping the intensity of the action—until you're ready to don a buoyancy belt and plunge in over your head (as shown in illustration B).

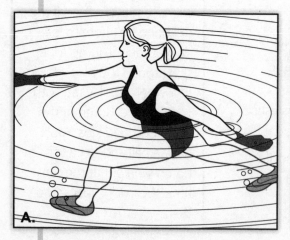

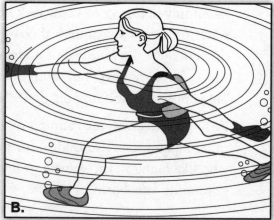

> Deep-Water Running

Essentially, deep-water running (a.k.a. aqua jogging) is simply jogging in water that's deep enough so that your feet can't touch bottom. But the first few times you jump into the pool, it's easy to forget that you're in there to run, not swim. So keep these guidelines in mind:

1. Begin with a brief warm-up, just as you would if you were running on dry land. Swim around gently or tread water for two to three minutes.

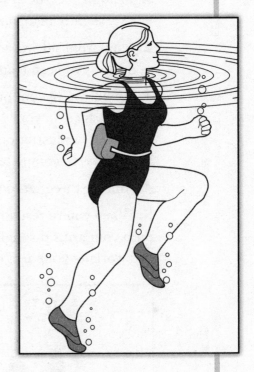

2. Keep your body erect in the water, with your shoulders back, your head held high, and your eyes looking straight ahead. Don't hunch over, and try not to lean forward.

3. Use the same basic form you use when you're running on land, only pull your knees up to about hip height and point your toes slightly.

4. Bend your arms at about 90 degrees, and swing them from the shoulders as you move forward. The faster you swing, the more you'll intensify your workout.

5. Keep your hands closed in loose fists, or flat with the palms turned inward. You want your hands to slice through the water, not cup it.

6. When you've finished your run, cool down the same way you warmed up: by swimming slowly or treading water for a few minutes.

Note: *In most cases, deep-water running is an excellent alternative for people injured in the "workout wars." But there are exceptions. In particular, jogging with a strained hip flexor is likely to cause discomfort. But regardless of the body part in question, if you feel any pain, speak with your doctor or physical therapist about other ways to stay in shape during your recovery.*

> Tick-Tock Hops

This bouncy item is a spin-off of a dry-land exercise known as mogul jumps. It couldn't be simpler, but boy, is it powerful! In addition to revving up your heartbeat, it works wonders at firming up your legs, abdomen, and rear end.

1. Stand in neck-deep water with your arms at your sides, your elbows slightly bent, and your hands formed into loose fists.

2. Jump from side to side (as shown in illustration A) 12 times, or as many as you can manage. Work up to three sets of 12 jumps each.

3. When you're comfortable jumping on both feet, bend your left knee, balance on your right leg, and perform the side-to-side hop (as shown in illustration B) 12 times. Then switch legs and repeat the process to complete a set.

4. Aim for three sets consisting of 12 jumps per leg.

5. When you're ready for an added challenge, cup your hands and push your arms through the water, thereby increasing resistance and working your arm muscles.

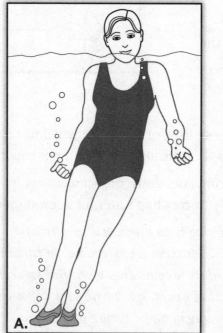 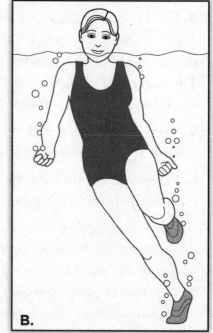

A.   B.

❯ Arm Exercises

Simply moving your arms as you walk or run through the water will build strength, but to ramp up the action, add these simple moves to your aquatic repertoire.

1. Wearing hand webs, stand in waist-deep water with your arms at your sides, your elbows close to your body, and your palms facing forward (as shown in illustration A).

2. Raise your forearms to the surface of the water, keeping your elbows close to your body and your wrists straight.

3. Turn your hands so the palms face downward, and push against the water until your arms are straight again.

4. Repeat, adding more repetitions until you can perform 12 to 15 rounds.

5. Advance to the next level by trading your webs for water weights (a.k.a. foam dumbbells), which create more resistance (as shown in illustration B). Again, start with your arms at your sides, gripping the bars of the weights with your palms facing up.

6. Raise your forearms to the water's surface, keeping your wrists straight and your elbows close to your body.

7. Turn the weights over so your palms are facing the bottom of the pool, and push downward until your arms are straight.

8. When you can do 12 to 15 repetitions comfortably, aim to complete two or three sets per session.

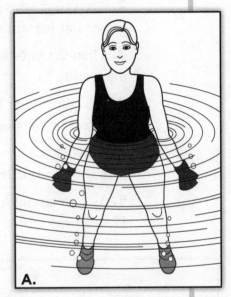

A.

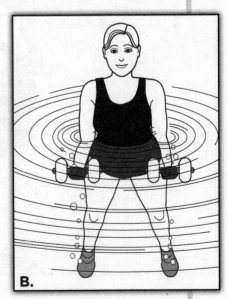

B.

> Pool Noodle Leg Lifts

These pliable foam cylinders weigh next to nothing. But thanks to the resistance created as you move them through the water, they make this simple exercise a real winner for every muscle in your legs.

1. Tie your pool noodle into a knot around one of your feet. Stand in waist-deep water with your back against the side of the pool.

2. Keep your arms pressed back against the pool's edge for balance. Raise your leg straight in front of you (as shown in illustration A).

3. Then flex your knee to about a 90-degree angle (as shown in illustration B).

4. Straighten your leg out, then return to the starting position with both feet on the pool's bottom. Repeat 12 to 15 times if you can.

5. Transfer the noodle to your other foot, and repeat the process with the opposite leg.

6. As your strength increases, build up to two or three sets of 12 to 15 repetitions per leg.

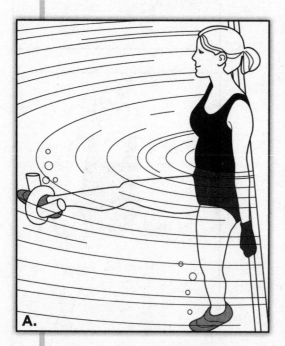

A.

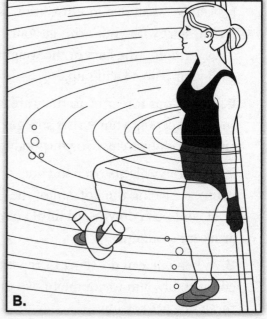

B.

> Cannonball

In this powerful lower-body shaper-upper, your pool noodle trades its resistance role for that of a buoyancy device. It keeps you afloat while your movements trim, tone, and firm your legs, hips, and core abdominal muscles.

1. Float in deep water with a noodle wrapped around your upper back, along your shoulder blades, and under your arms. Rest a hand on either end of the noodle to keep it in place.

2. Point your toes and extend your legs straight down toward the bottom of the pool (as shown in illustration A).

3. Tighten your stomach muscles as you raise your knees toward your chest, stopping at waist level (as shown in illustration B). Hold the position for two seconds, then straighten your legs back to starting position to complete one rep.

4. Do as many repetitions as you can until fatigued, working your way up to 20 per session.

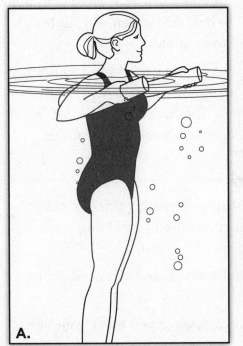

A.

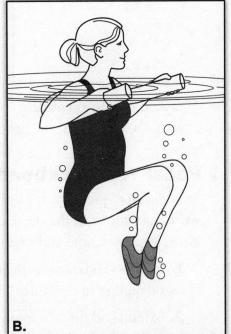

B.

Kickboard Climb

Your shoulders, abdominal muscles, and legs all get a dandy under-water workout with this movement.

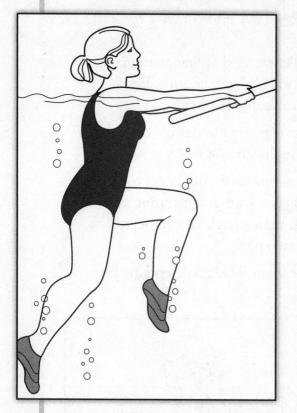

1. Stand in neck-deep water, with your hands, palms down, on a kickboard in front of you.

2. Bend forward from your hips and lean into the board.

3. Keeping your hands firmly in place, alternately raise each leg and bend it at the knee. Push your knee toward the kickboard, and lower it to the pool bottom—as if you were climbing stairs with an exaggerated motion.

4. Keep your stomach muscles taut and your arms stretched, pushing the kickboard away from your body to help strengthen all your body's core muscles.

5. Continue until you feel tired, then rest for 30 to 60 seconds and repeat. Aim to eventually "climb" for one minute, rest for 30 seconds, and repeat the process up to a total of three times.

Pedal Your Kickboard

In addition to giving you a great aerobic charge, this maneuver works just about all the muscles in your body, including your arms, legs, back, and abdomen.

1. Sit on a kickboard, with your arms at your sides and your legs dangling in the water.

2. Extend and flex alternating legs, while you move your arms from front to back in unison.

3. "Motor" your way around the pool for 60 seconds, or as close to it as you can before you're tired.

4. Aim to continue for one minute, then rest 30 seconds, and repeat the process up to three times. If you start to feel fatigued before completing your one-minute goal, go ahead and stop. Then, work up to a minute over time.

In the beginning, it can be tricky to get the rhythm right, but just imagine that you're pedaling a bicycle, and before you know it, you'll be zooming around the pool!

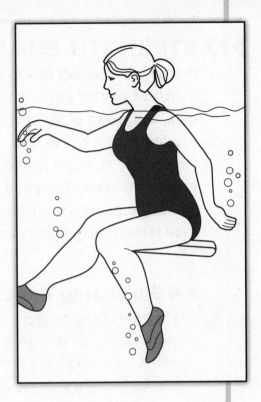

❯ Kickboard Push and Pull

This deceptively simple movement delivers dynamite results for your upper body in three easy steps.

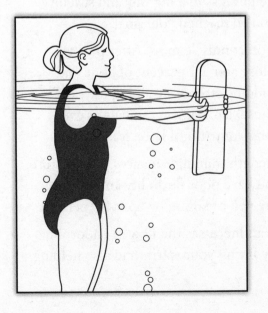

1. Stand in shoulder-deep water, holding a kickboard vertically against your chest, your feet hip distance apart.

2. Alternately push the board forward through the water as far as you can reach (as shown in the illustration). Then pull it back to your body.

3. Try to push and pull for 30 seconds, moving as rapidly as you can.

⟫⟫⟫ STRENGTH-BUILDING EXERCISES

If strength building (a.k.a. strength training) makes you think of a bunch of macho guys hefting monstrous barbells in a sweaty old gym, or a crowd of hip young professionals using high-tech machines in a highfalutin health club, think again. For one thing, you can get a mighty fine strength workout right at home, with no heavy weights or fancy equipment required. Keeping your muscles strong and in good working order is a must for anyone who wants to grow younger—or even retain basic mobility and independence in later years.

❯ 4 Surprising Benefits of Strength Training

The exercises in this section will do what the title implies: strengthen your muscles and tone your body. In the process, though, they'll deliver some delightful, youth-enhancing side effects—namely these:

1. Make you burn more calories—during and after your workout. In scientific lingo, the process is called physiologic homework, which means that your metabolism is boosted by as much as 15 percent and the ripple effect continues as you go about your daily routine. That can help you jump-start your weight loss in a big way and sustain your newfound slimness after you've reached your goal.

2. Increase bone density and protect muscle mass. After puberty, both men and women begin to lose about 1 percent of bone and muscle strength every year. By adding strength training to your routine (even long after menopause, ladies), you can halt or even reverse that loss, thereby reducing your risk of bone fractures.

3. Improve body mechanics. Strength training enhances your posture, balance, and coordination. If you have poor flexibility and balance, strength exercises can reduce the risk of falling by up to 40 percent

4. Boost your mood. Working out increases the flow of endorphins produced by your brain, thereby lifting your spirits and also helping you sleep better.

> How Much, How Often?

Fitness experts recommend doing strength exercises involving all of your major muscle groups at least twice a week. Always leave at least 24 hours between workouts to give your body tissues time to recover.

As for how much, in terms of both the number of exercises and the weight (if any) you use, they depend on your current physical condition and your goals. For example, do you want to shed pounds, dramatically increase your muscle strength, or merely get in better overall shape? For that reason, it's best to meet with a personal trainer who can help you map out a program that works best for you.

> A Shopper's Guide to Dumbbells

Most of the exercises in this section employ lightweight dumbbells. You'll want to purchase them in a local store, where you can try out all your options, with the help of the staff. Ultimately, you'll need to decide on two factors:

Style. Dumbbells come in a variety of shapes, colors, and materials. Make your selection based on your personal preference, but make sure the grip is comfortable to hold, or you'll be fatigued before you know it.

Weight. The classic rule of thumb is to start with a weight that you can lift only eight times. When you can raise it 12 to 15 times, move up to a heavier weight that you can lift only eight times. Again, stick with that poundage until you can raise it 12 to 15 times—and so on.

MIND OVER MYTH

MYTH: It's dangerous to exercise after you've had a hip or knee replacement.

REALITY: Hogwash! In fact, in order to take full advantage of the surgery, you need to stay physically active for the rest of your life. Otherwise, your muscles will grow weaker, greatly upping the odds that you'll take a tumble—and falls are the leading cause of repeat surgeries. Just one caveat: If you've had a joint repair or replacement, check with your orthopedic surgeon before doing any lower-body exercises or plunging into a joint-intensive sport such as skiing, jogging, or even tennis.

❯ Squats

In one sense, you perform this exercise every time you sit down in a chair and stand up again. When you subtract the furniture and fine-tune your technique a tad, you've got the easiest and most effective way to strengthen, tighten, and tone your entire lower body, from your calves to your rear end (a.k.a. gluteus maximus). But that's not all! Squats also improve your balance and increase your bone density—and they're tops for getting rid of cellulite and firming up those hard-to-whittle inner and outer thighs. There are dozens of variations on the squat theme, but this is the most basic:

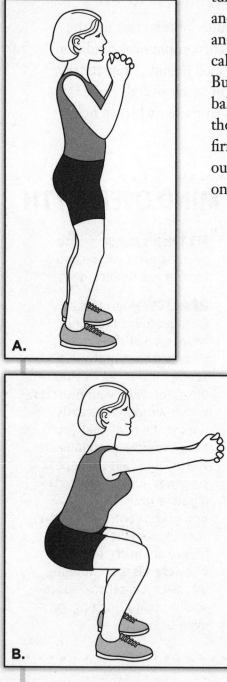

A.

B.

1. Stand up straight, with your knees relaxed, your feet spaced slightly wider than your hips, and your toes turned out slightly. Hold your hands in front of you in a prayer-like position (as shown in illustration A) and inhale.

2. Bend your knees, with your hips back, as though you were going to sit in a chair. Extend your arms to help maintain balance as you slowly lower your rear end. Hold your breath and look straight in front of you, keeping your back straight and your upper body still, so that your legs are doing all the work.

3. Aim for the position shown in illustration B, with your thighs parallel to the floor. Don't let your rear sink below your knees or your knees reach in front of your toes.

4. Stand up slowly by pushing with your heels and, again, using only your legs. Exhale as you rise, keeping your abdominal muscles tight and your back straight.

Start with whatever number of repetitions you can manage comfortably, but work toward three sets of 10 to 15 squats per set. Throughout, maintain a slow pace by counting to three as you go down and three on the way back up.

❯ Squats with Weight

Once you've mastered the basic squat, expand the action by adding weight. This way, in addition to giving your lower body a workout, you'll strengthen your legs, hands, forearms, and back. There's no need to buy a medicine ball or other formal equipment. Instead, just fill a plastic jug with sand or water to give it the weight you want. Start with whatever you can lift with no effort and gradually increase the amount of filling as your muscles get stronger.

1. Begin in the same position you would for a regular squat, with your knees relaxed, your feet spaced slightly wider than your hips, and your toes turned out slightly. But this time, add the jug, holding it in both hands, close to your body.

2. Then, as you lower your body, push the jug out, extending your arms until they're parallel to the floor.

3. As you return to a standing position, slowly bring the weight back toward your chest.

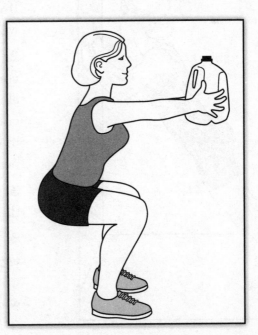

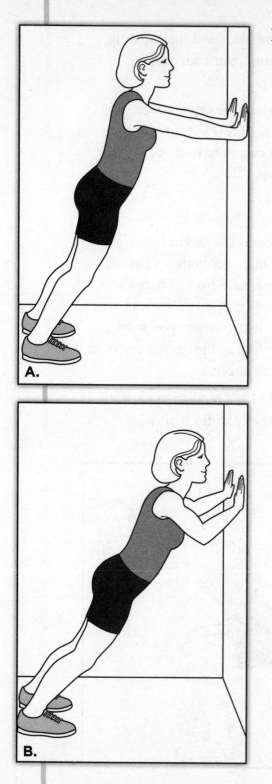

A.

B.

❯ Wall Push-Ups

In fitness, you hear a lot about strengthening your body's "core." This area encompasses your trunk—from waist to chest, front, sides, and back. Its muscles work in unison to support your spinal column. The best for shoring up this area is the old-fashioned push-up. But, it can take some work to perfect that technique. So ease into it with wall push-ups. Even if you never progress beyond this level, your core and your whole body will benefit in a major way.

1. Stand at arms' length from a solid vertical surface, with your arms straight in front of you, shoulder width apart, and no higher than shoulder level. Put both palms on the wall (as shown in illustration A). If you're stretching to reach the wall, you're too far away.

2. Keeping your back straight and your feet flat on the floor, bend your elbows and lean toward the wall until your nose almost touches it (as shown in illustration B). Don't let your body bend at the hips!

3. Hold the position for a second, then push back to your starting point.

4. Do 10 repetitions, then rest until you're ready for 10 more. Over time, work up to two sets of 20 to 25 reps, with just a short break in between.

❯ Bent-Knee Push-Ups

Once you've conquered wall push-ups, you're ready for this final step on the road to the real deal.

1. Kneeling on a carpet or non-skid exercise mat, lean forward so that your hands are flat on the floor, slightly more than shoulder width apart, with your arms upright, your spine straight, and your lower legs pointing upward (as shown in illustration A). Your feet can be crossed or not—that's your call. In the beginning, your knees should be slightly behind your hips; the farther back you move them, the more challenging the exercise becomes.

2. Keeping your stomach muscles tight, lower your upper body until it almost touches the floor (as shown in illustration B).

3. Push up from the floor, keeping your body stable. Be sure to keep your lower back straight; letting it sag could easily lead to injury.

4. Repeat as many times as you can, and then rest for at least two minutes.

5. Work toward a goal of five sets of 20 repetitions each.

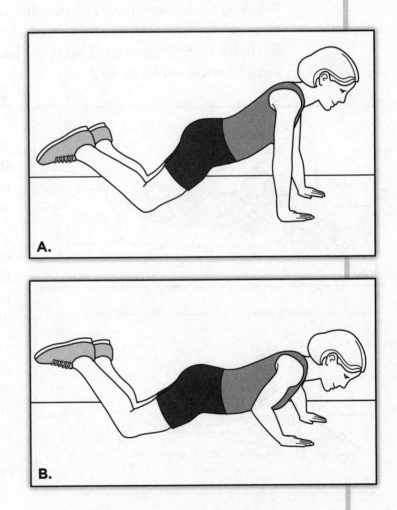

A.

B.

❯ Bridges

There are few exercises if any that are more effective at strengthening the backs of your thighs and slimming that notoriously troublesome sitting area than bridges. What's more, they're also simple to do and easy on your joints. Here's the drill:

1. Lie on your back and bend your knees, keeping your knees hip distance apart, your feet flat, and your shins perpendicular to the floor (as shown in illustration A). Your feet should be as close to your bottom as you can get them without causing any knee pain.

2. Pull your stomach in toward your spine, and slowly lift your torso off the floor until you've formed a bridge with your body (as shown in illustration B). Your upper back, head, and shoulders should remain on the ground.

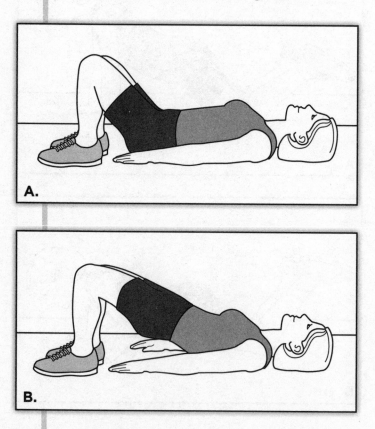

A.

B.

3. Slowly return your body to the floor, and repeat the move. Aim to perform two to three sets of 15 to 20 repetitions.

Rather than concentrating on raising your hips, focus on pushing your heels into the floor. The reactive force will automatically make your posterior come up. To ensure effective results and prevent injury, be sure to keep your torso in a straight line as you raise and lower it.

❯ Roll-Ups

Like many other exercises, sit-ups have a zillion and one variations. But, according to the experts at *Fitness* magazine and researchers at Auburn University, the Pilates roll-up is the most beneficial of all. Not only do roll-ups engage more muscles than traditional sit-ups (or crunches), but they've been found to be 30 percent more effective at strengthening abdominal muscles—and abolishing dreaded belly fat—than bent-knee sit-ups. So what are you waiting for?

1. Lie on your back, with your legs straight, arms stretched above your head, and shoulders down (as shown in illustration A).

2. With your back flat, inhale as you gradually lift your arms toward the ceiling.

3. Slowly roll forward, exhaling, as you peel your spine off the mat. Keep your head straight, your eyes focused forward, and your stomach muscles tight.

4. Inhale again as you stretch out over your legs (as shown in illustration B).

5. Exhale and slowly roll back down to the floor, and assume your starting position.

6. Without pausing, inhale as you roll up to begin the second repetition. Do as many reps as you can, working up to 10 per session.

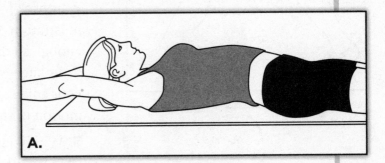

A.

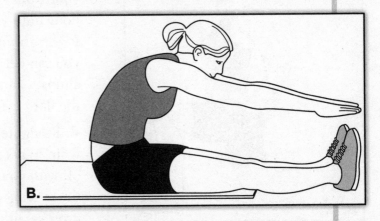

B.

› Forward Lunge

When it comes to versatility, lunges can't be beat. There are numerous variations on the theme, but the place to start—and remain, if you like—is with the basic forward lunge. It can slim down and tone up your lower body, increase muscle tissue, strengthen your core, make your hips more flexible, and help improve your balance. There's just one "but": In order to accomplish optimum results, and avoid possible injury, you need to proceed in exactly the right way.

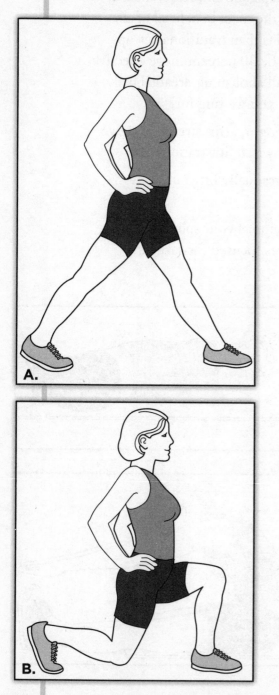

1. Standing with your feet together and your hands on your hips, tighten your core muscles to stabilize your spine.

2. Take a long step forward, keeping your back foot in place (as shown in illustration A). Make sure you step far enough so that the middle of your front knee will be directly above your ankle during the downward motion in step 3.

3. With your back straight, bend your front knee and lower your body until your front thigh is parallel to the ground (or as close to it as you can get) and your back knee almost—but not quite—touches the floor (as shown in illustration B).

4. Straighten your legs to bring your body erect again. Then push off with your front foot to return to the starting position, and repeat the process with your other leg forward.

5. Aim for one set of 8 to 12 reps with each leg.

When you're fully comfortable with this routine, you can increase the strengthening action by holding a dumbbell in each hand throughout the exercise (see "A Shopper's Guide to Dumbells" on page 257).

❯ Biceps Curls

Here's another ultra-simple—but oh-so-beneficial—move that'll tone and strengthen your biceps (maybe in time for sleeveless-dress season).

1. Stand with your feet shoulder width apart, holding a dumbbell in each hand, with your arms hanging straight down at your sides (as shown in illustration A).

2. Bend your right arm and exhale as you curl the weight upward toward your shoulder, keeping your elbow close to your side (as shown in illustration B). Then inhale as you slowly lower the weight to the starting position.

3. Repeat the procedure using your left arm, to complete one rep.

4. Aim to perform two or three sets of 15 reps. Work up to it if you need to start out more slowly.

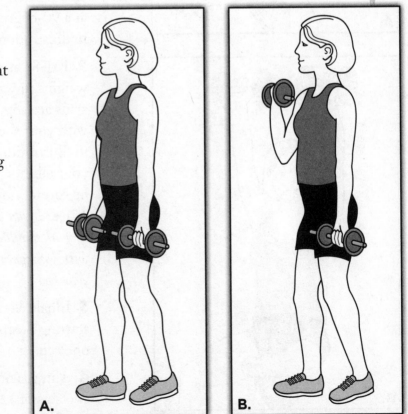

A.

B.

❯ Seated Overhead Press

Contrary to what a lot of folks think, lifting weights is not just for macho musclemen. For anyone of any age, working with hand weights is an excellent—and easy—way to gain strength in virtually every part of your body. This is one of the simplest moves for keeping your shoulders strong and supple.

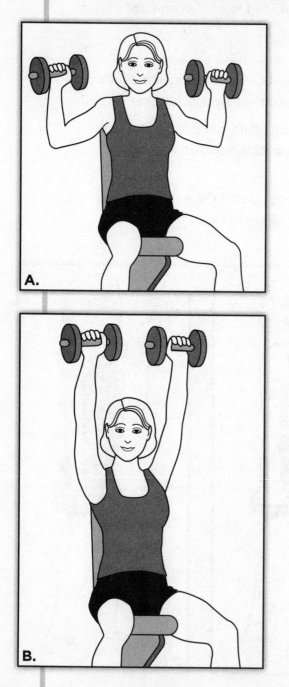

1. Sit straight up on a bench or chair that supports your back, holding a dumbbell or similar weight in each hand, with your palms facing outward and your elbows bent upward at a 90-degree angle (as shown in illustration A).

2. Exhale as you push the weights upward until your arms are straight and in line with your shoulders (as shown in illustration B). Don't lock your elbows into position, and be careful not to arch your back. **Note:** *If you experience discomfort in your shoulders, do the exercise with your palms facing in toward your body.*

3. Inhale as you return to the starting position to complete one rep.

4. Aim to complete one or two sets of 12 to 16 reps each.

❯ Lateral Arm Raise

Your shoulder and arm muscles benefit from this easy strength routine.

1. Sit up tall on an armless chair or stool, with your feet flat on the floor, approximately shoulder width apart. Hold a dumbbell in each hand, with your arms straight down at your sides and your palms facing inward (as shown in illustration A).

2. Inhale gradually, then slowly exhale as you raise both arms to the sides until they are shoulder height (as shown in illustration B).

3. Hold it for one second, inhale, then exhale as you slowly lower your arms to the starting position.

4. Pause for a second or two, then repeat as many times as you can while maintaining good form. Aim for two or three sets of six to eight reps. **Note:** *Throughout this process, keep your back straight so you don't injure yourself.*

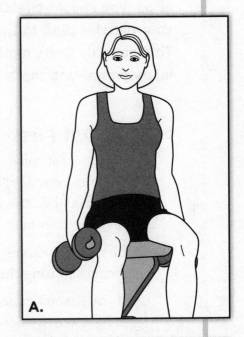

A.

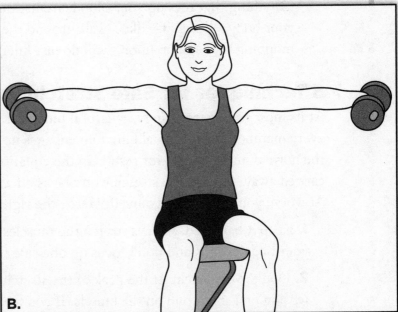

B.

>>> FLEXIBILITY

Serious fitness buffs make a big deal about stretching their muscles as part of their workout routines. But even if you don't formally exercise at all, you should stretch your body every day. As you grow older, your muscles tend to tighten and pull onto your skeletal structure. That not only limits motion in your joints, but also makes you more injury prone—and that's not how to grow younger, to put it mildly!

❯ Work Out First—Stretch Later

Contrary to what some so-called experts may tell you, the best time to do stretching exercises is after you've performed any aerobic or strength routine. That's because you can stretch more effectively—and more safely—when your muscles are warm. Also, follow these two guidelines:

- Be sure to focus especially on stretching the muscles you used the most during the activity you've just engaged in.

- If you haven't done a workout, warm up with 5 to 10 minutes of light activity before you begin your stretching exercises. (Anything that revs up your blood circulation and loosens up your body a little bit—like a walk around the block, or even mopping the kitchen floor—will do just fine.)

❯ 5 Techniques for Safe Stretching

At its most basic, stretching is a natural movement that just about every member of the animal kingdom engages in. But when you add the normal human quest for results to the equation, it's easy to get carried away. At best, the stretch won't be as effective as it should be. At worst, you could hurt yourself. Here's the right way to go about it:

1. Keep it balanced. Always stretch the muscles on both sides of your body evenly, and don't focus on one side more than the other.

2. Don't overstretch. At the peak of the stretch, you should feel mild tension or a slight pull on the muscle. If you feel pain, back off.

3. Take it slow and easy. Always stretch slowly and evenly. Hold the stretch for 15 to 30 seconds, then release just as slowly.

4. Keep it smooth. Never bounce or jerk during a stretch.

5. Don't hold your breath. Flexibility exercises should be relaxing.

Note: *If you have any health conditions, talk to your doctor about which movements are best for you and which ones you should avoid.*

❯ Do Your Chores...

And increase your flexibility at the same time. Consider this sampling of everyday household chores that provide stretching options galore:

Loosen your hips on laundry day. Sit on the floor with the bottoms of your feet together, and place a basket of clothes at arm's length in front of you so that you must gently lean forward to reach it. Stay in this position, breathing evenly, as you pull each garment out, fold it, and set it aside. This'll ease tension in your hip flexors and stretch your muscles.

Straddle a bench and stretch your legs. Again, set your basket at arm's length in front of you. But this time, sit straddling an ottoman or bench. Keep your back straight as you reach for the items inside the basket. This move loosens both your hips and legs.

Stretch and clean. As you dust ceiling light fixtures, bookshelves, or other high places, concentrate on using your shoulders and upper arms to do the work. You'll know you're doing it right if you feel the stretch in the sides of your torso as you reach up with your arms.

Do the vacuum torso twist.
Instead of pushing the machine with your arms, turn and stretch your torso as you move. Your hips, abdomen, and both upper and lower back will reap big benefits.

> " Exercise? I get it on the golf course. When I see my friends collapse, I run for the paramedics.
>
> —Red Skelton (1913–1997) "

❯ Neck Twist

There are hundreds of exercises that will help you grow younger and stay in good health. But this one—as ultra-simple as it is—could actually save your life. If that statement sounds way-out wacko, think about this: If you can't turn your neck freely, you can't get an adequate view of your surroundings as you're driving a car, riding a bicycle, or even navigating through a crowded room.

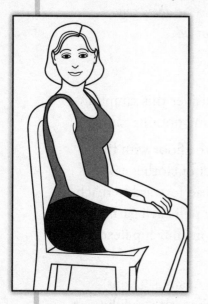

1. Sit straight up in a chair, with your feet flat on the floor, shoulder width apart.

2. Keeping your spine flat against the chair back and your shoulders facing forward, slowly turn your head to look over your shoulder. Hold the position for 10 to 30 seconds, then carefully return to the starting position. Repeat the twisting process on the other side to complete one rep.

3. Do six to eight reps. Rest briefly, then do a second set. That's all there is to it!

❯ Chin Drop

This equally simple companion to the neck twist above stretches both your neck and your shoulders.

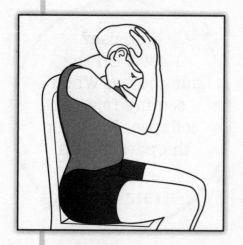

1. Place the palms of both of your hands on top of your head, with your elbows bent. Make sure your back is straight and your head is forward.

2. Using the weight of your arms, gently push your chin downward until you feel a definite, but comfortable, stretch in your neck and shoulders.

3. Take five deep breaths, inhaling and exhaling slowly. Relax and focus on releasing any tension in your upper back. Slowly raise your head to the starting position. Repeat two to four times.

> Lat Stretch

Over time, the muscles that connect your upper arms to your middle and lower back (a.k.a. your latissimus dorsi) tend to shorten and tighten as a result of overuse, poor posture, or both. The result can cause anything from simple discomfort when you reach overhead to debilitating pain that makes you feel years older than you are. The good news is that stretching your lats daily with a simple exercise like this one can relieve soreness, increase your mobility, and help prevent injuries.

1. Choose a sturdy countertop or table that's about the height of your upper thighs. Stand an arm's length away, with your feet hip width apart and your arms down. Tighten your ab muscles to stabilize your spine, and pull your shoulder blades down and back. Keep your chest lifted and your chin tilted up slightly.

2. Put your hands on the table, keeping your arms straight, your knees bent slightly, and your legs directly under your hips (as shown in illustration A).

3. Lean back into your hips, straighten your legs, and lower your body toward the ground (as shown in illustration B). Keep your back straight and your chin tucked into your neck so that your head doesn't drop toward the floor. Hold the position for 15 to 30 seconds. Repeat two to four times.

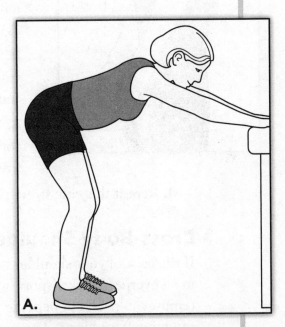

A.

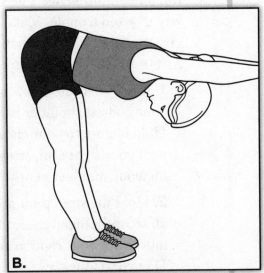

B.

> Arm Opener

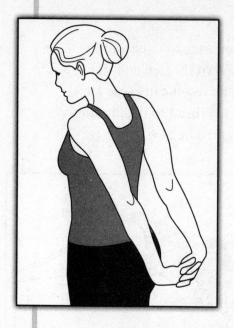

With one simple movement, this winner stretches muscles and boosts flexibility in your arms, chest, and shoulders.

1. Stand straight with your feet comfortably apart. Interlace your hands behind your tailbone, with your knuckles facing down, as shown in the illustration.

2. Looking straight ahead while keeping your arms loose, gently pull your arms up and as far away from your tailbone as you can.

3. When you feel a definite—but still comfortable—stretch, hold the position for five full breaths in and out. Then release.

4. Repeat this easy stretch two to four times for best results.

> Cross-Body Shoulder Stretch

If the back of your shoulder is tight, and you play golf or participate in an overhead racket sport like tennis, you're all but begging for rotator cuff problems. The simple way to avoid trouble: Make this guaranteed flexibility enhancer part of your regular routine.

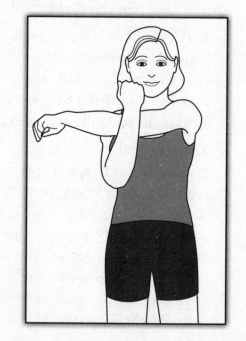

1. Bring your left arm across your body at shoulder height. Hold it close to your chest with your right arm, stretching your shoulder gently.

2. Hold the stretch for about 30 seconds, then repeat the move with your right arm. Do two to four reps.

› Overhead Triceps Stretch

As its name implies, this exercise enhances the flexibility of your upper arms, focusing on the triceps muscles on the back side.

1. Stand comfortably in a natural position with your feet hip width apart and your shoulders rolled down and back.

2. Extend your left arm toward the ceiling, keeping your shoulder below your ear. Bend your elbow, and put your left hand on your back with your palm facing in (as shown in illustration A).

3. Reach up with your right hand. Put your fingers on your left arm, just above the elbow (as shown in illustration B). Very gently push downward. Don't force it, and don't make any bouncing motions! Hold the position for 15 to 30 seconds. Repeat two to four times, trying to stretch a little farther each time. Don't push yourself to progress too quickly—if this stretch feels painful, take it back a notch.

4. Switch arm positions, and repeat the procedure.

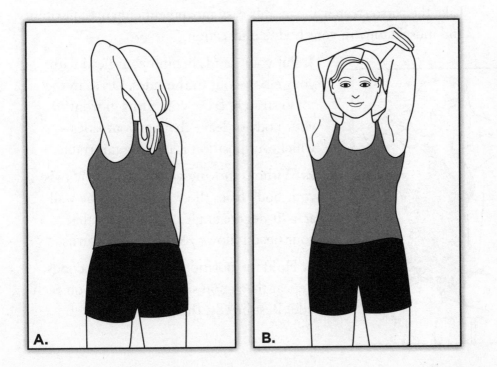

A. B.

❯ Torso Stretch

As its name implies, this movement stretches (and helps slim) your body's hips and waist.

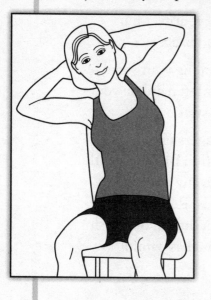

1. Put your hands behind your head with your elbows out to the side. If you find it more comfortable, you can either cross your arms in front of your body or leave them at your sides.

2. Keeping your head facing forward, lean to one side, bending your body at the waist. Hold the position for five seconds.

3. Return to the starting position, and repeat on the other side to complete one rep.

4. Perform six to eight reps. Rest for 30 to 60 seconds, then do a second set.

❯ Torso Twist

Like the torso stretch above, this easy movement enhances flexibility and muscle tone in your body's midsection.

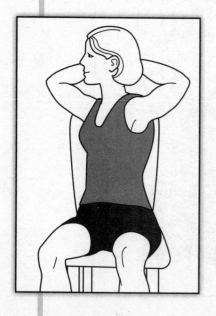

1. Put your hands behind your head with your elbows out to the sides. Or, as in the torso stretch, cross your arms in front of your body or leave them at your sides—whichever position is more comfortable.

2. Without moving your hips, slowly twist your body from the waist to face the wall at a 90-degree angle, making sure that your head follows your body as it turns.

3. Hold the position for 10 to 30 seconds. Repeat the action six to eight times on each side. Rest briefly, then do a second set.

❯ Seated March

Thanks to the fact that many of us spend
so much time sitting on our butts, tight hips
have become a major epidemic. Over time,
that can greatly hinder your mobility. Fortunately, there are a number of simple exercises
that can help keep—or get—those essential
body parts flexible, including this winner.

1. Sit in a chair with your feet flat on
the floor, shoulder width apart.

2. Raise one knee as high as your comfort
level allows. Return to the starting
position, and repeat with the other leg.

3. March 12 to 16 times—six to eight times
per leg. Rest briefly, then do a second set.

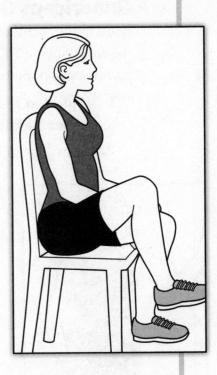

❯ Prone Hip Stretch

This companion to the seated march is an excellent mobility enhancer.

1. Lie on your back on the floor, with your legs straight, or as close to
it as you can get them.

2. Bend your right leg, and put your hands on the back of your right
thigh just below your knee.

3. Gently pull your thigh toward your chest as far as you can.

4. Hold the position for 20 seconds, then slowly straighten your

leg and lower it to
the floor. Repeat
with your left leg.

5. Do two or three
reps, working
toward holding
the stretch for a
full 30 seconds.

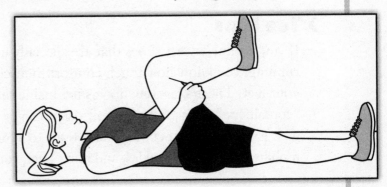

❯ Quadriceps Stretch

In addition to stretching your quadriceps muscles, which run along the front of your thighs, this simple movement also strengthens the hamstrings on the back of your thighs.

1. Stand 12 to 18 inches from a wall, with your left hand against the surface for support and your arm slightly bent.

2. Grasp your right ankle with your right hand. Gently pull your heel up and back, until you feel a stretch in the front of your thigh. (If you can't reach your ankle, grab your sock or pant leg instead.) Keep your left leg bent just a little bit to avoid injury on that side.

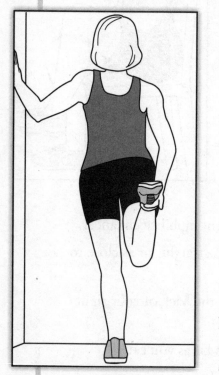

3. Hold the position for two to three seconds, standing tall and looking straight ahead. Your knee should be facing the floor and your ankle aligned with it—not turned to the side.

4. Let go of your ankle, and slowly return your foot to the floor. Repeat the move six to eight times. Then reverse your position and perform the exercise six to eight times with your left leg.

5. Rest briefly, then do a second set.

Note: *With practice, you should be able to perform this exercise standing on one foot with no support—thereby enhancing your balance as well as your flexibility.*

❯ Toe Fans

If you routinely wear shoes that are specially designed for walking or running, you know how much comfort their cushioned support gives your feet. There's just one downside: Inside those cushy, high-tech "containers," your joints and soft tissue can't move around in a normal way. Eventually, that confinement leads to a loss of flexibility as well as mobility in your feet, ankles, and toes. Then your lower extremities may become stiff, weak, or painful. Simply spending quality time in your bare feet can help alleviate or avoid problems. So can simple stretching exercises like the ones on this page.

1. Stand with your bare feet on the floor, parallel to each other, shoulder distance apart. Then simply lift your toes, and lower them. Repeat four times.

2. Lift and lower your toes in the same manner, but this time, while they're up, spread your toes as wide as you can. Again, repeat the action four additional times to complete one full repetition.

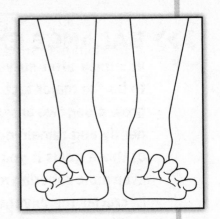

▶ Rock 'Em and Raise 'Em

The combined actions of this duo stretch and strengthen your ankles and feet.

1. With your feet parallel, rock onto the outer edges (as shown in illustration A). Then roll onto the inner edges. Repeat four times, or as many as you'd like until you feel a comforting looseness and free movement in your lower reaches.

2. Keeping your left foot flat, lift your right heel, so you're on the ball of your right foot (as shown in illustration B). Then slowly lower your heel back down to the floor. Repeat the move a total of eight times.

3. Then do a second set of eight, with one variation: While your heel is lifted, roll the ball of your foot from side to side.

4. Switch sides, and repeat the full routine once again with your left foot.

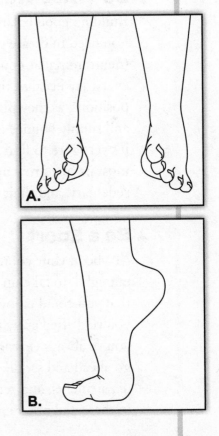

A.

B.

⟫⟫ BALANCE EXERCISES

In survey after survey, when people are asked what they consider to be the major factors in maintaining a good quality of life as they grow older, two answers rank at the top of the charts: living independently and remaining active. Of course, you can't accomplish either of those goals if you can't stay steady on your feet. Here's another, even more sobering reason that retaining—or regaining—good balance is crucial for anyone who wants to grow younger: Falling is the leading cause of ER visits and accidental deaths in people over the age of 65. For those 75 and older, falls account for a full 70 percent of accidental deaths. Need I say more?

❯ So What Went Wrong?

Building good balance is like learning to play a musical instrument: You need to create certain pathways between your brain and muscles (neuromuscular connections, in scientific lingo). Children do this every day because they are constantly putting themselves into unstable positions, as they play hopscotch, ride bikes and scooters, walk on stilts, and simply bounce around on playground equipment. Consequently, it's very rare to find a child who doesn't have excellent balance. Once most people grow up—especially in this day and age—they become sedentary, and their neuromuscular connections get rusty.

❯ Be a Sport

Maybe in your younger days you were lucky enough—or farsighted enough—to take up a balance-enhancing sport like skating or skiing that you could enjoy well into old age. If not, start now! Likewise, if you've drifted away from a beloved pastime like horseback riding—or you've always yearned to learn but didn't have the time or spare cash—go ahead and saddle up. Community colleges, municipal recreation departments, and senior groups throughout the country offer lessons in these and other sports that are specifically aimed at the over-50 set.

> Two, Four, Six, Eight...

We need to coordinate. Let me explain: Good balance and general body coordination go hand in hand. Any sport or activity that demands good coordination also helps improve your balance. Ballroom dancing is a champ in this regard (see "May I Have This Dance?" on page 245). According to sports analysts, these are also winners:

- Diving
- Golf
- Skeet shooting
- Fencing
- Lawn bowling
- Squash

According to recent research, one of the most effective balance-coordination boosters of all is a simple game of catch. Most of the academic studies have focused on controlled experiments in which the subjects throw and catch a lightweight medicine ball. But simply tossing a baseball (or any kind of ball) back and forth will do the trick. No doubt it'll bring back some mighty happy memories to boot.

> Try a Class Act

Both yoga and tai chi earn top marks for improving balance, flexibility, and muscle strength. Plus, taking part in an ongoing class will give you a chance to mix and mingle with your fellow students. As we'll see coming up in Chapter 8, social interaction is a crucial component in the art of growing younger. Do yourself a favor and check out classes in your area. If you have any chronic health issues, investigate your options, and check with your doctor before you sign up.

Fountain of Youth
LEAPIN' LINIMENT!

When you first take up any new sport, you're bound to wind up with some discomfort in your muscles or joints. A gentle rubdown with this recipe will put you back in action.

 2 egg whites
 ½ cup of apple cider vinegar*
 ¼ cup of olive oil

Mix all of the ingredients thoroughly. Massage the lotion into the painful areas, and wipe off the excess with a soft cotton cloth. (Be careful not to get any of the stuff on sheets, clothes, or upholstery fabric!)
*Use the pure, unfiltered kind— not the processed stuff in the salad dressing aisle.

Good Balance Is Habit-Forming

Or to put it another way, good habits can make for better balance. Regularly engaging in sports and performing exercises like the ones in this chapter are no-fail ways to improve your stability. But so are a whole lot of balance challenges that you can work into your daily routine. Consider these, for instance:

Stand on one foot. Do this every chance you get—for example, when you're talking on the phone; brushing your teeth; preparing food in the kitchen; waiting for a bus; or standing in line at the bank, supermarket, or post office. If you happen to be holding something in your hand, so much the better. For example, at the grocery store, you might take a bag of oranges out of your cart and hold it by the top while you wait for your turn to check out.

Walk the line. When you're on a fairly quiet street, with no traffic whizzing by, step along on the curb instead of the sidewalk itself—as most of us did as kids. You can also practice this feat at home. For instance, follow a single plank in a wood floor or a straight line of kitchen floor tiles.

Play one-legged pickup. When you drop your keys, a coin, or other small object, bend over and pick it up while keeping one leg slightly raised behind you. As your balance improves, up the challenge by lifting your leg higher.

Ride 'em, cowboy! Passenger, rather. Whenever you're riding on a trolley, train, or subway, assume a wide stance, with your knees slightly bent (as if you were surfing) and without holding on to a railing or overhead strap. Instead, tighten your leg and core muscles to keep yourself from falling. Do, however, stay within easy reach of a seat back or other firm support in case the vehicle lurches!

Note: *Granted, when you do any of these maneuvers in a public place, you're likely to get some strange looks or even quizzical comments. Just think of it as an excuse to strike up a conversation. Who knows? You just might wind up with better balance and some new friends.*

❯ Sit to Stand

If your balance isn't quite as steady as it once was, this sit-to-stand exercise belongs on your daily schedule. For as simple as it sounds (and is), it's one of the best, and most gentle, ways to strengthen all the muscles that keep you moving along securely in an upright position.

1. Sit toward the front of a firm chair, such as a wooden dining chair, so that your heels are lined up with the front of the seat.

2. Inhale, then exhale as you stand up, using your rear end and leg muscles. Keep your spine straight and your arms extended downward at your sides. If it's absolutely necessary to retain your balance, you can rest your hands lightly on the chair arms or seat, but try your best not to put any weight on them! (Try imagining that there's a helium-filled balloon in the center of your head, just above your eyes, and it's pulling you up.)

3. Sit back down in the same manner (without using your hands for balance, if you can) to complete one repetition. Do 5 to 10 repetitions twice per day—that is, in addition to using the technique every time you rise from a chair in the course of your normal activity. The more you practice this move, and the ones at left (see "Good Balance Is Habit-Forming"), the more your balance will improve!

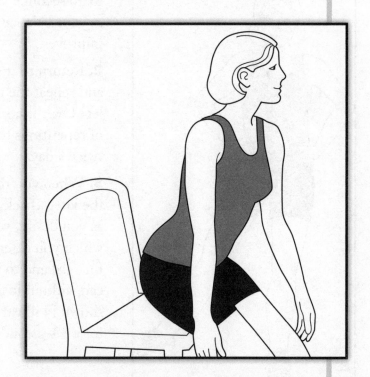

❯ Single-Leg Balance

Standing on one leg is another classic, and highly effective, way to improve your stability. In the beginning, perform this exercise within easy reaching distance of a wall or the back of a chair so you can reach out to catch your balance if necessary.

1. Stand with your feet hip width apart and your weight evenly distributed. With your hands on your hips, lift your left foot off the floor and bend your leg back at the knee (as shown in illustration A). Hold the position as long as you can, working up to 30 seconds as your balance improves.

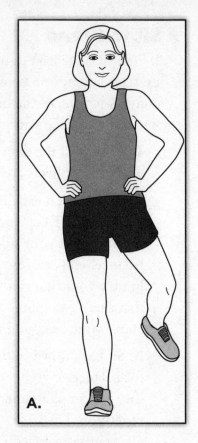

A.

2. Return to the starting position and repeat the process with your right leg. Over time, increase the number of repetitions to 10 to 15 once or twice a day.

3. When you're comfortable with the knees-back position, alternate it, as you desire, with a variation in which you extend your raised foot forward and to the side as far as you can without losing your balance (as shown in illustration B). Again, aim for a 30-second hold time.

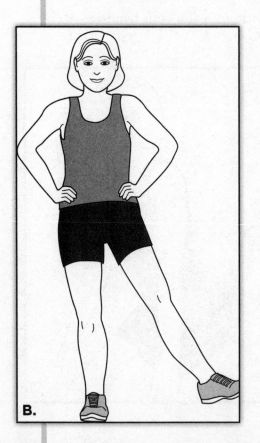

B.

❯ Single-Leg Balance with Weight

As I mentioned in the strength section (see page 256), the addition of hand weights can intensify the effect of almost any exercise—and those in the balance category are no exception.

1. Stand with your feet hip width apart and your weight distributed evenly. Hold a dumbbell in your left hand, at waist level or a little above, with your palm facing upward (as shown in illustration A).

2. Lift your right foot off the floor, and bend your leg back at the knee (as shown in illustration B). Hold the position for as long as you can, aiming for 30 seconds.

3. Return to the starting position and repeat the action using your left foot. As with the single-leg balance exercise at left, your goal should be one or two sets of 10 to 15 reps each.

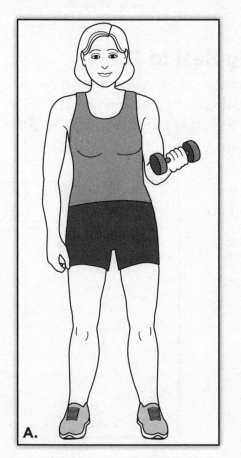

A.

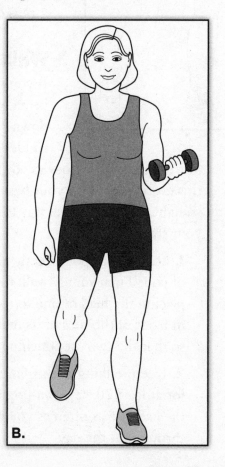

B.

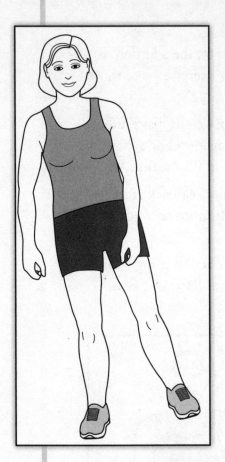

❯ Weight Shifts

When you're ready to try more formal balance exercises, start with weight shifts.

1. Stand with your feet hip width apart and your weight evenly distributed on both legs.

2. Shift your weight to the right, and lift your left foot off the floor, keeping both legs straight, but not locking your knees. Hold the position as long you can while remaining steady, eventually working up to 30 seconds.

3. Return to the starting position and repeat the process with your right foot. Do as many repetitions as you can, aiming for 10 to 15 reps once or twice a day.

❯ Walking Heel to Toe

If you've ever tried to walk across a balance beam, you already have this movement down pat. For all of you who haven't been so lucky, simply pretend there is an invisible line of tape on the floor as you practice this exercise, and try your best to walk straight. It's a top-notch way to improve your stability.

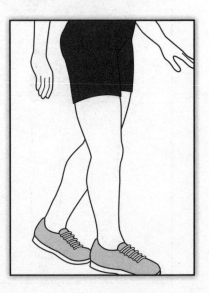

1. Focus on a spot directly ahead of you. Then simply walk forward, placing the heel of one foot directly in front of the toes of its mate so that the two are touching.

2. Keep walking in this fashion for at least 20 steps, and repeat the exercise as often as you can throughout the day.

❯ Balance Walk

To intensify the simple heel-to-toe maneuver you just learned, ramp up the action by adding your arms to the mix with this balance walk:

1. Raise your arms to shoulder height (as shown in illustration A).

2. Focusing on a spot directly ahead of you, walk in a straight line, placing one foot in front of the other—but with each step, lift your back leg (as shown in illustration B). Pause for one second before stepping forward.

3. Repeat, alternating legs, for a total of 20 steps. Perform this maneuver as often as you can throughout the day. Feel free to sneak it in as you're simply walking to the kitchen or down the hallway.

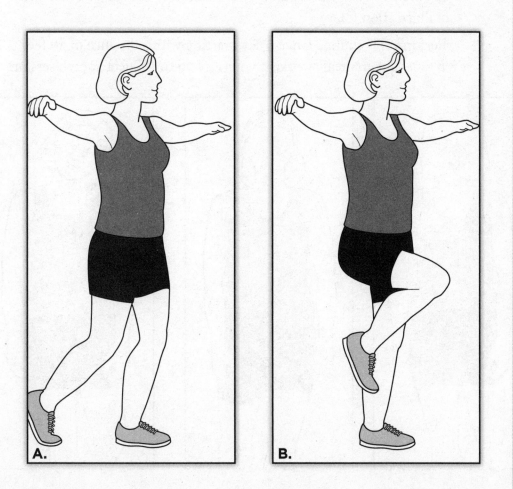

A.　　　　　B.

❯ Head-for-Balance Walk

This routine may sound like a piece of cake, but it's actually very tricky to stroll along in this manner without weaving back and forth, or even falling. In fact, for the first time or two, consider having someone nearby to lend a helping hand if you stumble.

1. Walk ahead in your normal pace for about 50 feet (or as far as you can go in a firm, straight line). Turn your head to the left and then to the right with alternate steps (as shown in illustration A).

2. Next, walk while moving your head up and down (as shown in illustration B). Again, strive to go 50 feet or so—but do not feel discouraged if you can't get that far just yet!

3. Finally, walk while tipping your head from side to side (as shown in illustration C).

Perform this routine twice a day, starting with a distance of 50 feet each time and gradually working your way up to 100 feet at each session.

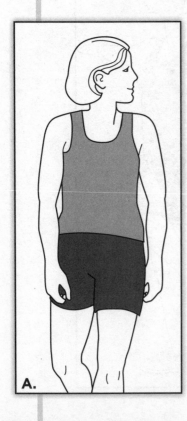

A.

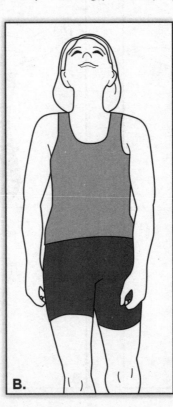

B.

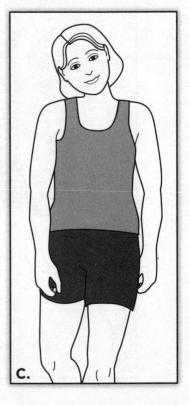

C.

❯ Stork Turn

This is not only a great balance exercise, but it also enhances flexibility in your torso. For that reason (attention, golfers!), it's an ideal way to create a bit of game-improving separation between the upper and lower body.

1. Stand up straight and place both hands on top of a golf club or similar support in front of you. (A length of pipe, a wooden dowel, or a broom handle cut to the right length will all work fine.)

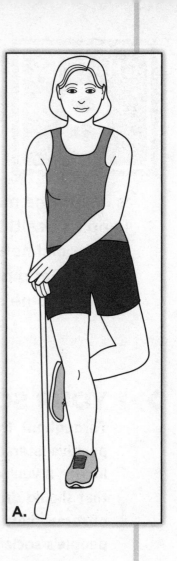

A.

2. Lift your left leg and hook your foot behind your right knee (as shown in illustration A).

3. Keeping your shoulders and torso stationary, rotate the raised knee across your right leg (as shown in illustration B). Repeat 10 to 15 times, or as many as you can manage while keeping your balance and your upper-body position.

4. Switch leg positions and repeat the motion in the opposite direction, again for up to 10 to 15 times. Perform two or three sets.

5. When you can successfully complete the full routine, you can move on to the unsupported version for a bigger challenge: Gently cross your arms, put your hands on your shoulders, and repeat the movements you just learned above.

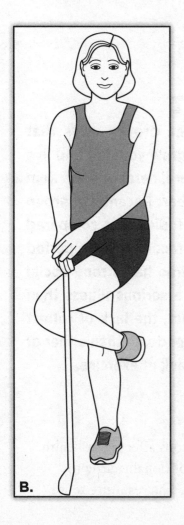

B.

In Good Company

CHAPTER 8

Medical science is now proving what the oldest members of our population have always known: A strong social network (as the scientific crowd likes to call it) is one of the most important factors in living a longer, happier, healthier life. So, you may ask, exactly what does this "social network" consist of? And how does it work its magic? Good questions. You'll find the answers coming up—and some of them might surprise you.

>>> YOUR SOCIAL SAFETY NET

Throughout this book, I've been touting the proven ways that positive interaction with others can help you grow younger and live longer. If you're still not convinced on that score, here's a news item that should drive the point home loud and clear: Recently, a group of researchers examined the results of 148 studies that compared people's social inclinations with their health records over a period of more than seven years. The result: Folks who had strong social ties were 50 percent more likely to survive a serious illness than those who were not so well connected. In fact, the lack of robust relationships presented a stronger risk factor for death than either of two infamous health destroyers: obesity and lack of exercise.

> Ways and Means

No one knows precisely why your social affiliations affect your health. Some psychologists reckon that when you're emotionally close to family or friends, you feel responsible for them. The resulting sense of purpose encourages you to take better care of yourself. That theory may account for part of the equation, but judging from both scientific and anecdotal evidence, there's a lot more to it than that. For example, interacting in a positive way with your fellow earthlings—human and otherwise—has been shown to:

Boost your spirits when you're feeling down, and over the longer term, help you raise your level of happiness. And, as we saw in Chapter 4, when it comes to growing younger, a happy, upbeat attitude is the closest thing there is to a magic bullet.

Lower your stress level by triggering your brain to release endorphins and other calming, feel-good chemicals.

Bypass dementia, in part by increasing your body's supply of brain-derived neurotrophic factor (BDNF), a protein that helps keep your brain cells functioning in high gear—no matter how old you are.

❯ On a More Concrete Level...

People who care about you can provide the moral support you need when you're trying to lose weight or kick an unhealthy habit, such as smoking or excessive drinking. This is especially true when your supporters have conquered the same demons themselves. Likewise, when you're recovering from surgery, an accident, or an illness, a "posse" of family, friends, and kindly neighbors is worth its weight in gold. Being surrounded by folks who cheerfully pitch in to run errands, do household chores, cook healthy meals, and encourage you to get plenty of health-restoring exercise will help put you back in action more quickly. Depending on the nature and severity of your condition, it could even save your life!

> " Love seems the swiftest, but it is the slowest of all growths. No man or woman really knows what perfect love is until they have been married a quarter of a century.
>
> —Mark Twain (1835–1910) "

❯ The Bedrock of All Social Networks

Without a doubt, the strongest support system of all is a strong, happy marriage. If you're in one, you already know that. Chances are you've also heard about the scads of studies showing that people who are happily married tend to live longer and stay healthier. But here's a trio of specific research findings that make the point loud and clear:

- Happily married people are less likely to die from heart disease, stroke, and cancer—and to recover when they do fall victim to any of those conditions. One study involving cancer cures found that in terms of statistical recovery rates, being happily married was comparable to the patients being 10 years younger than they actually were.

- One 20-year study of a nationally representative sampling found that being in a happy marriage was directly associated with better health habits, such as getting enough high-quality sleep, having regular medical checkups, drinking less, and getting more exercise.

- In psychiatric research, marital status is the number one factor for predicting depression. In fact, in one study, rates of major depression were nine times higher in unmarried men than in those who were cheerfully wedded.

MIND OVER MYTH

MYTH: Solitude is bad for your health.

REALITY: Not by a long shot. What's unhealthy is *feeling* isolated and lonely, not the simple fact of being alone. People naturally differ greatly in their desire for social interaction. Some folks crave the constant stimulation and companionship they find in group settings, while others are content within a small circle of friends and loved ones. Studies have shown that people who perceived themselves to be lonely—no matter the reason—had higher rates of mortality, even if they were married and had plenty of friends or relatives close by. The bottom line: When it comes to youth-enhancing social networks, it's the quality of your connections that matters—not the quantity of them.

❯ A Ring Is Not a Cure-All

While being happily married can work wonders for your health and well-being, the flip side is also true: A union that's not so cheery can take a major toll on your body's workings. And the problems between you and your mate don't have to be big ones. The chronic stress engendered by moderate discontent can impair your immune system enough to wipe out the advantages of your marital state. According to many researchers, this appears to be especially true for women.

One example: Scientists at the University of Pittsburgh conducted a long-term study designed to pinpoint the factors responsible for women's increased risk of heart disease after menopause. The finding: Women who saw their marriages as "highly satisfying" were far less likely to suffer from heart problems than their unwedded counterparts were. But ladies who gave their situations anything less than a five-star rating fared no better on the heart-health scale than unmarried women of the same age.

Centenarian SECRETS 100

Researchers have found that engaging in sex at least several times a week can make you look from four to seven years younger. But here's the *really* good news: Other studies have shown that having a regular romp in the hay doesn't just appear to turn back the clock—it can actually make you live longer. On top of that, the typical 30-minute tussle between the sheets burns about 200 calories and tones your muscles to boot. So, to quote Gus Kahn's classic lyrics, "Don't forget folks, that's what you get folks, for makin' whoopee!"

This news should be cause for celebration if you happen to be in a marriage that's drifting along okay but has lost the zip it once had. How so? Because there's a good chance that with just a little bit of conscious effort, you and your partner can bring back the magic connection and get on the high road to longer, healthier lives.

❯ Watch Your Language!

Over time, the youthful glow can fade from any marriage—and when you're caught up in the whirlwind of day-to-day life, the light can start

Rejuvenating Recipe
LIBIDO-LIFTING SMOOTHIE

Chocolate plays a starring role in this delicious aphrodisiac, releasing a potent load of dopamine, the brain's pleasure chemical. It's backed up by a supporting cast that delivers the romance-enhancing trio of vitamin B, vitamin D, and zinc, along with L-arginine, an amino acid that promotes healthy blood flow to the sex organs.

- **1 ¼ cups of milk**
- **¼ cup of plain yogurt (preferably Greek)**
- **1 frozen banana**
- **1 tbsp. of natural peanut butter**
- **1 tbsp. of unsweetened cocoa powder**
- **Handful of ice cubes**

Mix the ingredients in a blender until smooth. Pour the potion into a glass, drink it, and enjoy!

Yield: *1 serving*

to dim without you even noticing a change. But it doesn't have to. Simply being careful about the words you use can help keep the fire burning bright— or revive one that's flickering.

Play nice. The happiest couples have an agreement that they will not get mean, nasty, or short-tempered—no matter what. Even during arguments, they stay calm and treat each other with respect. The result is a feeling of trust, emotional safety, and love.

Say "thank you" often. As we saw in Chapter 4, cultivating an attitude of gratitude is one of the surest ways to a happier, younger you. It's also a no-fail way to firm up a marriage because every time you utter those magic words, you remind yourself of your partner's good qualities and inject a booster shot of positive energy into your relationship. To power up the impact, focus your comment on the doer of the deed—not on yourself. For example, don't say, "Thanks for cooking dinner tonight, honey; I was too tired to face a stove." Instead, say something like, "You make the most delicious burgers; it was thoughtful of you to cook dinner tonight."

Accentuate the positive. In addition to freely expressing your thanks, heed Thumper the bunny's classic advice: "If you can't say something nice, don't say nothing at all." That's not always easy, but marriage researchers tell us that every day, happy couples make at least five times as many positive statements to and about each other as they do negative ones—even when they're having a disagreement.

❯ 2 Ways to Ensure Domestic Tranquility

Whenever you encounter blustery waves in the normally calm sea of your marriage, hearken to these two pieces of advice from couples who have weathered more than half a century together:

1. Be secretly supportive. You might think that when your spouse is going through a challenging period, showing your support by (for instance) cooking special meals, running time-consuming errands, or taking on a bigger share of the household chores will shore up your connection. Not so. Psychologists tell us that overt support makes the recipient feel obligated, which increases stress in the relationship. So instead, buoy your mate up with more subtle gestures, such as stocking the fridge with favorite snacks or drinks, tidying up a cluttered work space, or planting a bed of beautiful flowers in a can't-miss location.

2. Lay your differences on the table. No two human beings agree on everything. What matters in a marriage is not how many differences you and your spouse have, but how you handle them. Happy couples face issues head on and look for ways to work around them—rather than dismissing them as irrelevant or (even worse) pretending they don't exist.

Say It with Music

It's no secret that sex and exercise trigger your brain to release happiness-boosting endorphins. But here's something you might not know: Listening to a favorite song does exactly the same thing. So if you're looking for a super-simple way to raise the happiness level of your marriage, put together a list of tunes you both love, and enjoy them together as often as you can—whether you play them on your home stereo, plunk them out on the piano, or seek out live venues where you know you'll be able to say, "Darling, they're playing our song."

Tick-Tock **TURN BACK the CLOCK**

⟫⟫⟫ WHAT EMPTY NEST?

A generation ago, one of the most pressing issues facing middle-aged couples was the "empty nest syndrome." As the last child left for college, these folks had to adjust to the change from a household bustling with activity to one where they had only each other for company. My, how times change! Today, nearly 40 percent of young adults between the ages of 18 and 34 are living with their parents. That's the highest percentage since 1940. Here's another shocker: Roughly 85 percent of college grads come back to roost, rather than taking wing after graduation, as most of their counterparts did in the past several decades. In these pages, I'll share some top-notch strategies for living life in the family fast lane—without losing your mind, your marriage, or your precious relationship with your offspring.

⟩ Dollars and Sense

"Boomerangers," as they're often called, return home for various reasons, but the most common factor by far can be summed up in one word: money. Or rather, the lack of it. Today, it's a rare scholar who *doesn't* leave college burdened with more debt than folks in previous generations ever dreamed of, including student loans, unpaid credit card bills, and often a car loan, too. Add to that the high cost of rent in many cities, and you've got way more outgo than most recent grads can even think of handling. Your challenge as a parent is to grant safe haven to your nestlings while gently nudging them toward independence.

⟩ Look to the Future

You'll avoid a whole lot of headaches and heartache if you establish some firm guidelines right from the get-go. (Look at it as the empty nest equivalent of a prenuptial agreement.) Of course, the details will vary, depending on such factors as your child's current debt load and whether he already has a paycheck or is still searching for that first job. These are some of the key issues to consider—and put in writing:

The goal. Living at home for a while after college can give a young person the foundation he needs to find a job, start a business, save for a down payment on a house, or simply get out of debt and onto sound financial footing. So sit down with your child and discuss his goals, then decide how you can work together to make them a reality.

The job search. Your recent graduate may be so eager to get her career rolling that you don't have to give this category a second's thought. On the other hand, someone who's not such a hard charger may let your warm welcome lull her into feeling that she's back in Mom and Dad's loving arms for keeps. In that case, you need to offer some strong encouragement, or even a little tough love. Insist that she spend a certain amount of time each day actively looking for work, even it means signing on with a temp agency. Granted, the pay isn't great, but anyone with basic business skills and a positive, professional attitude is all but guaranteed steady employment. Plus, you never know when a temp gig, or the people you meet there, may lead to "The Dream Job."

Move-out day. Set a target date that's based on your child's current income (if any) and his current debt load. Of course, you can always extend the time frame if you need to, but unless you put a firm deadline in place, your cohabitation could stretch on for years.

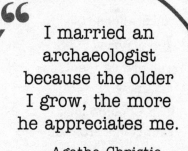

> " I married an archaeologist because the older I grow, the more he appreciates me.
>
> —Agatha Christie (1890–1976) "

❯ Keys to a Happy Home Front

In addition to helping your offspring gear up for his personal Independence Day (see "Look to the Future," at left), there are a couple of other matters that need to be settled at the very beginning of your cohabitation. Namely these two important ones:

- Chores. If you could use a little help around the old homestead (and who can't?), now's the time to speak up! But whatever jobs you choose to hand over, be careful you don't become so dependent on your resident worker that you let her stay stretch on much longer than it really should!

- Code of conduct. The teenager who left your home is returning as a full-fledged adult, but that doesn't mean you have to put up with behavior that drives you nuts. For instance, if you won't tolerate smoking, blaring loud "music," or opposite-sex sleepover guests, say so in no uncertain terms. You can decide what the acceptable limits are in your household, but no matter how strict or lenient they may be, it's crucial to set them from the very beginning.

❯ The Question of Rent

It goes without saying (I hope) that if having another mouth to feed poses a financial burden on you, then you should definitely insist that your returning offspring contribute to the family's expenses. But when money takes second place to the child's

---

Fountain of Youth

VANILLA BATH BLEND

It's a proven fact that any major change in our lives, either positive or negative, causes stress. That means no matter how much you enjoy having young John or Mary back in the fold, there are bound to be times when you feel so tense and stressed out that you want to scream. Don't scream. Instead, relax with this terrific softening tub-time treat.

> 1 cup of almond oil
>
> ½ cup of honey
>
> ½ cup of mild liquid soap (unscented)
>
> 1 tbsp. of pure vanilla extract (not artificial)

Mix the ingredients together in a jar with a tight-fitting lid. To use the formula, shake the jar gently to mix, and pour ¼ cup under running bathwater. Settle back, and dream of simpler times.

future welfare, psychological and financial experts differ on whether treating your boomeranger as a paying tenant is helpful or not. Only you can make the final decision on whether to charge your child rent but these are the two schools of thought:

1. When a child pays a certain amount each month for rent, food, and utilities, it helps instill a sense of financial responsibility and, ultimately, a smoother entry into "real life." If you simply don't feel right about accepting money from your child, you can always deposit the payments into an interest-bearing account and offer it as a housewarming gift when Junior finally moves into his own digs.

2. If your budget allows, it's better to let your recent graduate focus her full income and any other monetary resources on paying off debt and saving money for the future. The sooner she builds a good credit history and the more cash she's able to sock away, the sooner she'll be able to fly the coop and settle into a nest of her own. This does not mean giving your grown-up "baby" a free ride. It simply means that you let her pay for her keep by bartering her services instead of forking out cold, hard cash. For instance, you might have her spend a specific number of hours per week cooking family meals, doing yard and garden chores, or running errands in exchange for not having to hand over a portion of her paycheck. Ultimately, you can sit down and discuss with her the duties she would most like to take on, and come up with a plan that works for everyone.

What's Old Is New

There's nothing new about grown children living at home. In fact, before the end of World War II, young men and women rarely left the nest until they were married—and many couples stayed on with one set of in-laws, even after they'd had a baby or two of their own. Not until well into the 1950s did it become common for young, single adults to set up housekeeping, either alone or with roommates.

❯ Prepare for Takeoff

Before your child moves out on her own, sit down with her to discuss the basics of budgeting and setting up a realistic spending plan. If you don't feel fiscally savvy enough to do this job yourself, take her to see a professional financial planner. When it comes to budgets, one "size" does not fit all, so tailor the final product to suit your child's circumstances. Just make sure you include at least these nine basic categories:

- Housing
- Transportation
- Savings
- Utilities
- Groceries
- Personal care
- Health insurance
- Entertainment
- Clothing and its upkeep

> " You know you're getting old when all the names in your black book have M.D. after them.
> —Arnold Palmer (1929–2016 "

❯ Save Up or Pay Down?

Just as professional money managers differ on the question of boomerangers paying rent, they also disagree on financial priorities. Some planners say that paying off credit cards and other debts should rank at the very top of the list. Others insist that recent grads should begin saving at least something for their retirement, even if it means taking longer to trim the charge-card balances (presuming, of course, that the accounts are in good standing). This argument carries a lot of weight, especially for young folks who are gainfully employed and are eligible for either 401(k) or 403(b) plans at work. For instance, if a person in his early 20s sets aside $4,000 a year starting now, he could find himself with a seven-figure nest egg by the time he's ready to retire!

❯ Don't Discard the Cards!

Once folks have paid off a large amount of credit card debt, they're often tempted to cut up the cards and toss them out. Well, don't let your boomeranger do that! (And don't you do it with your cards either.) Why? Because the key to getting a home mortgage or a business loan is having a good credit score. And the surest route to a healthy number is to use major credit cards regularly and pay the bills on time—without fail.

You might think that perhaps you could accomplish the same thing by maintaining a good payment record with utility companies, local businesses, or your landlord, but that's not the case at all. Major credit card companies report their customers' transactions to the national credit data banks every single month, while most utility companies, independent stores, and rental agencies only report the negative information—for instance, when a bill remains unpaid for so long that it goes to a collection agency.

The bottom line: Your boomeranger should keep her cards, but make sure she is using them responsibly. If she sticks to her budget and pays off her bills on time, she can build valuable credit that will make it possible for her to get out from under your wing—and give you back your empty nest!

Stay on Track

Whatever you do, don't jeopardize your own long-term financial security for the sake of your adult children. Continue to invest as much money as possible for your retirement, and save for shorter-term goals, too. Don't forget, your youngsters have many more years than you do to get on the right financial track. If that sounds hard-hearted, think of it this way: If you shortchange yourself now, a few years down the road, you may end up having to depend on your kids for money—and that's definitely not the way to grow younger!

Tick-Tock TURN BACK the CLOCK

How-To Help for Harried Caregivers

More than 10 million Americans (mostly women) are caring for family members who have dementia—and that's often on top of running busy households and holding down demanding jobs. If you're one of those heroes, you know that it's all too easy to get so caught up in the daily whirlwind that you neglect your own health. Well, don't do it! Remember, if you don't take good care of yourself, you can't do much for anyone else. So consider this your own personal Tender Lovin' Toolkit.

Do what Mom always told you. Eat right, get a good eight hours of sleep each night, don't smoke, and get plenty of fresh air and regular exercise. (If you think you don't possibly have time to work *that* into your day, check out Chapter 7, "Get a Move On.")

Take a mental health day. Everyone needs a break now and then. If you work, call in sick. If you're based out of your house, simply devote the day to yourself—even if that means calling in a substitute caregiver. And what should you do with your very own day? Whatever you want. Go to a movie or an art exhibit. Take a walk in the park. Curl up on the couch and read a murder mystery. Or simply sit around and do nothing. Then, when stressful moments come up, think back to that quiet time. (And, when remembering your mental health day no longer reenergizes you, it's time to take another one!)

Stay connected. Having friends and other supportive people around you is crucial to good mental and physical health. In fact, you may find that being under a lot of strain makes you feel the need to be more social, even if you're the solitary type by nature. According to recent scientific research, being under stress causes your body to produce a hormone called oxytocin, which promotes a desire to connect with other people.

Granted, when you're caught up in a whirlwind of caregiving activity, it's hard to remain socially active. But whether you volunteer in your community, join a bridge club, or become more involved in your church, the lift to your health and spirits will pay off in big dividends for you *and* your loved one.

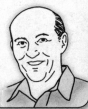

⇢≫ GATHER THE FAM

It's probably no coincidence that, over the past few decades, as life has gotten faster, more complex, and less certain, one very positive trend has emerged: a steadily rising number of family reunions. Each year, more and more families are holding these gatherings—and, in many cases, re-cementing bonds that have been broken for years. If you haven't yet dipped your toe into these delightful waters, you've come to the right place. In this section, I'll give you some pointers on getting your gang together—and having a whole lot of fun in the process.

≫ 3 Steps to Getting the Show on the Road

If the mere thought of staging a family reunion makes you break out in a cold sweat, relax. Here's all you need to do to get the ball rolling:

1. Cast your net. Even the smallest family tree can have a whole lot of branches (and twigs). So the first step in reunion planning is to decide whom you want to include in the event. For instance, which side of the family are you inviting—Mom's, Dad's, or both? Do you want to include only close relatives or all of the descendants of a particular ancestor? Just keep in mind that with every branch of the tree, you add scads of potential attendees (and scads of potential expenses). If this is your first attempt at holding a reunion, you can head off a passel of problems by keeping it on the small side.

2. Set the date—but only after you've consulted your intended guests. After all, it won't be much of a reunion if no one can make it! Just pick up the phone or send out an e-mail to your relatives and give them a choice of several dates that are open on your calendar. Make your

> " Happiness is having a large, loving, caring, close-knit family in another city.
>
> —George Burns (1896–1996) "

final decision based upon what works the best for the most people. As for how long the shindig should last, that's entirely up to you—it can be anywhere from an afternoon or evening to a week or more. A good rule of thumb, though, is that the farther folks have to travel to reach the location, the longer the reunion should be.

3. Send the invitations. You can call your guests on the phone, mail printed invitations, send a group e-mail, or even do all of the above. As for the timing, the earlier you issue your announcement, the bigger the crowd you're likely to draw. And if folks will have to travel far, or pay for rooms at a hotel or resort, send the invitations at least a year before the event. That way, anyone who needs to will have time to save up the necessary cash.

❯ Break the Ice

Suddenly finding yourself in a room full of people you haven't seen in years—even if they are your own flesh and blood—can feel mighty uncomfortable. In fact, it can feel downright icy, which is precisely why the term *icebreaker* was coined. There are a zillion of these silly games, but they all serve the same purpose: to make people laugh, relax, and start talking to one another. These are a few of my favorite icebreakers:

I know you! Ask each guest to send you a photograph of himself as a baby or a very young child, with nothing in the picture that could

---

Keep It Simple

The perfect "beginner's reunion" is a picnic or barbecue in your backyard or at a nearby park. It's fairly inexpensive, easy to plan, and simple to host. As the years go by (presuming you stick with this basic format), you can rotate the event among the homes of various family members, or find the ideal park and make it the permanent site. If that's not quite your style, then consider dinner and a reception at a good restaurant or hotel, a full-day or dinner cruise on a chartered boat, or a family camping trip—provided your clan is the outdoorsy type.

Tick-Tock
**TURN
BACK** the
CLOCK

provide a clue to his identity. (Make sure the person's name is written on the back.) Display all of the photos on a table or mount them on a poster board, and have everyone try to guess who each subject is.

Liar! Give each person a sheet of paper or an index card, and tell her to write down three statements about herself: one that's true and two that are complete fabrications. Then each person in turn stands up and reads her three sentences, and the rest of the group tries to guess which statement is true. If you want to fool the most people, make your true statement the most outrageous stunt you've ever pulled, or the strangest thing that's ever happened to you. For instance, "I once collided head on with John Wayne in the doorway to a hotel lobby." And use more realistic statements for your lies. Perhaps, "For three years running, I sold more Girl Scout cookies than anyone else in my troop."

Who am I? Gather as many index cards as there are reunion guests, and on each card, write the name of a famous person, either living or dead. Pin or tape a card on each guest's back (but, without him seeing the name, of course!). Then everyone has to guess his "identity" by going around the room asking yes-or-no questions of the other guests. Needless to say, the beginning queries are no-brainers ("Am I a man?"; "Am I still alive?"). But, trust me, the going gets trickier—and funnier—fast!

Hello, my name is... Of course, the best icebreaker of all is to provide name tags for all guests to fill out and wear as soon as they arrive.

Centenarian SECRETS 100

An ultra-simple way to start making folks feel at ease—and find out more about your far-flung family at the same time—is to buy an extra-large, detailed map of the United States (and whatever other countries your kin may live in). Mount the map on cardboard, or for a more lasting memento, have a picture framer dry-mount it on foam board. Then have each family member write his name on a small piece of paper and pin it to the spot that marks his home, sweet home.

❯ 3 Winning Themes

Having a theme for your reunion is a great way to get everyone involved in the action. It also simplifies the planning process by providing a focus for food, games, invitations, and just about every other aspect of the festivities. Here are just a few examples to spark your imagination:

1. Birthday party. This is a perfect choice if, for instance, Grandma is turning a milestone number of 90 or even 100 years old. Serve ice cream and a huge birthday cake with candles. Pass out party hats and play classic birthday party games, such as musical chairs and pin the tail on the donkey. Decorate with balloons and streamers, and bring in a magician or clown to entertain the guests. And, as the highlight of the occasion, organize a "This Is Your Life" slideshow for the birthday girl or boy.

2. Special holiday. For many families, certain holidays hold significance. Maybe your clan claims St. Patrick's Day, Oktoberfest, Mardi Gras, or the Fourth of July as sacred "territory." If that's the case, then pull out all the stops. Choose the menu, music, and decorations to suit the occasion, and have all the guests dress in appropriate costumes.

3. Western hoedown. For some reason, this is one of the most popular reunion themes of all. (I guess there's a little Roy Rogers or Dale Evans in all of us!) Hold the gathering at a park or dude ranch. Or, if your timing's right and there's a rodeo in town, take the whole gang out to holler "Ride 'em, cowboy!" And don't forget

Keep in Touch!

A family reunion can provide just the nudge we need to tighten the ties that bind. But make sure they don't come loose again once the festivities are over. One way to keep in touch with your kith and kin is to launch a family website or Facebook page. But consider taking two more steps:

Send out a family newsletter several times a year, in either electronic or printed form. You can even issue a special edition when an extra-big story hits the news wires.

Prepare a family directory that includes full contact information plus birthdays, anniversaries, and any other important dates. Keep at least one printed version— just in case your computer crashes, taking all your data with it.

to specify the mandatory dress: cowboy boots, ten-gallon hats, and blue jeans. Serve campfire chow, including baked beans, barbecued ribs, and corn on the cob. Hire a fiddler and a square-dance caller and do-si-do the night away, or simply sit around the campfire (or the stereo) and harmonize on cowboy classics like "Home on the Range" and "Tumbling Tumbleweeds."

❯ The Roots of Us All

The rising popularity of family reunions goes hand in glove with another healthy trend: More and more folks are diving into the past in search of their families' origins. Thanks to the Internet, genealogical research is easier than ever. A simple search for "genealogy" will bring up literally hundreds, if not thousands, of highly helpful sites. You can also buy software to help you organize your family tree. But, especially if you're new to the root-tracing game, one of the best—and the most enjoyable—ways to learn about your personal history is at a family reunion. For best results, let the guests know in advance that you want to focus on your family tree. That way, they can come equipped to share whatever knowledge they have.

- Make a large chart showing all of the family members that you know of, along with all the information you have in the way of birth and death dates, marriages, and so forth. Hang the chart on a wall or put it on a table, and ask each guest to fill in whatever additional information he knows, including people who may be missing, as well as dates or special events.

- Ask people to bring photographs or family mementos, and have a show-and-tell session. (Remember the ones we used to have in grade school?) After the session, create an attractive display to let people examine the items at their leisure.

- Set aside a separate table for any photographs or paintings you may have that show ancestors you can't identify. If you're lucky, maybe someone else will know exactly who these folks are. And if you're really lucky, you'll also get some dandy stories to add to your growing library of family lore.

- Interview older members of the family, recording them on video, audio, or both. Ask questions that may trigger memories, but as much as you can, let the "star" do most of the talking. Go gently, though: If a question appears to cause distress or even anguish, change the subject ASAP. After all, a reunion is supposed to be fun.

- Encourage everyone, young and old, to share family stories and legends that they've heard over the years. You won't believe some of the stuff folks come up with.

>>> FRIENDS FOREVER

Once upon a time, most folks never moved far from the place where they were born. As a result, they had a built-in network of extended family and lifelong friends who gathered to celebrate good times, shared the load when the going got tough, and lent a willing hand with chores ranging from babysitting to barn raising. Today—as most of us know all too well—few people stay in one place very long. According to Census Bureau stats, the average American moves 11 times during his life, and that figure is a drop in the bucket for many of us. In short, never has it been more prudent to heed the advice of a favorite Girl Scout song: "Make new friends but keep the old. One is silver, the other is gold." Coming up, I'll share some surefire tips on accomplishing both of those feats.

> Getting to Know You

It's an unpleasant fact of life that the older you get, the harder it is to build new, solid friendships. During your grade-school through college years, being in close proximity to your peers makes it a given that you'll meet congenial classmates who wind up being your bosom buddies. Likewise, parents of young children have friend-making opportunities galore as they cheer on their kids' Little League teams or ferry their future ballerinas to dance class. Later on—especially for single folks who are either retired or work from home—it can take some initiative to meet potential friends. Here are six ways to launch your search:

Volunteer. Anything from delivering Meals on Wheels to staffing a library book sale can help you get socially connected while you do a good deed at the same time. But if you choose your venue carefully, it could also launch you on a "second prime" career or avocation (see Chapter 9 for more on that score).

Sign up for a class. Ideally, choose one that's informal and also interactive—such as cooking, quilting, or hands-on horticulture. You'll stand a much better chance of getting to know your fellow students than you would in a classroom lecture setting.

Play a sport. Join a bowling league or hiking club. Take golf, tennis, or kayaking lessons. Whatever suits your fancy will introduce you to plenty of would-be playing partners—and help you grow younger and healthier in the process.

Go to church. It's a guaranteed way to meet like-minded people, especially if you sign up for a discussion or study group.

Take a group tour. Even if you're unmarried, don't limit yourself to singles' tours. Rather, choose one with destinations or activities that appeal to you for their own sake—maybe a theater and shopping tour to New York, or a wildlife-watching trek to a national park. After all, you want to have more in common with your potential pals than mere singlehood!

Get a dog. Almost any kind of pet can work wonders for your physical and mental health (see "Furry Family Members" on page 313). But a people- and dog-friendly canine is the strongest social magnet you could ever hope to find—provided, that is, you get out and walk him on a regular basis.

> **"** It is more fun to talk with someone who doesn't use long, difficult words but rather short, easy ones like 'What about lunch?'
>
> —Winnie-the-Pooh, quoted by A. A. Milne (1882–1956) **"**

It's a Date!

You never know when someone will cross your path and ignite a spark that says, "This could be a friend." Instead of saying, "Let's get together sometime," make solid plans. If you don't have your calendar with you, or you need to coordinate with your spouse's schedule, just pick a date at random. When you get home, call to confirm, changing the day and time if needed.

Grow Your Friendship

An acquaintance doesn't become a friend overnight. It takes time and sharing to create a real bond. When you're caught up in a whirlwind of work, family, and daily chores, that kind of time can be a real challenge to find. One solution: When you're building a new friendship, find ways to share your daily routines. For example, walk your dogs at the same time, shop for groceries, run your errands together, or help each other plant and tend your gardens. Just as drops of water eventually fill a bucket, each experience and shared memory will help cement your friendship.

Be Spontaneous

Nothing nudges a budding friendship along (or keeps an old one strong) like sitting down at home over drinks, snacks, or a delicious meal. Make it a point to keep your pantry and fridge stocked with food and beverages that you can pull out and serve on the spur of the moment. For example, make up a batch or two of the Baked Ham Sandwiches (at left) and stash 'em in the freezer. That way, after a round of shopping (or a round of golf), you'll always be ready to say, "Let's go back to my house for lunch."

> That's Entertainment!

Don't limit your get-togethers to spur-of-the-moment invitations (see "Be Spontaneous," at left). Whether you've just relocated and are aiming to make pals in your new hometown, or you want to keep longtime relationships alive and well, kick your mission into high gear by entertaining every chance you get. Don't get me wrong—that doesn't have to mean holding big, organized parties. Just be alert for opportunities to have people over. For example:

- After a productive Saturday of chores and errands, ask your neighbors and their kids over for a serve-yourself dessert party of ice cream and multiple toppings.

- A crucial World Series game, Monday Night Football, the final round of the Masters golf tournament—or just about any other televised sporting event—provides the perfect excuse for serving up hot chili and cold beer to your fellow fans.

- When visitors arrive from out of town, welcome them with a backyard barbecue and invite a handful of friends (new or old) to join you.

Centenarian SECRETS 100

In these days of e-mail, social media posts, and on-the-run cell-phone calls, a handwritten note is a memento to cherish—and a fat, newsy letter is worth its weight in platinum. Every once in a while, sit down and pen a greeting to a friend who's far away, even if it's only "I'm thinking of you" on the back of a postcard. And if it portrays a place that brings back joyful memories for the both of you, so much the better!

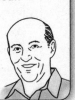

Give Thanks!

After you spend time with an old friend, whether you shared a long vacation away, a casual dinner, or a walk in the country, let her know you enjoyed her company. Even if you see her almost every day, drop her an e-mail or call her and say, "Thank you for the good time we had. I'm glad we're friends."

- On a neighbor's moving day, show up with a movable feast of finger food and drinks, and spread it all out on the packing crates.
- Wish vacationers off on a special trip with hors d'oeuvres and wine.

❯ 3 Timely Tips to Liven Up Your Friendship...

And grow younger in the process. Just like longtime careers or marriages, longtime friendships sometimes lapse into ho-hum routines. If you sense that happening in your life, here's a roundup of ways you can help put the sparkle back in your golden relationship—and the youth back in your heart.

1. Dip into a friend's interest that you've never tried. Go along to the ballet or a baseball game; try waterskiing or hot-air ballooning, even if you've never thought you'd like it. Who knows? You might discover that you love your pal's pastime! Either way, the experience will give you another shared memory to carry through the years.

2. Keep your childhood spirit alive. Remember all the adventures you've had with your best pal? Resolve to have another one every so often. Learn a new sport together, jaunt off to a place you've never been, or check out that new art museum you've been hearing about.

3. Declare your own holidays. Any date that's significant to the two of you is a great excuse to celebrate friendship—and life. Hold a yearly party on the anniversary of the day you started first grade together. Honor the birthday of your teenage idol, or the date of your favorite historic event. Or stage an annual festival with a floating date—maybe the day the first roses bloom in your garden, or the first day a snowfall arrives that's deep enough for making snow angels or a snowman.

❯ Class Acts

Just like a family reunion (see "Gather the Fam" on page 301), a class reunion provides a golden opportunity to renew old friendships and forge new ones. Simply showing up can be barrel-loads of fun, but being part of the planning process will give you a chance to cement bonds even more firmly as you work with fellow alums to orchestrate the extravaganza. If you attended a large college or university, the best way to throw your hat in the ring is to contact the chairman of the planning committee for your class's next get-together. The alumni office can put you in touch—and may even have your fellow grad's e-mail address listed on the "upcoming reunions" section of its website.

❯ Think Outside the Classroom

When the topic of reunions comes up, high school as well as college graduating classes most often spring to mind. But it can also be fun—and often a whole lot simpler—to reunite any bunch of people who were once close but have drifted apart. For example:

- Your old Girl Scout troop
- A tour group that bonded during a long cruise (or adventure)
- Former coworkers from a memorable job or volunteer project
- The kids you played with day after day in your old neighborhood
- The parents of your Little Leaguers' teammates

The list could go on . . . and on. But you get the picture.

Plan Ahead

When planning your own reunion, the details will vary depending on the size of your group, how far its members have spread, and the nature of the festivities you have in mind. But for a successful reunion, make sure to start early. The more elaborate the goings-on will be, the more lead time you'll need. You'll want to start planning at least 12 to 16 months ahead of your intended date. And if you want to book a prime venue, you may need to reserve it even further in advance.

Tick-Tock **TURN BACK the CLOCK**

Lose the Solo Holiday Blues

It's probably safe to say that for most of us, as the old song says, "There's no place like home for the holidays." But what do you do when you're living far away from home and simply can't get there to celebrate with family and old friends? Here's what:

When you know in advance that you can't make the trip, compensate.

- Rally other stay-behinds in your neighborhood or apartment building and enjoy an "Orphans' Thanksgiving."

- Call a children's hospital, nursing home, or hospice and ask if they can use a volunteer for the day.

- Or be shameless: Call a neighbor or coworker you like and announce that you'll be alone for the holiday. It's almost guaranteed that you'll be invited to dinner. If not, keep trying until you hear a friendly "Come join us!"

When the unexpected happens—say, an unpredicted blizzard leaves you stranded in your house for Christmas, or your Thanksgiving hostess has to cancel plans at the last minute—view it as a chance to indulge yourself.

- Cook your favorite dinner or take yourself to a good restaurant. Curl up with a book. Put on some soothing music and soak in a hot bubble bath. Make a big bowl of popcorn and watch a favorite movie.

- Or head outside with your camera. You just might discover that when you're alone, you're in very good company.

Plan for the best, prepare for the worst. At winter holiday time, Mother Nature can leave you stranded and alone due to closed airports or unsafe blizzard conditions.

- Go ahead and make plans for travel and merriment, but also create a solo survival kit that'll get you happily through your involuntary solitude.

- For example, stash away some favorite comfort food, a few bottles of good wine, and a selection of books and DVDs you've been wanting to dig into.

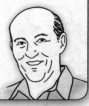

FURRY FAMILY MEMBERS

For the past quarter century, study after study has shown that pet owners generally feel happier, healthier, and more independent and secure than folks who don't have an animal in the household. Back in Chapter 3, you discovered some of the specific ways that pets deliver their health-enhancing magic (see "The Doggone Purr-fect Secrets to a Healthy Heart" on page 98). In this section, you'll find helpful tips on choosing the best pet for you and making the most of Rover and Fluffy's companionship.

No Surprises, Please!

No matter how eager you may be to offer the gift of companionship, resist the urge to give a puppy, kitten, or other pet to anyone. At best, you'll be depriving the giftee of the ability to select her own mate. (Like a marriage or a human friendship, the person-pet bond is a matter between two unique individuals, and for the relationship to really "click," the chemistry has to be just right.) At worst, the animal could be rejected by the recipient and wind up on death row in a shelter. Plus, the flurry of activity on holidays can be traumatic for an animal who's new to the household. The occasion can even end in tragedy if—as often happens—the critter gobbles up an iconic, but toxic, ingredient of the festivities, like chocolate, tinsel, wrapping paper, or ribbon.

The win-win solution: Buy a gift certificate from a shelter and present that to your friend or relative so she can choose her own pal. If it turns out she doesn't want a pet at all, you will still have made a tax-deductible contribution to a noble cause—and possibly also saved a life!

> "Don't accept your dog's admiration as conclusive evidence that you are wonderful.
>
> —Ann Landers (1918–2002)"

MIND OVER MYTH

MYTH: Big dogs need more care than small ones and are not good for small homes.

REALITY: On the contrary! Some of the smallest breeds are the most high-strung, energetic, and vocal dogs of all, and require extensive (and often very expensive) grooming sessions. Many popular midsize breeds, including both golden and Labrador retrievers, need to do plenty of running. Conversely, giant breeds, such as Saint Bernards and Great Danes, don't need as much strenuous exercise and can thrive in tiny apartments. What's more, the big guys tend to be as quiet as dormice except when they have a good reason to bark. **Note:** *The bigger a dog is, the more you'll have to spend on food, toys, treats, and vet bills. While size alone should not determine your choice of a canine companion, it's an important consideration if your budget is limited.*

❯ Bigger Is Not Better

Don't get me wrong! The fact that many people have misconceptions about the role of size in dog selection (see Mind Over Myth, at left) does not mean that a large dog is better than a small one. Far from it! When you're deciding on what kind of dog to get, size should not be your only consideration. Instead, take some time to ponder the personalities of the folks in your family, the things you like to do, and the patience you have for such chores as bathing and grooming. Then do some research into various breeds of dogs and choose the one that best suits your situation and energy level. Or "interview" shelter dogs with those criteria in mind. There are also some excellent books on how to select the right dog, so check your local bookstore or search online.

❯ Choose Your Partner

If you've already found the dog or cat of your dreams, you can skip this tip. But if you're thinking of adopting a four-legged pal—and you're not sure whether to opt for an adult or a baby, this advice can help you make the right call.

Cat or kitten? Bear in mind that our feline friends commonly live well into their teens and, sometimes, even into their early 20s.

So if you're not sure you can make that kind of long-term pet commitment, don't even think of getting a kitten. Instead, adopt an older animal from a shelter or rescue group. An adult feline is also your best bet in any of these circumstances:

- You lack the patience to put up with a kitten's curious nature and almost nonstop, high-speed antics—and the damage they can cause around the old homestead.

- You don't have the time or inclination for training a young animal. Even if your kitty got some basic grounding at her mama's knee, chances are you will still need to spend some time teaching her the fine points of using a litter box and scratching post.

- Your household includes youngsters under six years of age. Kittens are fragile, and young children usually don't have sufficient muscle control to handle them safely—or to protect themselves from the kitty's playful scratching and nipping.

Dog or puppy? Although any living creature you bring into your home does demand attention, puppies are just about the most labor-intensive pets of all (at least among the critters most folks choose to have around the house). If you don't have the time or patience for responsibilities like housebreaking, obedience training, and frequent trips to the vet's office for puppy shots—or if you want a companion for young children—take the same route I suggested for family felines above, and get a mature, kid-loving dog from an animal shelter or rescue group.

Centenarian SECRETS 100

Having trouble deciding what kind of dog or cat is best for you? Or maybe you're not really sure you want a pet at all. In that case, do some paws-on research: Offer to pet-sit for traveling friends and family. It's an ideal way to "test-drive" your options before you make a firm decision about the species, breed, and age of your potential BFF. It's also a good way to enjoy the benefits of animal companionship through the years without making a long-term commitment.

❯ 3 Pleasing Places to Mix & Mingle with Your Dog

Walking your pooch—especially in an urban neighborhood—is a guaranteed way to meet new people. But there are also plenty of places that will bring you in contact with dogs and their humans, thereby giving you both the chance to build lasting friendships. For example:

1. Training classes. In every community, you can find professional trainers who offer group classes at levels from puppy kindergarten through advanced obedience and agility instruction. You'll have a chance to master valuable training skills and meet kindred spirits who are doing the same thing.

2. Resorts and camps. These places are springing up all over the country. Some provide residential training programs for dogs and their owners. Others feature planned activities, like those you'd find on a cruise ship. Still others have a more laid-back atmosphere, allowing you and your pal to interact with fellow vacationers on your own terms.

3. Outdoor cafés. Many restaurants that have outdoor seating facilities for humans are also pet-friendly (provided, of course, that the critters are calm and well socialized). Some of these places even offer special menu options for their canine customers.

Park with Caution

An off-leash dog park can provide a terrific opportunity for you and your dog to play and interact with other dogs and owners alike. Just make sure you choose your venue with care. If at all possible, look for a securely gated, members-only park, where you know that all the human attendees are responsible and the dogs are friendly, healthy, and up to date on all their essential vaccines. In a casual, come-one-come-all setting, you could be asking for trouble, ranging from dirty conditions to possibly fatal dogfights.

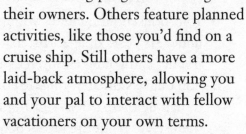

❯ Playtime Kitty Style

It's well documented that cats who stay inside are healthier and live longer than their counterparts who roam outdoors. But for an indoor feline to be happy and well adjusted, she needs to indulge her natural instincts for hunting. Helping her do that will also give you a chance to get off the couch and give a NEAT boost to your day (see "Don't Commit Suicide by Sitting!" on page 234). These pastimes can also help solve or head off some major problems. For instance, when Fluffy spends a little time romping and pouncing each day, she's a lot less likely to turn her energy (and claws) loose on your furniture and draperies. She'll also get some good exercise that will keep her muscles toned and her weight down—that's just as important for her health as it is for yours! Here are a few feline festivities:

The search is on. Gather up a bunch of orphan socks and rub each one with a cat-pleasing substance like peanut butter, meat, cheese, or catnip. Turn each sock inside out so that nothing greasy or oily gets onto your carpets. Then scatter the scented lures all around the house. Your kitty will have a ball tracking her "prey" and then pouncing on it.

Paper bag playground. Lay two flat-bottom paper bags on the floor, with the openings facing each other a few inches apart. When your cat goes into one of the sacks to investigate, scratch the bottom with your fingers. Like any self-respecting feline, she'll pounce at the invisible "prey" on the other side of the paper wall and start to scuffle with it. At that point, you scratch the bottom of the other bag. This should cause kitty to fly out of the first sack and into the second.

Roller Derby, kitty style. This ultra-simple game reminds me of the Roller Derby shows on television. All you need to do is put your cat and a Ping-Pong ball in the bathtub (with no water, of course!). Then stand back and enjoy the show as Kitty makes the ball sail around the curves and up and down the sides of the tub.

Connect Online

Tick-Tock **TURN BACK the CLOCK**

It should come as no surprise that social networking sites catering to pet owners are popping up all over the Internet. They are by no means a replacement for personal interaction with your fellow pet "parents," but they can be highly useful for comparing notes, sharing tips, and making plans to get together for canine playdates. A search for "pet networking sites" will bring up scads of them.

>>> FOOD FOR FAMILY & FRIENDS

Whether you're planning a family reunion, entertaining lifelong pals, or building a network of friends in a new town, one of the most effective ways to ensure a good time can be spelled out in four letters: F-O-O-D. And that's exactly what this section is all about.

>> ONE-POT WINNERS

> Gone for the Day Casserole

Don't let a jam-packed schedule keep you from accepting potluck party invitations. With this recipe at your disposal, you can just toss the ingredients into a slow cooker before you leave in the morning.* Then, when you get back, all you need to do is pour the finished product into a travel-worthy serving dish and take off for the shindig.

1 cup of uncooked wild rice, rinsed and drained	1 garlic clove, minced
	½ cup of slivered almonds
1 cup of chopped celery	3 beef bouillon cubes
1 cup of chopped carrots	2 ½ tsp. of seasoned salt
2 cans (4 oz. each) of sliced mushrooms, drained	2 lbs. of boneless round steak cut into 1-inch cubes**
1 large onion, chopped	3 cups of water

Add all of the ingredients to your slow cooker in the order listed. Cover and cook on low for 6 to 8 hours, or until the rice is tender. Stir thoroughly before pouring the mixture into a serving dish.

To save precious morning time, you can do all the food prep the night before and stash the ingredients in the fridge. Take them out as soon as you wake up, so everything can come to room temperature while you get ready.

**Or substitute skinned chicken legs or wings.*

Yield: *12 servings*

➤ Easy Cowboy Chili

There are almost as many chili recipes as there are stars in the West Texas sky. But this version is one of the simplest to make—and it's sure to leave your guests hootin' and hollerin' for more!

4 lbs. of lean ground beef or turkey	2 cups of beer
3 tbsp. of vegetable oil	¾ cup of Cowboy Chili Seasoning Mix (see below)
2 cans (28 oz. each) of diced tomatoes with juice	2 cans (29 oz. each) of pinto beans, rinsed (optional)
2 cans (15 oz. each) of tomato sauce	

In a large, heavy pot, brown the meat in the oil, stirring occasionally. Add the remaining ingredients, except for the beans, and stir. Bring to a boil; cover, and simmer for 45 minutes. Add the beans, if desired. Cover and simmer for another 15 to 20 minutes.

Yield: *15–20 servings*

➤ Cowboy Chili Seasoning Mix

Don't let the name fool you. While this blend is ideal for any kind of chili, it also gives a delightful kick to taco meat, grilled burgers, or meat loaf. To make it, simply combine all of these ingredients:

¼ cup of ground red chili pepper or cayenne	2 tsp. of dried oregano
¼ cup of paprika	2 tsp. of salt
2 tbsp. of dried minced onion	1 tsp. of dried red pepper, crushed
4 tsp. of cumin seeds	1 tsp. of garlic powder

Combine all of the ingredients, and store the mixture in a container with a tight-fitting lid, away from light and heat. The rule of thumb is to use 3 tablespoons of the seasoning per pound of meat, but (as with any seasonings) let your taste buds be your guide.

Yield: *3/4 cup*

❯ New England Boiled Dinner

Cowboy chili isn't the only single-pot recipe with deep historic roots. This one—again with countless variations—has been comforting Yankee families and their guests for more than three centuries.

6 lbs. of corned-beef brisket	1 medium turnip, quartered
8 small onions	1 medium cabbage,
6 medium potatoes	quartered and cored
6 small carrots	Prepared horseradish
5 small parsnips	Spicy brown mustard

Cover the meat with cold water and boil gently for three to five hours, until done. Skim off the excess fat, and add all of the vegetables except the cabbage. Boil, uncovered, for 20 minutes. Add cabbage, and continue cooking until the cabbage is soft. Then transfer the meat to a large platter, and surround it with the vegetables. Serve bowls of horseradish and mustard on the side, so diners can choose their condiment(s).

Yield: *6–8 servings*

Accept Substitutions

It's frustrating, all right: You're in a hurry to whip up a potluck casserole when you discover that you're fresh out of the herbs you need. Well, don't get all hot and bothered. And don't spend valuable time rushing off to the store because there's a good chance you have perfect stand-ins close at hand. Here's the lowdown:

- You can substitute mild-flavored herbs like parsley and chives for any other kind at any time.
- To substitute dried herbs when a recipe calls for fresh ones, simply use one-third to one-half of the measured amount suggested.
- If a recipe specifies dried herbs, but you only have fresh ones, just double or triple the amount. Fresh herbs are milder and smoother in taste, so in this case, more is always better.

Tick-Tock
**TURN
BACK** the
CLOCK

Scalloped Potatoes with Broccoli and Ham

Other one-dish dinners don't come any more well rounded—or more satisfying—than this classic delicious dish.

1 large yellow onion, chopped

1 tbsp. of extra virgin olive oil

2 ½ cups of milk

¼ cup of all-purpose flour

Salt and freshly ground
    black pepper to taste

4 cups of sliced potatoes

3 cups of chopped broccoli

1 lb. of boiled or baked ham,
    cut into 1-inch cubes

1 tbsp. of Dijon mustard

Grease a shallow 2-quart casserole with olive oil or cooking spray, and set aside. In a heavy saucepan, cook the onion in the oil over moderate heat for about 5 minutes, or until golden. Combine the milk, flour, salt, and pepper in a bowl. Pour the mixture into the pan and cook, stirring, until thickened, for about 3 minutes. Spread half of the potatoes in the casserole, then top with the broccoli and half of the sauce. Arrange the ham cubes on top, dot with mustard, and add the remaining potatoes and sauce. Cover tightly with aluminum foil and bake at 400°F for 40 to 45 minutes, or until the potatoes are just tender. Remove the foil, and bake for another 15 minutes, or until the taters are lightly browned.

Yield: *4 servings*

Bag the Oil

When a recipe calls for a lightly oiled or greased pot, skillet, or griddle, you can use an aerosol cooking spray. But unless you're really careful, it's easy to pull the "trigger" farther than you intend and wind up with an overly oiled pan. So instead, try this old-time trick: Fill a small square of clean cotton cloth with salt, bring up the corners, and tie them to form a bag. Dip it in oil, and wipe it over the bottom of the pan. You'll get just the right amount of slickness.

❯ Four-Bean Hamburger Bake

This hearty casserole is tailor-made for a winter potluck—and you won't find a dish that's happier to travel, that's for sure.

8 oz. of lean ground beef

½ cup of chopped onion

1 can (16 oz.) of baked beans

1 cup of canned cannellini beans, rinsed and drained

1 cup of canned pinto beans, rinsed and drained

1 cup of red kidney beans, rinsed and drained

6 tbsp. of barbecue sauce

6 tbsp. of pure maple syrup

3 tsp. of spicy brown mustard

Salt and freshly ground black pepper to taste

Sauté the ground beef and onion in a large, heavy skillet for 4 to 5 minutes over medium-high heat. Stir in the remaining ingredients, and bring the mixture to a boil. Transfer it to a Dutch oven or heavy-duty casserole dish, and bake at 400°F for 20 to 30 minutes, or until it is bubbly. Stir occasionally during cooking time. Then, let cool, and dig in.

Yield: *4 servings*

> "
> I cook with wine. Sometimes I even add it to the food.
> —W. C. Fields (1880–1946)
> "

▶▶ SIMPLE SNACKS & DELICIOUS DIPS

❯ Vanishing Blue Cheese Herb Spread

Why "vanishing," you ask? Well, because when you serve this delectable spread at a get-together, it will immediately start to disappear before your very eyes!

¼ cup of walnuts

2 tbsp. of chopped chives

2 tbsp. of chopped fresh parsley

½ cup of crumbled blue cheese

1 package (8 oz.) of cream cheese, cold

Finely chop the first three ingredients in a food processor, and pour the mix into a small bowl. Stir in the blue cheese and set aside. Put the cream cheese in the bowl of the food processor, and process until smooth. Add the herb-nut mixture, and process until thoroughly blended. Serve the spread in a pretty bowl, surrounded by crackers, melba toast rounds, or raw vegetables. Or use it as a topping for finger-size ham or chicken sandwiches. **Note:** *You can make this blend up to three days ahead of time and store it, tightly covered, in the refrigerator. Let it cool before serving.*

Yield: *About 2 ½ cups*

> Fabulous Fruit Salsa

This tasty sweet-and-tart combination makes a dandy dipping partner for tortilla chips or a tangy topping for chicken tenders.

½ ripe avocado

½ ripe mango

2 tbsp. of fresh lime juice

½ fresh cantaloupe, cut into ¼-inch pieces

2 tomatillos, with outer husks removed, cut into ¼-inch pieces

1 nectarine, peeled and cut into ¼-inch pieces

½ cup of chopped red onion

2 tbsp. of fresh cilantro

½ tsp. of minced jalapeño

Mash the avocado and mango together in a bowl, and blend in the lime juice. Stir in the remaining ingredients and mix thoroughly. If you're taking your salsa on the road, transfer it to a tightly sealed traveling container. Give it another quick stir before serving.

Yield: *About 3 cups*

> Fondue with Fortitude

After a day of skiing or an evening of Christmas caroling, cheese fondue is just what the doctor ordered for a warm-up snack. Unfortunately, though, if it isn't stirred frequently, it can scorch on the bottom—making it less than ideal for a longer party. Enter this altered version: It has many of the same flavors as traditional fondue, but it can be kept warm for a much longer period with no unpleasant side (or bottom) effects.

1 tbsp. of unsalted butter	1 package (8 oz.) of
1 small onion, chopped	shredded Swiss cheese
1 tbsp. of brandy	½ cup of freshly grated
1 cup of mayonnaise	Parmesan cheese

Melt the butter in a small skillet over medium heat. Add the onion

---

Dip Those Veggies!

And in some cases, give them a little TLC first. Many vegetables, like baby carrots and cherry tomatoes, simply need to be cleaned before you arrange them around a bowl of dip. But these types require a little pre-treatment to perk up their flavor and appearance:

- Broccoli and cauliflower. Cut the florets into bite-size pieces. Cook in a large saucepan of lightly salted water for about 1 minute—no longer!
- Potatoes. Look for tiny, marble-size new potatoes—a combo of red, white, and blue varieties looks especially festive. Scrub them well, and then cook them in a pan of lightly salted water for about 15 minutes, or until tender when pierced with the tip of a small knife.

In each case, drain the water from the pan, and immediately rinse the veggies under cold running water to stop the cooking process. Spread the pieces on paper towels and pat completely dry. When they're cool, wrap in fresh paper towels, and refrigerate in Ziploc® plastic bags for up to 24 hours.

Tick-Tock
TURN BACK the **CLOCK**

and cook, stirring frequently, until the onion is translucent (about 3 minutes). Remove from the heat, stir in the brandy, and set aside. Mix the mayo and cheeses in a bowl, and stir in the cooked onion. Transfer to a 1-quart casserole or heat-proof serving dish. Bake in the center of the oven at 350°F for about 30 minutes, or until the dip is bubbly. **Note:** *You can prepare the dip up to one day ahead of time and store it, uncooked and covered, in the refrigerator. If the dip is chilled before cooking, increase the oven time accordingly.*

Yield: *About 3 cups*

> Marinated Olives

With a stash of these tasty (and healthy) tidbits in your pantry, you'll always be ready for unexpected guests. They beat anything you'll find in a fancy food shop—and they couldn't be simpler to make.

4 cups of assorted olives (such as kalamata, manzanilla, pimiento-stuffed)

2 garlic cloves, minced

1 tbsp. of lemon peel, cut into thin strips

1 tbsp. of orange peel, cut into thin strips

1 tbsp. of red pepper, cut into thin strips

1 sprig of fresh oregano or 1 tbsp. of dried

¼ tsp. of dried red-pepper flakes (optional)

½ cup of extra virgin olive oil

½ cup of balsamic vinegar

Drain off any brining liquid, rinse the olives, and put them in a large jar that has a tight-fitting lid. Add the next six ingredients. Whisk the oil and vinegar in a bowl, and pour just enough of the mixture into the jar to cover the olives. Put the lid on the jar and shake it to mix the contents. Then stash it in the refrigerator. You can use the olives right away if you really need to, but they'll reach their peak of flavor after two weeks or so. When you're ready to serve, place the olives in a few colorful bowls, and set them out for your guests to enjoy.

Yield: *About 1 quart*

❯ Pub-Style Cheese Spread

This spicy spread is a well-loved staple in English pubs. It's best when aged for at least a week in the fridge.

1 lb. of white cheddar cheese, grated

½ cup of beer*

4 tbsp. of unsalted butter, softened

**2 tbsp. of finely chopped
   fresh parsley**

1 tbsp. of grated sweet onion

1 tsp. of lemon juice

½ tsp. of dry mustard

3 garlic cloves, peeled and halved

Combine all of the ingredients except the garlic in a blender or food processor and blend until smooth. Spoon one-third of the mixture into a jar that has an airtight cover. Push two garlic halves into the surface. Add another third of the mixture, followed by two more garlic halves. Finish with the remaining cheese blend and garlic. Cut a circle of wax paper to the size of the jar's interior, and lay the paper over the cheese mixture. Close the jar tightly and stash it in the refrigerator. Let it age in the fridge for at least seven days, and remove the garlic slivers before serving with crackers or bread. * *For a more sophisticated version (like that served in proper English clubs), substitute ½ cup of brandy or cognac.*

Yield: *2 cups*

>> DELECTABLE DESSERTS

> Chocolate–Peanut Butter Fudge

The fudge fans in your crowd will love this easier-than-pie treat!

3 ½ cups of sugar	1 tbsp. of white vinegar
1 ½ cups of evaporated milk	3 cups of peanut butter
½ cup of butter	1 cup of marshmallow cream
¼ cup of corn syrup	1 cup of chocolate chips

In a large saucepan, cook the first five ingredients over medium heat, stirring constantly until the mixture comes to a full boil. Add the peanut butter and marshmallow cream, and stir until smooth. Pour half of the hot batter into a bowl, and stir in the chocolate chips. Spread the mixture into a 9-by-9-inch pan lined with wax paper, and top it with the remaining batter. Let the dessert cool, and cut the fudge into squares.

Yield: *9–12 squares*

> Fast and Easy Fruit-Torte Bars

This crowd pleaser goes together in a snap—thanks to a trio of handy packaged ingredients.

1 can (21 oz.) of apple pie filling	1 box (15 oz.) of lemon cake mix
2 cans (8 oz. each) of crushed pineapple with juice	½ cup of butter, cut into bits
	Whipped cream*

Layer the pie filling and pineapple in a greased 10-by-15-inch pan. Sprinkle the cake mix on top, and dot with the butter bits. Bake at 375°F for 45 minutes, or until golden brown. Top with whipped cream and cut into squares. * *Use freshly whipped if possible, but in a pinch, the canned kind will do.*

Yield: *10–12 squares*

❯ Raspberry Brownies

Who doesn't love brownies? Serve these up at your next party, or take them to a potluck function, and get ready for a round of applause.

1 cup (8 oz.) of unsalted butter

4 oz. of unsweetened chocolate

2 cups of sugar

1 tsp. of pure vanilla extract

1 tsp. of salt

4 eggs

1 cup of unbleached all-purpose flour

2 cups of chopped walnuts

1 cup of raspberry preserves

Melt the butter and chocolate in a large, heavy saucepan over low heat, stirring occasionally. Remove the pan from the heat and mix in the sugar, vanilla, and salt. Add the eggs, one at a time, mixing well after each one. Add the flour and then beat until smooth. Then stir in the walnuts.

Pour half of the batter into a greased 9-by-13-inch baking pan, and freeze for 30 minutes. Spread a layer of preserves on top. Pour in the remaining batter, and gently smooth it over the preserves. Bake at 350°F for 40 to 45 minutes. Cool the pan on a wire rack for 10 minutes before cutting the brownies.* Let them cool completely before serving (or wrapping for transport to your destination). * *Because they're rich, you may want to cut them into roughly 1-inch squares.*
Yield: *16 1-inch squares*

❯ Chilly Minty Marvel

With this creamy peppermint confection stashed in the freezer, you'll always be prepared to issue a spur-of-the-moment invitation for coffee and homemade dessert. Plus, your guests will love it!

1 ½ cups of chocolate wafer crumbs	1 can (14 oz.) of sweetened condensed milk
¼ cup of butter, melted	1 cup of crushed peppermint candies
¼ cup of sugar	3 drops of red food coloring (optional)
1 package (8 oz.) of cream cheese, softened	2 cups of heavy cream, whipped
	10–14 whole peppermint candies

Combine the first three ingredients in a small bowl. Press the mixture onto the bottom and 2 inches up the sides of a greased 8-inch springform pan. Set it in the refrigerator to chill. In a large bowl, beat the cream cheese until smooth, and then gradually beat in the milk, followed by the crushed candies. Add the food coloring, if desired. Fold in the whipped cream, then spoon the mixture into the crust. Cover and freeze the treat for at least eight hours or up to one month. Remove from the freezer 10 minutes before serving, and garnish the top with the whole candies.

Yield: *10–14 servings*

❯ Old-Time Vinegar & Molasses Taffy

Taffy pulls were popular forms of entertainment back in the Roaring Twenties—which is when this recipe originated.

2 cups of molasses	1 tbsp. of butter
1 cup of sugar	1 tsp. of white or apple cider vinegar

Combine all of the ingredients in a saucepan and boil for about 20 minutes, stirring constantly. Then beat the mixture by hand until it's smooth and creamy, and pour it into a buttered 8-by-8-inch pan. When the batter is cool enough to handle, pull it into long strips until the candy is satiny and light-colored. Cut the strips into desired lengths. Wrap individual pieces in wax paper, and store them in an airtight container for easy enjoyment.

Yield: *About 1 pound*

❯ Pumpkin Cheesecake

Instead of ending your Thanksgiving feast with the usual pumpkin pie, try this variation on the theme. It just might become a new fixture at your holiday table.

2 tbsp. of unsalted butter, softened (for pan)

⅓ cup of gingersnap crumbs

4 packages (8 oz. each) of cream cheese, at room temperature

1 ½ cups of firmly packed dark brown sugar

5 eggs

¼ cup of all-purpose flour

1 tsp. of allspice

1 tsp. of ground cinnamon

¼ tsp. of ground ginger

¼ tsp. of salt

1 can (15 oz.) of 100% pure pumpkin (not pie mix)

Pure maple syrup and walnut halves for garnish

Unsweetened whipped cream (optional)

Grease a 9-inch springform pan with the butter, then sprinkle the gingersnap crumbs into the pan, and shake to coat the bottom and sides evenly. Beat the cream cheese in a large bowl until fluffy. Gradually beat in the brown sugar. Add the eggs, one at a time, mixing thoroughly after each addition. Sift in the flour, spices, and salt, and blend well. Beat in the canned pumpkin.

Pour the batter into the pan. Bake at 325°F (in the center of the oven) for 1 ½ to 1 ¾ hours. Cool on a wire rack for 60 minutes, then carefully remove the ring from the pan and let the cake finish cooling to room temperature. Refrigerate, covered, until chilled. Brush the top with maple syrup, and garnish with walnuts.

Serve the whipped cream on the side, if desired.

Yield: *14–16 servings*

> " The only time to eat diet food is while you're waiting for the steak to cook.
>
> —Julia Child (1912–2004) "

❯ Applejack-Spiked Baked Apples

These apples are true potluck superstars. They travel well, and whether they're served warm, at room temp, or even cold, they never fail to win rave reviews from party guests.

¼ cup of finely chopped dates

¼ cup of finely chopped pecans
  or walnuts

3 tbsp. of unsalted butter, softened

4 large baking apples, cored*

⅓ cup of pure maple syrup

¼ cup of water

⅓ cup of applejack

1 tsp. of pure vanilla extract

¼ tsp. of ground cinnamon

Mix the dates, nuts, and ½ tablespoon of the butter in a small bowl. Stuff the mixture into the apples to within a ¼ inch or so of the tops. Arrange the filled apples in a large pie pan. Bring the maple syrup, water, and remaining butter to a boil in a small saucepan. Let the mixture boil briefly, then remove it from the heat and stir in the remaining ingredients. Pour the blend over the apples and bake at 375°F for about 50 minutes, basting every 10 minutes. Remove from the oven and let cool. Continue basting periodically with the pan juices.

Core apples a little on the wide side. Then peel the upper third of each one to prevent them from bursting. Trim bottoms so they sit flat in the pan.

Yield: *4 servings*

Dodge Dish Dilemmas

A potluck party gives you a great opportunity to showcase your favorite recipes—not to mention your cooking talent. There's only one potential downside: forgetting to take your dish home at the end of the festivities. There are two ways to avoid that problem:

1. Prepare your food in a disposable foil pan, or pack it in an attractive plastic serving dish (or a plastic plate, depending on the nature of the food), and don't give it another thought.

2. Buy a nice new ceramic dish or plate, or a sturdy glass storage container, and leave it behind (with a note) as a hostess gift.

❯ Gingerbread Christmas Cookies

You'll win raves with these spicy delights at a Christmas cookie swap.
Just be sure to make extras to leave under the tree for Santa!

½ cup of molasses	3 cups of all-purpose flour
½ cup of sugar	½ tsp. of baking soda
½ cup of vegetable shortening	½ tsp. of ground cinnamon
1 ½ tsp. of white vinegar	½ tsp. of ground ginger
1 large egg, well beaten	¼ tsp. of salt

Combine the first four ingredients in a saucepan and bring to a
boil. Cool, add the egg, and stir well to blend. Sift the dry ingredients
into a bowl. Add them to the wet ingredients and mix well. Chill for
at least 2 hours. Roll the dough out on a lightly floured surface to
about ⅛ inch thick or to your desired thickness.* Use your favorite
Christmas cookie cutters, then put the cut dough onto greased cookie
sheets (use a spatula for the transfer process so the cookies keep their
shapes). Bake at 375°F for 8 to 10 minutes. Let them cool completely
before decorating them with your favorite frosting. * *This recipe is also
excellent for making gingerbread houses. In that case, roll the dough out to
¼ to ½ inch thickness and cut it into whatever shapes your pattern calls for.*
Yield: *About 36 cookies*

A Light and Sweet Holiday Treat

It seems that between Thanksgiving and New Year's Day, the heavy,
calorie-laden desserts never stop coming. So at your next winter holiday
gathering, offer your guests a change of pace with a seasonal fruit salad
featuring pears, tart apples, and grapes topped with a dressing made
from 2 parts honey to 1 part balsamic vinegar. It makes an especially
useful addition to a buffet because, thanks to the vinegar, it can sit
on the serving table for the duration without the fruit turning brown.

Tick-Tock
**TURN
BACK** the
CLOCK

CHAPTER 9

Declare Your Independence

It's probably safe to say that there is not a person on the planet who doesn't want to go on living independently right up until the final curtain falls. In large part, of course, your ability to do that depends on your physical condition. But there are three other factors that determine to what degree you can live a full, rich, independent life: a healthy financial picture; emotional well-being; and a safe, secure home front.

 GET ON A FIRM FINANCIAL FOOTING

Depending on whose statistics you read, anywhere from 72 to 80 percent of Americans plan to work beyond their retirement age. For some, the official reason falls firmly into the category of emotional and physical independence: Either they find their jobs highly satisfying and want to stay on as long as possible, or they've cast their sights on a whole new career and can't wait to charge down that path. But many other folks must continue gainful employment as long as possible because Social Security, pension plans, or investment income won't provide sufficient funds to make ends meet. Regardless of which category you fall into, the tips in this section will help.

Hire a Navigator

You can't just meander along the road to financial independence. Getting there takes careful planning, a fair amount of discipline—and an in-depth knowledge of all your investment options. Your best navigator for the journey is a professional financial planner (see "How to Choose a Financial Planner" on page 340). The right one can help you achieve your objectives, regardless of your specific needs, which could include any of these:

- Saving for retirement
- Rolling over a pension or IRA
- Handling a sizable inheritance or other financial windfall
- Preparing for a marriage or divorce
- Dealing financially with the death of a spouse
- Caring for aging parents or a disabled child
- Buying or selling a business, or passing on a family-owned enterprise
- Coping with a financial crisis such as a layoff, natural disaster, or serious illness

❯ Solving the Social Security Puzzle

As you move toward your 60s, one of the biggest financial decisions you need to make is when to sign up for Social Security retirement benefits. You can start receiving checks at age 62, but the longer you wait between then and age 70, the higher the payments will be. These are the three age-related milestones to reckon with:

Age 62. The advantage of claiming now is (of course) that you'll receive payments for the longest possible time. On the downside,

---

Another Reason to Wait

If you're still on the fence about when to start collecting Social Security, consider this financial fact: Each year that you hold off until age 70, your benefit increases by as much as 8 percent. Your chances of finding *guaranteed* income growth at that level anyplace else are virtually nil. Just make sure you've got some other resources to fully cover your living expenses—you don't want to shortchange yourself today for the sake of a higher payout somewhere down the road.

Tick-Tock
TURN BACK the **CLOCK**

the checks will be smaller, and if you're still working, your monthly payment will be reduced by as much as one dollar for every two dollars you earn above a specified amount.

Your full retirement age. This is the age that Social Security uses to calculate your base benefit amount (that's the key headline number listed on your Social Security yearly statement). When you reach that milestone depends on the year you were born; that detail, too, appears on your statement. If you wait to claim your benefits until after you've passed this threshold, then you will receive your base amount each month, *and* you can continue to work without facing any penalty.

Age 70. After you reach your seven-decade mark, your payment amount stops increasing, so there is no advantage to waiting any longer.

❯ 2 Points to Ponder Before You Sign Up

Within the framework created by the three key milestones (see "Solving the Social Security Puzzle," at left), the ideal age for tapping into this income stream depends on your individual circumstances. If you've turned 62, and you need additional cash to make ends meet, by all means, start the flow now. Otherwise, consider these two factors before you make your decision:

Get a Handle on the Pennies

We've all heard the saying "Take care of the pennies, and the dollars will take care of themselves." But to fully appreciate—and act on—the wisdom of that advice, you need to know where a lot of those dollars are going. So try this trick: Each day for several months, write down every single expenditure you make. That includes the latte you get on your way to work and the chocolate-peppermint wafer you buy for a quarter at the drugstore checkout, as well as larger amounts for things like gas, groceries, and utility bills. At the end of your designated time frame, cast a cold eye on the numbers. When you realize—for example—how much that daily latte is setting you back, suddenly the pot of java brewing in the company break room may look a lot more appealing!

Except when you're engaged in a snowballing campaign (see "Demolish Credit Card Debt," at right), never pay only the minimum amount due on your credit card. Typically, it's 2 to 3 percent of the outstanding balance, so it could take years, or decades, to pay off. That's exactly what the banks want. The longer you take to repay the charges, the more they earn in interest—and the more you wind up paying for the stuff you bought. Instead, try to pay as much as you possibly can each month—even if it means scrimping elsewhere. And remember: You don't need to wait until the statement arrives. If you find yourself with extra cash during the billing cycle, simply mail in a check, with a cover note requesting payment to your account.

1. How many more years you think you'll have ahead of you. Just make a rough estimate, based on your current age; your family's longevity history; any medical conditions you have; and any risk factors such as smoking, obesity, or a sedentary lifestyle. The longer you expect to live, the more sense it makes to hold out for the larger payments.

2. When you intend to stop working. If you're earning enough money to easily cover your living expenses, you're better off waiting until your full retirement age or—better yet—70 if possible.

▶ Demolish Credit Card Debt

While any debt can be a hindrance to your future security, few hang a darker cloud over your financial and emotional independence than a mountain of credit card bills. There's no more liberating feeling in the world than finding yourself free of those miserable monthly payments. So do everything you can to win the battle of the balances. If you have two or more accounts to pay off, use a technique the financial gurus call "snowballing." This means that you pay the minimum amounts due on all your cards but one—which you attack with the highest payments you can possibly afford each month. When you've zeroed out that balance, move to another card. As your debt decreases, the amount of money you have to pay it off increases. Hence the name of the game: Your payments snowball until you've defeated your debt.

❯ Which Card Comes First?

The answer depends on a number of factors, including your current credit standing and your financial goals, but here are the options:

The one with the highest interest rate. Taking direct aim at this card would seem like a no-brainer. And it does make sense from a simple debt-reduction standpoint.

The one with the lowest balance. Paying off a full account—regardless of the interest you're paying—can give you a mighty powerful incentive to keep up the good fight.

The one that's closest to being maxed out. The reasoning here is that your FICO® Score (see "Why Care a Fig about FICO?" below) is based in part on how close you are to the credit limit on each of your cards. Paying off the account that has the least available credit will give an instant boost to your score—and a healthy FICO number is essential for getting a mortgage or business loan.

❯ A Better Kind of Debt

While the amount you owe on your home mortgage may be a lot higher than your combined credit card balances, it shouldn't pose nearly as big a threat to your financial or emotional independence. In fact, as long as you're up to date on your payments—and not struggling to make them on time—a home mortgage is actually a good thing. That's true for several reasons:

It's a secured loan, which means that it's backed up by a tangible piece of property—which, most likely, is increasing in value every year.

Why Care a Fig about FICO?

Your FICO Score is the criterion that most lenders use when they decide whether to approve your credit request, what terms to offer, and whether to increase your credit limit once your account is established. The score's calculated monthly based on a variety of info, including credit card payment history and more. Some credit card companies automatically include your FICO® Score with your monthly statement, but you can also learn where you stand by checking www.myfico.com or viewing your latest credit report at www.annualcreditreport.com.

The interest rate is all but guaranteed to be a lot lower than that on any of your credit card accounts—and the interest is tax deductible to boot.

Owning your home (even if it is technically shared by your mortgage lender) gives you the kind of emotional and physical security you don't have when you're renting. Think about it: At any time, a landlord can come along and say, "I've decided to sell the building, so you'll have to move."

❯ 2 Factors before Refinancing

Refinancing your home may seem like a dandy way to build financial independence. And sometimes it can be helpful. At other times, it's not such a good deal. Of course, much of your decision depends on how much lower the new rate would be. But these factors matter too:

MIND OVER MYTH

MYTH: A reverse mortgage is a financial boon for senior homeowners.

REALITY: Not necessarily. Simply put, this is a home equity loan that does not have to be paid back until the owner of the property dies and the property is sold. It can be ideal for folks who are barely getting by on Social Security, but there are serious downsides, such as:

- Loan fees and closing costs can be expensive.
- You must pay for homeowner's insurance and taxes in a timely manner, or risk having to repay the loan early.
- In most cases, interest rates are variable and could rise significantly over time.
- Interest can't be written off until the loan is repaid.
- The equity in your home is depleted—reducing the assets you can pass on.

1. How long you plan to remain in your current home. Bear in mind that you will have to pay the same origination fees and closing costs that you paid when you got your original mortgage. That could add at least several thousand dollars to your loan balance. If you intend to move within the next two years or so, you may be better off sticking with the higher interest rate (and a higher tax deduction).

2. Your overall debt load. If you can use the money you'll save each month to pay off credit card balances or other higher-interest loans, go for it. Just make sure you devote that extra cash to the cause and not simply fritter it away.

▶ Simple Ways to Save Big Bucks

The less money you shell out each month, the more you have to invest in your future independence. And since there are so many ways to drop bushels of bucks these days, you have a lot of options for cutting back—without depriving yourself of things that really matter to you and your family. For starters, consider each of these categories:

Food. Simply by eating out less frequently than you probably do now, you could save a bundle. Plus, when you tote your lunch to work or cook dinner at home, you know exactly what's going into your body—and that can actually lead to a longer life (see "Nothin' Beats Home Cookin'!" on page 174).

Automotive. Selling one or more cars that you don't need is an obvious way to trim costs. So is trading in a high-maintenance gas-guzzler for an easier keeper. But regardless of the kind of vehicle you have, you can make your outgo drop dramatically merely by leaving the buggy at home more often (see "Walk More, Spend Less" on page 241).

Housing. Downsizing your domicile can be the most effective cost-cutting caper of all. This is especially true if your plans call for relocation and you opt for a smaller house in a less expensive area. But de-cluttering your current digs can also result in major savings, whether you plan to stay put for the long haul or move on when you bid your current employer adieu. (More on both fronts coming up.)

> " All I can
> say about life
> is, 'Oh God,
> enjoy it!'
>
> —Bob Newhart
> (b.1929) "

How to Choose a Financial Planner

When it comes to retaining independence in all aspects of your life, a financial planner is just as important as a doctor or lawyer (see "Hire a Navigator" on page 333). So it's crucial that you find a pro who has a firm commitment to ethical behavior and high professional standards—and who puts your needs and interests first. Unlike the medical and legal professions, financial planning is not regulated by either federal or state governments, but these tips will help you make the best match:

Get personal recommendations from friends or coworkers. Other good sources are lawyers, accountants, insurance agents, and bankers, who often work with financial planners on behalf of their clients.

Contact the Financial Planning Association (FPA) to find a list of Certified Financial Planners™ (CFP®) in your area. These professionals must have three to five years in the field before passing a comprehensive certification examination. Once on board, they must ascribe to the FPA's code of ethics and other standards, and also stay current with the field through continuing education courses. Check www.plannersearch.org for more information.

Narrow the field. Many planners have minimum income as well as asset requirements; some specialize in certain areas, such as retirement or asset management; or they work with particular types of clients, such as small-business owners or retirees. So make sure to pinpoint pros who can address your needs.

Interview at least three candidates in person. Ask about each one's work experience, planning methods, and form(s) of compensation. Some planners earn commissions from companies whose financial products you buy. Others charge fees for their services, on an hourly, project, or percentage basis. Still others work for financial services firms.

Note: *Other credible designations to look for include Chartered Financial Consultant (ChFC®) and Personal Financial Specialist (PFS). These have their roots in particular financial disciplines such as insurance and accounting.*

READY, SET—REFIRE!

In recent years, *refire* has become a major buzzword in self-help circles. Simply put, the term means redirecting your interests or passions into a new career that allows you to make a living doing what you want, the way you want to do it—in other words, hanging on tight to your financial, emotional, and physical independence for as long as possible. That may entail continuing your current profession on a freelance or consulting basis. You could convert a longtime hobby into a moneymaking business or try something new. Whichever path you select, the timely tips in this section will help get you started on what's often called a second-prime venture.

❯ Take the First Steps

We've all heard stories about people who had chance encounters or out-of-the-blue happenstances that set them off on new careers in later life. But don't count on that happening. As long as possible before retirement time, start preparing for your future endeavors this way:

- Figure out how much money you'll have to make to supplement Social Security, pension, or investment income you expect to have. Always round up, because it's all but guaranteed that your living expenses will be higher than you anticipate.

- Decide on what area(s) of interest you want to pursue and learn as much as you can about not only the subject matter, but also what it takes to make it pay off financially.

- Pinpoint the marketable experience and abilities you can transfer to a new job or use to launch your own business.

> " When I stand before God at the end of my life, I would hope that I would not have a single bit of talent left, and could say, 'I used everything you gave me.'
>
> —Erma Bombeck (1927–1996) "

- If you plan to relocate when your current job ends, but you haven't chosen a destination, start researching your options—now. And be sure that opportunities for pursuing your areas of interest rank high on your list of criteria.

❯ Learn All about It

Whether you're leaning toward turning a current avocation into a full-time job or business, or you're contemplating a leap into an entirely new field, you've got a lot of resources at your disposal. For example:

Formal education. This can be anything from taking adult-ed classes at your local high school or community center to earning a second (or maybe first) degree at a college, university, or technical school. You can also find online tutorials, seminars, and even degree programs focused on just about any subject you can name.

Professional associations. Many of these groups offer associate memberships to people interested in joining the field, or they welcome visitors at their conventions and seminars. In most cases, their websites alone can give you a wealth of knowledge about the profession, what it takes to break into it, and where to learn more. So if you're thinking you'd like to become (let's say) a de-cluttering

---

It's Not Too Late to Bloom

Can't imagine launching a new career at your age? Maybe all you need is a role model. One of these, perhaps:

Anna Mary Robertson ("Grandma") Moses was 75 when she picked up a paintbrush for the very first time. She kept turning out her iconic scenes of rural life until shortly before her death at the age of 101.

Harlan Sanders worked as a farmer, salesman, riverboat pilot, and gas station owner before starting Kentucky Fried Chicken at age 65.

Laura Ingalls Wilder had spent decades as a farm wife and mother before she began writing about her childhood on the Great Plains. She was 65 when *Little House in the Big Woods* came out and 76 when the last title in the *Little House* series hit bookstore shelves.

Tick-Tock
**TURN
BACK** the
CLOCK

consultant, book indexer, animal trainer, or caterer, search the Internet for "professional organizations for [your area of interest]."

Volunteering. This is a win-win way to check out new directions. In fact, if income is not an issue, you could even make a whole second career of devoting your time to one or more causes that you care deeply about.

❯ Calculate Your Assets

When you're thinking of starting a business or looking for a position in a new line of work, your nonmonetary capital matters as much as ready cash. So sit down right now and list the assets you have in each of these categories:

- Your professional-level skill sets, including abilities you've gained in both present and past positions, as well as in volunteer work or life experience—for example, teaching, accounting, sales, customer service, or interior decorating.

- Your personal passions. After all, the whole idea of refirement is to enable you to wake up looking forward to the day that lies ahead. Write down the things you love to do most and the subjects that fascinate you.

- Market segments you know well. For instance, maybe your work, leisure activities, or social connections have brought you into close, ongoing proximity to young mothers, real estate agents, dedicated flea-market shoppers, or the 60-plus set—which also happens to be the fastest-growing demographic in the country.

- Friends who share your interests and might want to join you in starting and running a business.

Prepare for Peace of Mind

One of the surest ways to retain your emotional, mental, and physical independence throughout your life is to plan ahead for the day when you're no longer here. For example, making your funeral and burial arrangements now will ensure that you can go about the business of living life to the fullest—knowing that you've lifted a huge burden from your family members' backs. The same goes for executing these documents:

A will stipulates who will receive your property at your death and designates an executor to carry out your wishes. It also allows you to name a guardian for minor children and to specify funeral arrangements. Your will goes into effect only when you die—then, it usually goes through the public probate process.

A living trust remains private and takes effect as soon as you create it. You call the shots until you die, become incapacitated, or choose to relinquish control to a chosen "successor." You can distribute property while you're still living, arrange for its distribution upon your death, or designate a later time. A trust can be used to plan for disability, and it can be a highly effective vehicle for saving taxes.

Power of attorney (PoA). This document gives permission to another person to make decisions on your behalf, either in specific areas or over all of your medical and financial affairs. There are two types: A durable PoA grants ongoing authority to your agent; while a conditional PoA kicks in only at the onset of a specified event, such as a military deployment or disabling illness.

Advance medical directive. In this document, you can express your wishes related to life support and other medical treatments should you become unable to communicate.

It is a good idea to start making arrangements early. Once you have thought about and decided on who you would like to be responsible for carrying out your wishes (whether it is an executor of your will, guardians assigned to care for children, a successor, or anyone you would like to leave property, money, or other personal items to), it is important to sit down and go over the details. Once everything has been finalized and discussed, make sure to file all your important documents in a secure place for safekeeping, and let your loved ones know where your directives are stored.

⟫ CAN THE CANTANKEROUS CLUTTER

What, you may ask, has clutter got to do with your independence? Plenty! Cluttered surroundings may be costing you money that you could direct toward achieving financial independence. Plus, clutter can actually speed up your aging process, delivering a knockout punch to your emotional and physical independence. That is because it can send your stress-hormone producers into overdrive and, as we've seen in this book, they play a leading role in bringing on just about every debilitating condition under the sun. Conversely, ridding your home of excessive stuff is one of the easiest ways to give your mental, physical, *and* financial well-being a great big boost.

⟩ 5 Ways Clutter Busts Your Bank Account

It's no secret that living in cluttered surroundings raises your stress level, but it also costs you cold, hard cash. That's money you could invest in your new career plans—or spend right now on such healthy ventures as a gym or swim club membership, or active getaways to (let's say) hike, sail, or ski. Consider these areas where your junk may be costing you big bucks:

1. You eat out frequently because your kitchen is such a mess that you don't want to make dinner or pack yourself a lunch.

2. You have to keep buying more clothes because you're gaining weight from either too many fast-food meals or clutter-caused stress—or both.

3. You're continuously buying duplicate stuff, ranging from food and clothes to tools, lightbulbs, and office supplies, because you can't find the ones you have.

> " A pessimist sees the difficulty in every opportunity; an optimist sees the opportunity in every difficulty.
>
> —Winston Churchill (1874–1965) "

If you're a natural-born pack rat, take the advice in "Divide and Conquer" (at right) one step further: Begin your de-cluttering campaign with the smallest drawer in your chosen room. Let's say it's your bedroom. Whether your target is the drawer in your nightstand, or the top one in your dresser, it shouldn't take you more than 10 or 15 minutes max to sort through the contents, pitch the junk, and put back the things that really belong there. Once you see how neat and orderly it looks, you'll be all fired up to tackle the rest of the room—and the house.

4. You're constantly paying late fees—and damaging your credit rating to boot—because you misplace your checkbook, your bills, or even the stamps to mail them.

5. You have so much stuff that it won't fit in your home, so each month you shell out rent for a storage unit.

Note: *Getting rid of those belongings you neither need nor want puts money in the bank account—that is, if you sell them on an online venue such as eBay or at a flea market or garage sale (see "A Winning Garage Sale" on page 357).*

▶ More Stuff Leads to an Older You

Consider these ways that clutter clobbers your mind and, in turn, your body:

- It distracts you from things that you need to focus on.

- It bombards your brain with extra stimuli, forcing your senses to work overtime and often disturbing your health-giving sleep.

- It makes it harder to relax, both mentally and physically.

- It constantly whispers to your subconscious that your work is never—and never can be—done.

- It triggers feelings of guilt and embarrassment, especially when unexpected visitors drop by your home or office.

- It can make you reluctant to invite folks over, so you deprive yourself of youth-enhancing social interaction.

- It sends your frustration skyrocketing when things like keys, bills, or important documents get buried in piles of junk.

❯ Set a Winning Strategy

A lot of de-cluttering "experts" lay down didactic—and highly unhealthy—rules about what to keep and what to pitch. Just ignore them. Remember: Your goal is to simplify your life and reduce your stress—not to deprive yourself of everything you hold dear. For example, if you truly love and appreciate the rich, natural sound of your LP records (as every professional musician I know does), don't let anyone talk you into transferring your collection to digital format and tossing your treasured vinyl in the interest of freeing up shelf space. Instead, follow this golden rule for every item you own: If you need it, use it, or love it, keep it. Otherwise, get rid of it (see "Categorizing Care" on page 348).

The same goes for your jam-packed to-do list. Keep the essentials and the things you love to do, but weed out the marginal stuff.

❯ Divide and Conquer

If your home is buried in stuff, there's no way you're going to sort it all out in one day—or even one week. And don't even try. If you do, you'll only send your stress level higher than it is already. Instead, start by choosing a single room to focus on. Which one is your call, but from a grow-younger standpoint, the bedroom is an excellent option—even if you're gearing up to start a home-based business. Why? Because a clutter-free bedroom will not only provide a

---

Wake Up and Ditch the Junk!

If you need still more convincing that de-cluttering can make your life better, these two stats alone should give you a loud wake-up call:

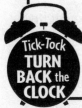

- On average, people spend one entire year of their lives looking for lost stuff. Imagine what you could do with an extra year!
- De-cluttering would eliminate 40 percent of housework in the average home. Less cleaning—sign me up!

Centenarian SECRETS

If you don't believe that an uncluttered, serene, sleep-inducing bedroom can help you live a longer, happier life, consider these facts: Scientists tell us that routinely getting sufficient, high-quality sleep extends your life by 8 to 10 years. As for the happier part, on the Greek island of Ikaria (where residents routinely live well past the century mark), more than 80 percent of people between the ages of 65 and 100 are still having sex several times a week—without the aid of enhancement drugs. For more on how to get your fair share of shut-eye, see "Good Health—Sleep on It!" starting on page 200.

peaceful place to start your day and a restful haven at the end of it, but it'll also promote better sleep and more health-giving sex. Plus, by tackling this important room first, you will realize just how wonderful your de-cluttered surroundings can be, and that will keep you motivated to conquer your office and then the rest of the house.

❯ Categorizing Care

As you move from room to room (or from drawer to drawer), make enough space for five boxes—or piles—depending on your preference and the size of the objects at hand. Then, as you grab each item, assign it to one of these categories:

- Trash—Get rid of unwanted junk.

- Keep—Put these items away as you sort through each room. Don't pile them up to create more work later.

- Donate or Sell—Give these to charity, or make some extra money by holding a garage sale.

- Recycle or Repurpose—Find a new use for these items, or pass them onto a new owner.

❯ Get Open for Business...

After your bedroom, your home office is most likely the next highest priority on your de-cluttering list. A neat, well-organized space will help you focus on all the elements involved in planning and carrying out your retirement strategy, from researching your career options to managing your finances. Whether your "office" occupies a section of kitchen counter or an entire spacious room, the basic procedure for making it shipshape is the same as it is for any other room (see "Categorizing Care," at left).

❯ And Stay Open!

When you've got a whole new stage of your life to get off and running, make sure you never have to waste time on a major office-sorting spree again. How? Whenever you've finished a particular chore, or you need a break from a longer project, take a quick look at your desktop and the surrounding territory. Grab anything you haven't used lately—or that has strayed into your office from someplace else—and put it back where it belongs. If you take this simple inventory every few days, office clutter will be a thing of the past.

❯ Build a Home Office

It's a common conundrum: Your kitchen-counter setup worked just fine when you only used it to pay the monthly bills. But now that you're looking to build a whole new lifestyle, you need more space—and you don't have a spare room to set up shop in. No problem! Build yourself an office using one of these simple methods:

Convert a closet. First, add as many shelves to your closet as you can to hold files and supplies, but leave space below them. Next, buy

MIND OVER MYTH

MYTH: In order to prevent financial fraud and identity theft, you need to shred all personal documents before you dispose of them.

REALITY: In most cases, you don't need to shred the entire thing—only the parts that contain your signature and sensitive information such as your Social Security number, account numbers, and maybe your name, address, and phone number. So what on earth has it got to do with de-cluttering? Well, just this: Unless you receive a steady stream of confidential documents, you can get rid of that bulky paper shredder that's sitting in the corner and replace it with a pair of shredder scissors (available via the Internet and in catalogs). They work like ordinary scissors, but they have five cutting blades instead of one, so they snip paper into very slender shreds quickly— and quietly.

a file cart on wheels (they're available in office-supply stores and on the Internet), and roll it into one side of the closet. Then find a rolling desk or worktable that can hold your computer, and tuck it in beside the cart. (These, too, are easy to find.) When you're ready for action, just roll your gear out into the great wide open. When you're finished, simply slide it back into "storage" until next time.

Use the "now you see it, now you don't" approach. No closet to spare? Then get a sturdy folding table that you can use for office work, and stash it in a closet or under a bed when it's off duty. For any downtime, reserve a space near your work area for files and work-in-progress materials that you can't finish in one sitting. A good-looking trunk or a basket with a lid on it will fill the bill, as will a small cabinet or chest of drawers that blends with your decor.

❯ 2 Ways to Make a Bedroom Closet Count

A home office that was formerly a bedroom has a built-in advantage: a closet. But to get the most out of that storage space, you need to organize it in just the right way. Fortunately, you have a couple of excellent options. Which one is better depends upon how much time and effort you're willing to spend on it.

1. Gut the current closet, removing all the hanging rods and built-in shelves. Then install wall-to-wall shelves that are 10 to 12 inches apart, from floor to ceiling. Either wood or vinyl-coated wire versions will work out fine.

2. Simply remove the hanging rod(s) and find a free-standing bookcase that fits under and/or beside the existing shelves.

❯ Beware of Going Paperless

You might think that keeping all of your data—from appointment dates to phone numbers—in digital format is a dandy way to cut clutter in your home office. That may be so, but it can be an even dandier way to mess up your plans (or worse). Remember that gadgets—especially small ones—are famous for vanishing or crashing when you need them most. So play it safe: Always keep paper copies of any information you cannot retrieve easily if the electronic data (such as unlisted phone numbers, or notes from your new-career brainstorming sessions) suddenly disappears.

'TIL WE DON'T MEET AGAIN

No matter how much storage space you have in your office—or anywhere else in your home—once-important papers that have outlived their usefulness are nothing but clutter. How long you need to keep various records varies greatly, but here's a rundown of the most common documents, along with their "expiration dates."

Type of Document	Keep them until ...
ATM receipts	You verify them on your bank statement
Credit card receipts	You verify them on your statement
Leases of any kind	Seven years after they expire
Pay stubs	You verify them on your W-2 form
Sales receipts	The warranty expires
Tax records/returns	Three years from the date you filed your return; seven years if you've filed a claim for a loss from worthless securities or bad-debt deduction
Vehicle records	You no longer own the vehicle
Veterinary records	The animal is no longer part of your household
Warranties and operating instructions	You no longer own the product
W-2 and 1099 forms	You retire completely and start receiving Social Security benefits

>>> THE DEAL WITH DOWNSIZING

Downsizing your home can be one of the most effective ways to gain financial, physical, and emotional independence. The fact is, though, that even if you've relocated many times, moving from larger quarters to smaller ones is never easy. And when the place you're moving out of has been your family's home for decades, downsizing can be one of the most stressful experiences of your life. The key to success is a positive attitude: Don't think of it as casting off generations' worth of cherished possessions. Instead, consider it a golden opportunity to weed out all the extraneous clutter in your life and focus on the things that really matter.

> Better Safe Than Sorry

Few things are more vitally important to your physical and emotional independence than the safety and security of your home. So when you are shopping for your new living quarters, keep these tips in mind:

Think ahead. You may be in great shape now, but there's bound to come a time when actions like climbing stairs, stepping into the bathtub, and stooping to retrieve heavy things from low shelves become accidents waiting to happen. So examine the new place for potential trouble spots. If everything is not senior-friendly now—indoors and out—make sure you can make alterations easily as needed.

Protect yourself. Guard against any "guests." Unless you're moving into a building that has a security system, have one installed. But do your homework before you choose a provider. Start by getting personal referrals from your neighbors or the local police.

> " In the central place of every heart there is a recording chamber; so long as it receives messages of beauty, hope, cheer, and courage, so long are you young.
>
> General Douglas MacArthur
> (1880–1964) "

❯ It's Never Too Soon to Start

If you've decided to move to smaller quarters in a couple of years, the time to begin downsizing is now—not a few weeks (or even a few months) before the moving van arrives. Here's why:

- The sooner you start, the less you'll have to deal with as your moving day approaches. Plus, you'll avoid having to make hasty decisions to toss out items you might regret losing later.

- The less stuff you have to pack up and transport, the easier—and less expensive—your move will be.

- You can take your time finding exactly the right home for any belongings you're sure you won't be taking, like your vintage boat or the dining table that's been in your family for generations.

- It's a lot easier on your physical and mental health. Even routine de-cluttering can be tiring work. Just the thought of clearing out an entire house on a tight deadline can make your stress hormones hit the stratosphere.

❯ Over My Dead Body!

Before you start sorting—and, if possible, before you start looking for your next home—make a list of the possessions that give you the greatest pleasure and the items that you simply refuse to leave behind. Keep your list handy as you sort through your belongings. Maybe it's your dad's photo album from World War II, the journal your mother kept when she was expecting you, or the souvenir plates you collected

---

Crunch the Numbers

As soon as you have your new home lined up, get a blueprint or drawing that indicates the exact dimensions of each room, including the garage and any other places you might use for storage. Don't forget to measure the height of the ceilings, as well as doorways and windows (including their height from the floor). Then go through your current house and measure each piece of furniture and any other large objects you might like to keep. Knowing which items can fit into your new rooms and which ones can't will make your decisions about what to keep a whole lot easier—and allow you to make the best use of your future space.

on road trips with your loved ones. Putting your priorities in writing will remind you that all of your belongings are not created equal. And if you love nothing better than sitting down at your piano and plunking out your favorite tunes, do everything you can to keep that baby as well, even if it means trading in your big couch for a smaller model, or making your coffee table double for dining.

❯ Don't Go It Alone

When your home is filled with things that bring back decades of memories, it can be mighty hard to start sorting through it all. To get going—and reduce stress—ask for help from a close friend or family member. Choose someone who knows your tastes, and be sure you can trust her to give you an honest, objective opinion about everything from how you really look in your bright-red dress to how likely you are to need half a dozen party platters in your new home. Above all, your sorting buddy should be able to make you laugh because—of course—laughter is the greatest stress reliever of all.

❯ Coming to Terms

The sorting categories for a large downsizing will be a little bit different than they are for routine de-cluttering (see "Categorizing Care" on page 348). In this case, in addition to your trusty boxes and bags, gather up a supply of labels or index cards to use for items that are too big to fit in cartons. You should have designated containers and tags marked Trash, Donate, Sell, Take Along, and Special Handling. That last category is for family heirlooms, treasured collections, or other prized possessions that you'll turn over to relatives, friends, or particular organizations.

Centenarian SECRETS 100

Before you part with anything that might have real historic value—say, your grandfather's collection of baseball memorabilia—have a dealer make an appraisal. It may include objects that the National Baseball Hall of Fame in Cooperstown would love to have, or that you might want to sell at auction or on eBay.

The Organizing Process

For routine de-cluttering, the normal procedure entails weeding out all the stuff you don't want and then organizing the keepers in whatever way works best for you. When you're downsizing for a move, you need to organize before, during, and after your sorting spree. To be specific:

Pack as you go. Before you start sorting, stock up on boxes, tape, and plenty of padding, such as bubble wrap and foam peanuts. Then, as you pinpoint items that you want to take with you but don't use every day, pack them up and set them aside. (Be sure to label each box with its contents and the room it belongs in.) If you can, designate a guest room or other little-used space as a "holding tank," where the boxes will be out of the way. Prime candidates for your early packing sessions include out-of-season clothes, seasonal or holiday decorations, photo albums, books, and artwork.

Give as you go. Assign separate areas for things that you will be donating to charity or giving away to friends or family—and keep the stuff flowing outta there. Not only will you lessen the chances of changing your mind about getting rid of the silver candlesticks you haven't used since 1985, but you'll also free up room to store the things you'll need to load onto the moving van. And take it from me: If your belongings are packed in boxes, they'll actually take up a lot more space than they did when they were hanging on the wall or sitting on shelves!

Fountain of Youth

PEPPERMINT FOOT SOAK

When manning a garage sale has left your dogs dog-tired, this minty footbath will pep 'em right up.

- ¼ cup of Epsom salts
- ¼ cup of sea salt
- 4 drops of liquid menthol (available in pharmacies)
- 4 drops of peppermint essential oil
- Warm water

Mix all of the ingredients in a foot-size basin. Then sit back, relax, and soak your tiredness away for good.

Don't sell as you go. Instead, as you come across potential garage sale fodder, move it to a certain area (maybe the garage, if there's room). If an item is too big to move easily, or you're still using it, attach a "Sell" label to it. Then go about your business as usual until it's time to set up shop.

❯ 5 Reasons to Leave It

When it comes to belongings that do not have great sentimental value, plan on selling or giving away any items that meet the following five criteria:

1. You won't need it in your future home. For instance, if you're moving to a condo or rental apartment where the management handles all maintenance chores, you won't need many tools.

2. It's not in good shape. If your coffee machine is showing serious signs of age, you may want to leave it behind and get a new one after the move.

3. You seldom use it. When push comes to shove, you can rent or borrow just about anything, from cocktail glasses to canoes.

Look High and Low

The best place to begin the weeding-out process is the basement or the attic because that's generally where most clutter piles up. And much of it's likely useless junk that you can toss without giving it a second thought. The instant results should spur you on to tackle the rest of your house. If you don't have a basement or attic, or you're not ready to tackle such a big area, start in a spare bedroom, closet, or other space that meets these two terms:

- It contains a lot of items that are being stored rather than displayed or used on a regular basis. Much of it is bound to be stuff that you won't even want to consider taking with you.

- For the most part, the things you'll be dealing with have little sentimental value. That will make your take-it-or-leave-it decisions easier and much less stressful.

Tick-Tock
TURN BACK the CLOCK

So why crowd your home and your life with stuff that you only haul out once in a blue moon?

4. It can be replaced. If you cast off your big roasting pan, you can always pick up a new one when your family suddenly announces they'll be joining you for the holidays. But it's a whole different ball game to part with a family heirloom, beloved antique, or original work of art, only to find out that it would have fit in your new home after all.

5. It's easier or cheaper to replace it than it is to move it. In this case, your decision depends largely on how far you're moving. If you're only headed across town, then by all means, take your brand-new kitchen trash can. On the other hand, if you're leaving Boston and are bound for Key West, forget it!

MIND OVER MYTH

MYTH: China is meant for special occasions, so you need to have a second set of "everyday" dishes on hand.

REALITY: You might have a set of beautiful kitchenware that you have always kept on display and another assortment of less-special versions that you actually use—but storage space in your new home will be at a premium. To downsize your dinnerware, just get rid of the so-so stuff, and use the bowls, plates, glasses, and so on that you really love! After all, that's what they were made for.

❯ A Winning Garage Sale

A garage sale is one of the best ways to get rid of the things you don't want. But like any other aspect of successful downsizing (or general de-cluttering), it takes some planning. The better you organize your event, the more stuff you'll sell—and the more money you'll have to spend in your new locale.

Well in advance of the sale, arrange for Goodwill, the Salvation Army, or another charity to come by and pick up whatever hasn't sold. And be sure you tell them the stuff is garage sale surplus because some groups won't accept anything that still has a price sticker on it.

10 Steps for a Longer, Happier, and Healthier Life!

By now, you should be all fired up and rarin' to grow younger! To help get the show on the road, let's recap your action plan:

1. Make healthy habits part of your daily routine. Keep your weight where it should be for your height and bone structure, get a good 40 winks each night, drink in moderation, and—above all—don't smoke!

2. Relieve aches and pains using natural remedies instead of commercial painkillers that can deliver side effects that'll age you fast.

3. Conquer chronic conditions that were once part and parcel of aging by adopting sensible eating habits, remaining physically active, and keeping toxic crud to a minimum in your daily environment.

4. Look on the bright side. Happy, optimistic folks have stronger immune systems, handle stress better—and even have fewer accidents.

5. Stay mentally active. Stimulate your brain every single day by (for example) reading, engaging in crafts or hobbies, working crossword puzzles, or playing Scrabble® with your pals.

6. Do as Mom always told you: Eat a balanced diet that's rich in all of those nutrients you need for good health.

7. Strive to look your best at all times by paying careful attention to your skin, your hair, and your wardrobe.

8. Keep your body moving, as Mother Nature intended—whether you choose to adopt a formal exercise routine, take up a sport, or simply work more movement into your daily routine.

9. Maintain strong social ties. Medical science has proven beyond a shadow of a doubt that this is one of the most important factors of all in growing younger and living longer. Conversely, the lack of robust relationships poses an even stronger health risk than obesity and lack of exercise.

10. Do all of the above consistently and cheerfully. That will enable you to achieve the results that this final chapter is all about: Keeping your physical, emotional, and financial independence your whole life long. Good luck, and God bless!

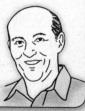

·>> INDEX

A

AA (Alcoholics
  Anonymous), 32
Acid reflux, 184
Acne, 216
Acupressure, 97
Acupuncture, 37, 45
Addiction, 33, 39.
  See also Alcohol use;
  Smoking
Adult children living
  at home
    finances and, 296–299
    setting guidelines for,
      294–296
Advance medical directive,
  344
Aerobic exercises
  arm exercises, 251
  cannonball, 253
  deep-water running,
    247, 249
  function of, 237
  kickboard exercises,
    254–255
  kids' games as, 247
  pool noodle leg lifts, 252
  tick-tock hops, 250
  variety in, 246
  walking in water, 248
Age spots, 211–212
AHAs (alpha-hydroxy
  acids), 192
Air fresheners, herbal, 92
Alcoholics Anonymous
  (AA), 32
Alcohol use
  cons and pros of, 27–28
  craving relief, 173, 184

drug interactions with,
  30–31
excessive, 28–29, 193
hangover cures, 31,
  32–33
migraines and, 73
myths, 28
One for the Road, 29
precautions for, 29–30
psoriasis and, 115
reducing, 30, 31–32
signs of addiction, 33
Allergens, 82
Allergies
  contact, 175
  as headache cause, 67
  as IBS cause, 113
Almond oil
  for hand and foot care,
    212, 213
  Sore Skin Solution, 175
Almonds, 101
Aloe vera gel
  Aloe-Blueberry
    Smoothie, 115
  for skin care, 201, 205
Alpha-hydroxy acids
  (AHAs), 192
Alzheimer's disease. *See also*
  Brain health
    misconceptions,
      144–145
    preventive strategies,
      3, 98
Anemia, 185
Angelica, 68, 69
Anthocyanins, 176–177
Anti-Aging Egg Salad, 178
Anti-Anxiety Nightcap, 141
Anti-Asthma Massage Oil, 83

Antibiotics, 20, 116
Antioxidants
  beverage sources, 98,
    182, 185
  food sources, 174–175
Anxiety
  Anti-Anxiety Nightcap,
    141
  as IBS cause, 113
  Incredible Comfort
    Cream, 139
  myths, 140
  remedies for, 139–142
  symptoms of, 138–139
Apples
  as antioxidant source,
    175
  Applejack-Spiked Baked
    Apples, 331
  for conjunctivitis relief,
    175
  for gout pain relief, 66
  health benefits of, 85–86,
    180
  Multinutrient Smoothie,
    158
  Sautéed Apples and
    Onions, 86
  Spinach-Apple Salad, 79
  weight loss and, 15
Arm exercises
  aerobic, 251
  strength training, 265–267
  stretches, 272–273
Aromatherapy
  as mood booster, 121
  for sleep problem relief, 25
  for weight loss, 14–15
Arrhythmia, 100–101
Arteriosclerosis, 181

Conjugated linoleic acid (CLA), 13
Conjunctivitis, 175
Constipation, 173
Cooking spray alternative, 321
Corned beef, 320
Cornmeal, for skin care, 199, 200
Cortisol, 22
Counseling, for smoking cessation, 37
Cowboy Chili Seasoning Mix, 319
Cranberries, cranberry juice
    as antioxidant source, 175
    for asthma relief, 85
    for healing cuts, 176
    for UTI relief, 189
Cravin'-Kickin' Oil Mix, 39
Cream of tartar, 108, 135
Credit card debt, 336–337
Credit cards, canceling, 299
Credit scores, 299, 337
Crohn's disease (CD), 111
Crow's-feet, 194
CT scans, 60
Cucumbers
    Beautifying Body Cleanser, 205
    in fortified vinegar, 171
    for hair care, 221, 222
Cumin, 33
Curcumin, 147, 173
Cuts and scrapes, 176
Cycling, 241–242

D

Dairy products, 164, 188. *See also* Buttermilk; Milk; Yogurt
Dancing, 144, 245

Dawn simulators, 150
Dead Sea salt water, 114
Deep-water running, 247, 249
Dehydration, 160. *See also* Hydration
Dementia. *See* Brain health
Depression
    back pain and, 52
    SAD, 149–152
    weight loss and, 5
Desserts
    Applejack-Spiked Baked Apples, 331
    Chilly Minty Marvel, 328–329
    Chocolate–Peanut Butter Fudge, 327
    Fast and Easy Fruit-Torte Bars, 327
    fruit salad, 332
    Gingerbread Christmas Cookies, 332
    Old-Time Vinegar & Molasses Taffy, 329
    Pumpkin Cheesecake, 330
    Raspberry Brownies, 328
De-Stressing Bath Blend, 133
Detox diets, 6
Diabetes
    preventive strategies, 3, 92–93, 233
    risk factors for, 90–91
    service dogs and, 94
    sleep problems and, 21
    symptoms of, 90, 224
    types of, 89, 94
Diarrhea, 188
Dietary fat, 12–13, 156
Diets. *See also* Eating habits; Nutrition
    detox, 6
    fat-free, 156

Mediterranean diet, 8–9, 48
    modern American diet, 82, 112, 148
    weight loss and, 6–10
Diet soda, 186–187
Dinnerware, 11, 357
Dip recipes. *See* Snacks and dips
Dirty Dozen list, 163
Divorce rates, 35
Doctor visits, 110
Dogs. *See* Pets; Service dogs
Downsizing
    choosing new home, 352
    garage sales, 357
    myths, 357
    sorting and organizing, 352–356
    what to leave behind, 356–357
Dried fruit
    Easy Energy Bars, 241
    migraines and, 73
Drinking glasses, 17
Dumbbells, buying, 257
Dysentery, 188

E

Earaches, 80
Easy Cowboy Chili, 319
Easy Energy Bars, 241
Eating habits
    arthritis and, 43, 47–48
    asthma and, 82–83
    autoimmune disorders and, 112
    for brain health, 147, 148
    cooking at home, 174
    food shopping and, 161–170
    gout and, 64, 65

Fingernail care, 216, 226–230

Fish and seafood, 147

Fish tanks, for anxiety relief, 142

Flaxseed, flaxseed oil
for arthritis pain relief, 47–48
as mood booster, 125
Multinutrient Smoothie, 158

Flexibility exercises. *See* Stretching (flexibility exercises)

Folate, 147

Fondue with Fortitude, 324–325

Food allergies, 113

Food as medicine. *See specific ailments or foods*

Food costs
eating out and, 339
losing weight and, 4
organic foods, 162–163

Food for entertaining
desserts, 327–332
one-pot meals, 318–322
sandwiches, 308
snacks and dips, 322–326

Food sensitivities, 67–68

Food shopping
expiration dates, 166–167
label terminology, 163, 165–166
organic food, 161–165
produce, 167–170
weight gain and, 17

Food supplements
for arthritis pain relief, 46
buying, 160
calcium, 159, 176
multivitamins, 158, 159–160

Foot care. *See also* Nail care
Peppermint Foot Soak, 355
rough or cracked skin, 212–215
for smelly feet, 215
stretching exercises, 276–277
Treat for Tired Feet, A, 244

Forgiveness, and happiness, 123

Four-Bean Hamburger Bake, 322

Fragrances, synthetic, 91, 93

Friendship. *See* Socialization

Fruit salad, 332

Fruits and vegetables. *See* Produce; *specific foods*

Fruit-Torte Bars, Fast and Easy, 327

Functional fitness, 237

Funeral arrangements, 344

Fungi
Candida albicans, 20
finger- or toenail, 229–230

G

Gallstones, 86

Garage sales, 357

Garlic, garlic oil
for asthma relief, 84–85
for hair care, 220
for nail care, 226
Triumphant Triad Tonic, 7

Gelatin, 229

Genealogy, 305–306

Genetically modified organisms (GMOs), 165

Genetics
autoimmune disease and, 111
gray hair and, 223
skin health and, 196

Geranium oil, 39, 127

Ginger
for anxiety relief, 142
for hand and foot care, 212
Hot Healing Liniment, 44
Migraine-Mashing Tea, 73
for migraine relief, 74
One for the Road, 29
Pain-Pulverizing Smoothie, 58
for pain relief, 44, 57
for skin care, 209
Sweet & Spicy Throat Cure, 187

Ginger ale, 29, 227

Gingerbread Christmas Cookies, 332

Glucosamine, 46

Glutathione, 102

Gluten
sensitivity or intolerance to, 79, 110
weight loss and, 6

GMOs (genetically modified organisms), 165

Golf, and back pain, 54

Gone for the Day Casserole, 318

Gout
causes of, 43, 62–64
Gout-Pain-Begone Paste, 65
myths, 63
preventive strategies, 64–65
remedies for, 65–66, 155, 180

therapy (HRT), 83, 146
Horseradish, 44, 211
Hot Healing Liniment, 44
Hot-pepper sauce, 11
Household chores
    for adult children at
      home, 296
    as exercise, 242–243, 269
HRT (hormone
    replacement therapy), 83,
    146
Hugs, 128
Human growth hormone, 22
Hydration
    for arthritis pain relief, 51
    in good nutrition, 161
    for headache relief, 137
    for minimizing wrinkles,
    193
Hypertension. *See* High
    blood pressure
Hyperthyroidism, 110
Hypothyroidism, 19

I

IBD (inflammatory bowel
    disease), 111–113
IBS (irritable bowel
    syndrome), 112–113
Icebreaker games, 302–303
Immune system boosters,
    116, 181, 184, 185
Inactivity physiology, 234
Income, and obesity, 4–5.
    See also Finances
Incredible Comfort Cream,
    139
Indigestion, 189
Inflammatory bowel disease
    (IBD), 111–113
Insect bites, 175
Insomnia. *See* Sleep problems

Insulin resistance, 91, 92
Iron, in eggs, 178
Iron overload, 100, 158
Irritable bowel syndrome
    (IBS), 112–113
Ischemic stroke, 104

J

Jars, sterilizing, 86–87
Joint pain. *See also*
    Arthritis
      apples for, 180
      Leapin' Liniment!, 279
      Leek Liniment, 136
      weight loss and, 3
Juniper oil, 139
Juvenile diabetes, 89, 94

K

Kale-Mustard Topper, 169
Kickboard exercises, 254–
    255
Kidney stones, 155, 184, 190
Kids' games, as exercise, 247
Kindness, and happiness,
    123
Kitchens, weight gain and,
    15–16, 17
Knuckles, cracking, 43
Kombu, 141

L

Lactose intolerance, 188
Lateral arm raise, 267
Lat stretch, 271
Laughter
    for asthma relief, 84
    immune function and,
    116
    as mood booster, 121,
    122–123

skin health and, 198
Lavender, lavender oil
    for anxiety relief, 140
    for asthma relief, 84, 87
    for back pain relief, 56
    for better sleep, 25
    floral vinegar bath, 206
    for migraine relief, 74
    as mood booster, 127
    for stress relief, 131
Leaky gut syndrome, 180
Leapin' Liniment!, 279
Leek Liniment, 136
Leek seeds, 225
Lemonade, 183–184
Lemon balm, 73
Lemon oil, 39
Lemons, lemon juice
    Beautifying Body
      Cleanser, 205
    Classic Lemonade, 184
    for hair care, 219, 221–222
    for hand and foot care,
      211–212, 215
    health benefits of, 184
    to lower blood
      pressure, 108
    for nail care, 226, 228
    for skin care, 209
    Sore Skin Solution, 175
L-glutamine, 46
Libido-Lifting Smoothie,
    292
Lights and lighting
    for SAD relief, 150, 151
    sleep problems and,
    24–25
    weight gain and, 16
Limes, lime juice
    for arthritis pain relief, 51
    for hand and foot care,
      212
    for headache relief, 137

Parsley
    for arthritis pain relief, 48
    for eye bag relief, 195
    footbath, 214
    health benefits of, 190
    Ticker Tune-Up Tonic, 98
Peanut Butter Fudge,
    Chocolate, 327
Peanut oil, 229
Pecans, 101
Pedometers, 240
Peppermint, peppermint
    oil. *See also* Mint
    for back pain relief, 57
    Chilly Minty Marvel,
        328–329
    in facial toner, 201
    as mood booster, 127
    Peppermint Foot Soak,
        355
    weight loss and, 15
Peppers, 43
Perfect Produce Cleaner,
    165
Perfluorooctanoic acid
    (PFOA), 19–20
Petroleum jelly, 201, 213
Pets
    choosing, 314–315
    giving as gift, 313
    health benefits of, 98–99,
        107
    myths, 314
    playing with, 316–317
    socialization and, 307,
        316, 317
PFOA (perfluorooctanoic
    acid), 19–20
PH balance, 112
Phthalates, 91, 93
Physical therapy, 52
Phytonutrients, 154,
    176–177

Pineapple juice, 196
Pistachios, 195
Plastics, 91, 93
PMS, 180, 181
Polyphenols, 98
Polyvinyl chloride (PVC), 19
Pomegranate juice, 190
Pool noodle leg lifts, 252
Pork fat, 80
Pork 'n' beans, 180
Potassium
    to lower blood pressure,
        107, 180
    overdose effects, 158
    for SAD relief, 151
Potatoes
    arthritis and, 43
    Beautifying Body
        Cleanser, 205
    for hair care, 224
    to lower blood pressure,
        108
    phytonutrients in, 176–
        177
    Scalloped Potatoes with
        Broccoli and Ham, 321
    serving with dip, 324
    for sour stomach relief,
        188
    Twice-Baked Potato
        Casserole, 106
Potluck dishes, 331
Power of attorney, 344
Prediabetes, 90
Processed meats, 73
Produce. *See also specific
    foods*
    canned, 169–170
    fresh, 167–168
    frozen, 168–169
    increasing intake of,
        168, 170–171
    limp vegetables, 167

organic, 161–164
Perfect Produce
    Cleaner, 165
Professional associations,
    342–343
Prostate problem relief
    parsley for, 190
    pumpkin seeds for, 177,
        186
Protein, in eggs, 178
Psoriasis, 113–115, 175
Pub-Style Cheese Spread,
    326
Pulse, and heart health, 96
Pumpkin Cheesecake, 330
Pumpkin seeds, 177, 186
Purines, 64
Push-ups, 260–261
PVC (polyvinyl chloride), 19

Q

Quadriceps stretch, 276
Quercetin, 183

R

RA (rheumatoid arthritis),
    42–43, 48
Rabbit tobacco, 26
Rashes, 175
Raspberries
    in fortified vinegar, 171
    Raspberry Brownies, 328
Raspberry leaves, 108
Rebound headaches, 68–69
Recipes. *See* Food for
    entertaining; *specific
    ailment, food, or recipe
    name*
Record-keeping, 351
Refire, 341–343
Rekindle Your Fire Bath, 151
Resveratrol, 48, 147